ANDREW PATTERSON

MY JOURNEY

BEYOND

THE SUMMIT

A STORY ABOUT THE TRANSFORMATIVE
POWER OF STEPPING INTO THE UNKNOWN

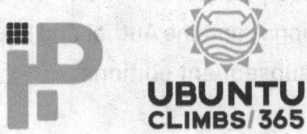

MY JOURNEY BEYOND THE SUMMIT

First Edition (2024)

ISBN: 978-0-7961-7396-6 (print), 978-0-7961-7386-7 (e-book)

©2024 by Andrew Patterson.

All rights reserved. No part of this publication may be reproduced, distributed, or transmitted in any form or by any means, including photocopying, recording, or other electronic or mechanical methods, without the prior written permission of the author, except in the case of brief quotations embodied in critical reviews and certain other noncommercial uses permitted by copyright law. For permission requests, write to the publisher at the address below.

39 Houston Street
Unit 001
Asheville, North Carolina
USA, 28801
email: ap@andrew365.com

Publisher: Imprint Publishing Pty
Editor: Matthew Hodges at Imprint Publishing Pty
Book and Cover Design: Imprint Publishing Pty
Cover Concept: Andrew Patterson
Printed in South Africa and USA

Disclaimer: Every effort has been made to ensure that all acknowledgements of copyrighted material and permissions from contributors are correctly cited within this publication. If any omissions or errors have occurred, they are unintentional, and the Author and Imprint Publishing PTY will endeavor to correct them in subsequent editions.

Table of Contents

Prologue		4
Chapter 1	The Day my World Imploded	8
Chapter 2	The Ingredients that Made it all Possible	17
Chapter 3	Turning an Idea Into Reality	32
Chapter 4	January - Taking the First Step into the Unknown	55
Chapter 5	January - Hell Week	76
Chapter 6	February - Building on Solid Foundations	135
Chapter 7	March - Don't you Get Bored?	116
Chapter 8	April - Learning the Harsh Reality of Extremes	143
Chapter 9	May - The Power of Perspective	166
Chapter 10	June - The Importance of Mental Well-Being	203
Chapter 11	June To July - Celebrating 100 Years of Madiba Magic	225
Chapter 12	An Education on Building A Legacy	252
Chapter 13	September - Unconditional Love	277
Chapter 14	October - Reaping Rewards	302
Chapter 15	November - The Perfect Storm	328
Chapter 16	December - 31 Days to Embed the Lessons	361
Chapter 17	Saying Goodbye to an old Friend and Mentor	397
Acknowledgements		407

To see photos related to Table Mountain, my training, and each month's challenge, please scan the QR code below!

PROLOGUE

It's so easy to become overwhelmed by the problems of the world or by the idea that our lives are not where they should be. I've felt that many times, have you? I don't claim to have all the answers, but I discovered two simple principles (and let's not confuse simple with easy) that helped me achieve fulfilment in the midst of life's worries and hardships.

They are:

1. Taking action in the face of discomfort
2. Ubuntu

Ubuntu is an African Philosophy that's usually translated as, "I am because you are."

This definition also resonates deeply with me:

Ubuntu is a collection of values and practices that African people view as the essence of what makes us human beings. While the nuances of these values and practices vary across different ethnic groups, they all point to one thing – an authentic individual human being is part of a larger and more significant relational, communal, societal, environmental, and spiritual world.

This resonates with me because it highlights two important interconnected principles: **be your best self, and think of your community and how to best serve them.**

This book details how I used these two principles to achieve fulfilment. I love the concept that, to experience something I've never had, I have to do something I've never done — especially when it's scary.

PROLOGUE

In June 2017, my life took an unexpected turn when I lost my job. It was a shock that inspired me to take an idea, and turn it into an initiative that would change more than just my own life. Determined to forge a new path outside of the corporate environment, I reshaped my perspective of the world and set out to create a life of purpose. As part of my mission, I embarked on an extraordinary endeavour: to climb Table Mountain in Cape Town every day for an entire year in 2018.

This audacious undertaking became known as 365 Ubuntu Climbs. The challenge was about harnessing the power of unity and addressing issues like the lack of housing and education in challenged communities. Motivated by my past experiences in fundraising, I recognized the potential of this extreme physical challenge. Completing the challenge would be the equivalent of climbing Mount Everest 71 times and would aim to capture people's attention and inspire them to participate and donate. I envisioned each climb as an opportunity to contribute just R1 a day (less than $0.10), illustrating how simple it was to make a meaningful impact. Rather than relying on major corporate sponsors, I took action, built trust, encouraged people to join and demonstrated how collective efforts can drive change. I invited donors to climb alongside me so they could experience the journey firsthand and claim their own part in this historic endeavour. Even my parents, my sister, and her family, who live in another province, made their way to Cape Town, embraced the challenge, and climbed on days 101/365 and 62/365, respectively.

I knew that by stepping into the public spotlight, I'd be subjecting my ideas and beliefs to scrutiny, especially as I was attempting something that had never been done before. I had no roadmap, no template, and pretty much everyone doubted my ability to complete such an ambitious goal, but my soul burned with determination. My physical perseverance, emotional fortitude, mental strength, and spiritual resolve were all stretched past their limits just to get to the 6-month mark. Having battled self-doubt all my life, the odds seemed stacked against me. But no matter what, I just had to wake up each day and focus on the steps at my feet. I had to ignore the future, embrace the present, and express gratitude for what was behind me. I had to dig deeper than I thought possible to get through the year.

The purpose of this book is to give you hope, shine a light on the possibilities in life, and share the experiences and lessons that shaped my body and mind in preparation for this outrageous goal. The idea was not a spontaneous act; but rather a culmination of 38 years of life and six months of meticulously planning and executing a training regimen that would increase my chances of success. Six years earlier, I suffered a serious injury on the same route, so to come out the other side of this challenge healthy, uninjured, and still able to walk without pain for the rest of my life, I had to prepare for the worst. So much could go wrong in 365 days.

Take this transformative journey with me as I show you how life is not just about the destination, but a series of moments all interlinked and worthy of your full attention. Every step, every challenge, and every encounter, had a profound impact on my growth and perspective. This is my story, and I hope that by sharing it, I can inspire you to passionately embrace your ideas and dreams. One magical thing that you'll discover, just as I did, is how unpredictable and serendipitous the journey can become.

In the shadowy corners of my story, the unknown lurked like a mysterious character, and taught me the art of surrender and how to look deep within for the truth. I was tested beyond my belief. I realise now that I DO want to be tested before I jump in because once you're in the pool — it's too late to complain about being wet. I learned to embrace the whims of the weather, and accepted that some days would be gruelling battles against nature's forces, which would put my safety at risk. I relinquished control, embraced the unpredictability, and found solace in the journey and its revelations. Surrendering to the unknown became a transformative practice, and allowed me to release the need for absolute certainty and trust.

I had to persevere and show extreme levels of grit as doubts and fatigue threatened to overwhelm me. I had to remind myself that I was discovering the power of resilience, and that true strength is forged in the face of adversity. Resilience alone is not enough. Adaptability, vulnerability, surrender, and consistency are vital to success.

Consistency is the bedrock that supports the towering mountain of our aspirations. Just as a mountain stands tall against the elements, it is the consistent force of our actions and mindset that form a solid foundation for our journey. With the steps we take, decisions we make, and challenges we overcome, we ascend higher towards our goals. Amidst the unpredictable terrain and changing conditions, consistency serves as our guide, and anchors us to the summit of achievement. By persistently pushing forward, adapting to the ever-changing landscape, and embracing vulnerability, we forge an unbreakable bond with the mountain of our destiny, conquering challenges and realising our full potential. These elements, as well as the actual elements, emerged as powerful teachers in my life, and moulded me into the person I am today.

This book also serves as a testament to the extraordinary achievements possible when we courageously pursue our dreams. It emphasises the significance of community, proving that even the seemingly craziest ideas, when rooted in love and Ubuntu, have the power to nurture collective growth and transform lives. May it inspire you to embark on your own transformative journey and discover the extraordinary magic that awaits **Beyond YOUR Summit**.

'It always seems impossible, until it's done'
– Nelson Mandela, 2001

CHAPTER 1
THE DAY MY WORLD IMPLODED

On the 22nd of June 2017 I woke up with a sickening feeling in the pit of my stomach. I tried to distract myself, but the gnawing was relentless and demanded my full attention. I had the feeling that my life was about to change in a way I could never imagine.

It had already been three weeks since I got laid off. Three weeks of driving to work closing out my notice period; painfully being asked, "what are you going to do?" Three weeks of panic in anticipation of having my future slate wiped clean. For three weeks I processed the shame of being deemed 'unworthy' by my company to fulfil a role I'd been doing for five years – a role I'd executed cleanly and without any poor performance reviews to my name.

We'd been told to apply for multiple positions, this way if we were unsuccessful with one, then there'd surely be another to fall back on. I chose not to apply for multiple roles. My thinking was that if I didn't get the 'promotion', then I wouldn't want to work in a company I'd lost respect for, and in an industry I was rapidly becoming disillusioned with. Mike Tyson said, "everyone has a plan until they get punched in the mouth," and this had certainly felt like one of his punches.

As the chaos unfolded, two choices appeared:

1. I could decide out of fear to apply for another role in the company that didn't fit my career path and which had me feeling unfulfilled. Or,
2. I could choose love and use this as an opportunity to reimagine a new vision for my life.

Receiving a retrenchment package as compensation meant I had the gift of time, financially it would give me a buffer. Having already been at a company in 2008 that was liquidated, I'd built a belief that if something was painful now, and it was managed effectively, then that pain would develop character and could become the bedrock of future opportunities.

The pain I experienced back in 2008 is what helped me choose love this time around, it inspired me to move forward, so I made the decision to process the retrenchment. It would've been disingenuous of me to take a role that didn't fulfil me, and it would've been unfair to take an opportunity away from someone else more enthusiastically committed to the company. But still, I look back and I cringe because I know, it's easier said than done to make the bold choice in a situation like this and to step gung-ho into a future of uncertainty with no clear path to follow. The truth is that it scared the hell out of me.

It was a rough time in my life. I painstakingly worked on a new vision by focusing on what I loved doing: hiking, mountains, spending time with people, and adding value to society. With the help of my powerhouse friend Lianne, I explored the possibility of starting a hiking tourism company, and I contemplated how I could support non-profits like Habitat for Humanity and DKMS Africa with the skills I had. DKMS Africa, prior to changing their name, was well known as The Sunflower Fund.

During that three-week period of introspection and decision-making, a special ray of light came to me in the form of a podcast launch, courtesy of my friend Andre. It was called 'Powerful Beyond Measure,' and I was invited to the breakfast launch. I gladly accepted, to support him and to hear more about it. I knew what it was like to put yourself out there and to do new things, so I appreciated and understood the power of support. I also made it a point to do this for others wherever I could.

At the launch, we had the most amazing group of human beings at our table which made me feel honoured to be there. As the day progressed, I was presented with an unexpected gift – an introduction to Astrid, a woman I'm incredibly proud to call a friend today.

Before I knew what was happening the universe began showing me some clues to something bigger. Puzzle piece number one took shape as Andre excitedly introduced me to another amazing person by the name of Lynne. Explaining his delight, he matched my love of hiking in the mountains around Cape Town, to the challenge she'd begun. She was climbing Table Mountain via Platteklip Gorge for 67 consecutive days, a feat that would culminate on Nelson Mandela's birthday. Lynne chose the number 67 because it had become tradition in South Africa to do something charitable for 67 minutes on Mandela's birthday, to commemorate his 67 years of public service.

I loved this!

I found the challenge fascinating because it ran all the way through the Cape's cold & wet winter, and I knew just how tough that route was with its unapologetically direct path up the front face to the top of the mountain. I enjoyed hearing how the first three days had gone, so we exchanged details. I'd hoped to offer my company and support by climbing with her on a day when the weather was bad, or on a day when she'd been struggling with motivation.

Now, although the plan was to meet up and synchronise our efforts, we never got around to it. However, that conversation dug the hole for another seedling

CHAPTER 1
THE DAY MY WORLD IMPLODED

idea to be planted. The next piece of the puzzle arrived at a catch-up dinner five days later with Patsy, a primary school friend. Patsy and I followed opposite paths in our careers – she worked in the alcohol industry before heading to Coca-Cola, then she decided to start her own business, and I left Coca-Cola to join the alcohol industry. It was fascinating listening to Patsy and the first-hand challenges experienced by entrepreneurs and those working from home. She highlighted the trials of getting out of bed early in the morning instead of snoozing and how this required added motivation. So, to build her resolve she entered half Ironman competitions. This required a strict training schedule to ensure not only survival from start to finish but also an enjoyable day of racing.

Patsy's journey got me thinking about winter and how my gym sessions dwindled as darkness, cold and wet conditions provided 'excuses' to remain in the sanctuary of my warm bed. If snoozing were a sport, I'd be world champion and with winter thrown into the mix, I just turned into a human hibernating bear. I started asking myself the hard questions, like...... *"What activities could I do for the next year to push my physical capabilities and to prevent hibernation?"*

It sure as hell wasn't going to be half an Ironman! And with that, I slipped this unsolved puzzle piece into my pocket with the others.

Right on cue, the next morning I snoozed and missed another gym session. A sign? Perhaps, nevertheless I got up, pulled myself together and set off for my seventh last drive into work, this time with an important conversation playing over in my mind. My brain had become a washing machine of ideas, desires, fears, and experiences, all churning around as it welcomed another one of my passions into the mix – my love for writing.

I'd been blogging for just over two years, largely thanks to the guidance and coaxing of my friends Lianne and Martelize. Lianne was an incredibly successful businesswoman who went on to become a Business Network Director at YPO – an organisation that harnessed the knowledge, influence and trust of the world's most innovative business leaders, to inspire others. Martelize was also an experienced radio host with her own blog whose influence was monumental on me. And while others may have initiated earlier conversations pushing me to write, the combination of Lianne and Martelize's encouragement forced me to take it seriously.

I proposed dinner to Martelize and she accepted my invitation as well as the opportunity to let me pick her brain about getting started on my blog which I'd decided to call Renaissance Guy. It was a tribute to my Latin teacher, Mr Wilson. He was our 'Mr Keatings' from the well-known movie Dead Poets Society, and I'd never forgotten his challenge to us.

'Dare to be renaissance men'

That challenge had always stuck with me and felt like the perfect fit to challenge the way I was thinking about living intentionally. Men of the renaissance era became painters, sculptors, poets, writers, scientists, philosophers, and were limitless in their capacities for development. They tried to embrace all available knowledge and developed themselves as fully as possible.

My friend Andre contacted me after reading my blog, 'Pray for Something Bad,' earnestly stating, "You need to write a book." It was a huge confidence boost for me, and hearing it from one of South Africa's most sought-after coaches for high-performing executives, CEOs, and marketers, gave it so much weight.

Seven months later, Andre's encouraging endorsement was still swirling around my head, only now I had so much more information to work with. The washing machine of ideas was in full force while heading to work, along the freeway, deep in thought. I passed the Good Hope Centre with Table Mountain looming large in front of me, and another question struck!

What should I write about?

This one really hit me hard and triggered one of the most memorable moments of my life. Immediately it was answered from within the deepest recesses of my mind. It was as if someone else had been present inside, taking control of my thoughts.

CHAPTER 1
THE DAY MY WORLD IMPLODED

The voice within said, **"Climb Table Mountain every single day for a year!!"**

Suddenly 37 years and 229 days of living collided in a life-changing instant, it was my own Big Bang moment, the rebirth of my inspiration, and it felt like the rocket fuel for my life's space shuttle had just been ignited.

What came to me was a simple idea; but it instantly set my soul on fire.

I'll never forget the 22nd of June 2017, 8 days before my last day of the corporate journey, when the stormiest weather in my life suddenly transformed into clear, blue skies. It wasn't just the concept of an intense mountain journey that blew my mind, it was also the understanding of how this would be my greatest physical, emotional, mental, and spiritual test. Committing to a year-long journey of daily Table Mountain summits would set the stage to raise money and awareness for organisations that tirelessly worked to empower those held back in life. The purpose and the intention behind the initiative would encourage others to be a part of the journey as well. This idea absolutely blew my mind, it impacted me physically, and it began to show.

The people driving next to me must have thought that I was insane as I slammed the steering wheel. My heart pounded with exhilaration and with the wildest smile on my face I screamed, 'No ways! It's such a simple idea! It can't be that simple?!'

As the minutes passed, I began to see how each puzzle piece linked up to make my idea a realistic possibility. This concept had:

- My desire for Personal Growth
- My love for writing
- My absolute passion for experiencing Nature
- A valuable contribution to society
- An intention to build communities
- A plan to empower others
- A brutal solution to my hibernation problem

- A powerful element of awareness that would show people how easy it was to give

I let the idea of 365 times in a row up Platteklip Gorge sink in again, this was the plan! I loved the route even though it had picked up a bad rap and got labelled as 'boring'. I thought it had some of the most spectacular paths that relentlessly snaked through the crack up the front face of the mountain. And as you approached the summit, you were flanked by towering cliffs on either side that conveyed a majestic aura that seemed to transport you to a mythical land. The relentless 'staircase' wound its way up the mountain looking like an impossible feat from afar.

Tackling Platteklip was the perfect sweet spot as a significant daily challenge that would ask serious questions of me, but at the same time, it wasn't an impossible act. For most people, doing it once provided an extreme sense of achievement – and rightly so.

My mind raced a million miles an hour as the benefits of this challenge continued to flow out into my consciousness, it was as if a dam wall had broken and everything that had once been contained, had now been released. As the most direct and 'easiest' route up Table Mountain, I loved the freedom it afforded me to invite donors to join and participate in challenging their own capabilities on any day they wished.

The challenge was extreme for me because I'd do it every day, but anyone else participating and climbing with me on a chosen day would share in the history of the climb that corresponded to just that day, for them it would be so much more manageable.

Participation and the company of others would be one of the greatest gifts I'd get to enjoy throughout the year while meeting new people and learning the value of Ubuntu. My mind was still racing and re-connected to a previous thought about the power of numbers. I used our company's figure of five thousand people to calculate what the result would be if each person donated R10 a month – that would be R50 000. Most of us paid R50 for parking each month – so using that as a benchmark, it quickly ramped the total up to R225 000!

That was just one company, so what if 50,000 Capetonians (1.11% of the population) pledged R1 per climb? I'm ashamed to admit this but I pulled out my phone to calculate it while driving. I didn't crash but I may as well have with the noise I made at the number. If 50,000 people gave R1 per day (R30 a month – which was also the price of a coffee in most cafes) it would add up to.... R1 500 000 every month!

EVERY MONTH?!

As if I wasn't excited enough, I started dreaming of the impact this could have on the companies on the receiving end of these funds. The number of houses we could build for the people who live in the shacks that line the highway on my way to my work. The number of new donors that could be added to the registry, that, thanks to DKMS Africa, would save the lives of many leukaemia sufferers. I loved the simplicity and the potential of this idea.

For the first time in my life, I stopped searching outside for clarity on what to do. Instead, I had patience and trusted things would happen as needed, I was rewarded with an idea that aligned with my internal compass, it touched my heart and resonated with my soul. I was able to focus on what I wanted and genuinely believed that something bigger was possible. This created a fertile mind ready to embrace and commit to one seriously insane idea.

More importantly though, this was the first time I'd ever had zero self-doubts in my abilities to complete a challenge. I couldn't explain it to you, I just knew that come rain, hail, wind, and heat, I was going to climb Table Mountain every single day in 2018.

I started sending voice notes on WhatsApp to my family, my friends and other group chats about my 'once in a lifetime' idea. Needless to say, their responses told a story – they couldn't quite believe what I was going to do.

I arrived at work a lighter man which was clearly visible to everyone. Then the questions started coming my way, so I explained my idea and spoke about what I'd be doing. It was great to see the reactions of disbelief, and even though I couldn't answer all the questions; nothing could douse the excitement that had begun to grow.

Some colleagues were still just finding out about my departure and came down to check in with me. The conversation started sombre and supportive, but as the news of my epic journey emerged, it ended with – 'holy shit! This is incredible – I'm a little bit jealous'.

Calamity was transformed into Celebration.

I'd been handed a test that was set up to challenge all my beliefs and everything I'd learned up until this point.

I was excited to find out what I was made of.

And I knew my life would never be the same.

'We may not be responsible for the world that created our minds, but we can take responsibility for the mind with which we create our world' ~ **Gabor Mate**

CHAPTER 2
THE INGREDIENTS THAT MADE IT ALL POSSIBLE

I am who I am because of the sum total of my experiences, good and bad. So how did I get here today? Well, allow me to give you some insight into the history of South Africa and the experiences that shaped me. I was 10 years old when Nelson Mandela was released from prison. 14 years old when we had our first free and fair elections for all. The New South Africa was born. I was part of the generation that saw the first integration between white and black students in schools.

Apartheid (literally translated *Apart hood*) was the name for the system of institutionalised racism against anyone 'not white'. I was too young to understand what the horrors of Apartheid meant for the majority of the population. At the age of 14, I had the privilege of witnessing Nelson Mandela speak at our all-boy school in Johannesburg – King Edward VII School (KES). I wish I'd known then how significant hearing him speak was, he was just ten metres away from me. I wish I could remember the wisdom he imparted on us that day. Sadly, I can't.

But thanks to the internet, I searched our school's website and found a copy of an article written in our school magazine that year. Someone else that day was paying close attention to the message he gave us.....

'With privilege, comes great responsibility'

I believe that was a seed planted in my young mind, it remained there all these years, waiting for the first rains before it would sprout. That rain came almost a quarter of a century later.

Life as a teenager was tumultuous, I couldn't comprehend the impact Nelson Mandela had on our country's peaceful transition – we were seconds away from a full-blown civil war, a fact I learned later on in a *Transformation Workshop*.

The *Truth & Reconciliation Committee* was headed up by Archbishop Desmond Tutu from 1995 to 1998. The purpose was to provide a safe space for victims of Apartheid to share stories of the abuse suffered and the brutal way in which many were arrested and still missing.

Perpetrators who were able to submit a compelling claim that they were acting under the 'law' of the government, were also allowed to apply for amnesty. Horror stories were revealed about what was done to freedom fighters and how inhumane their torture and treatment was. While painful to hear for all, many found peace in the finality of knowing what happened to their friends or family.

I remember sitting spellbound in front of the television, watching the stories and being deeply moved by the constant tears that Desmond Tutu cried day after day. The strength he and his colleagues needed to listen to the reports of atrocities across the country blew me away and still impacts me to this day.

CHAPTER 2
THE INGREDIENTS THAT MADE IT ALL POSSIBLE

Back then, I heard it – but I didn't understand or feel it. Much like watching a fictional movie. It felt like the difference between knowledge and wisdom, anyone could have knowledge, but wisdom was having the ability to understand a situation from another's perspective.

I was sensitive to what this system had done. As I grew older, I realised that I had benefited from it – and that it had favoured me because I was white. I struggled to fully understand it, how could I?

I hadn't personally experienced or listened to people who had endured years of suffering. Real suffering. Enforced suffering.

At the age of 22 I visited the recently opened Apartheid Museum near Gold Reef City, located in Johannesburg. I don't know what the pull was. I just know that on Youth Day, June 16th, 2002, I felt a call and drove there, on my own, to learn about our nation's past. I liken the experience to the time I visited Dachau Concentration Camp in Munich, Germany, three years later. Solemn, horrific, heartbreaking, and immensely painful. The difference was that this time it was my country where the injustices were inflicted, and it was my fellow countrymen that suffered.

The museum was incredibly well designed and offered a walking tour much like the World Trade Center's Ground Zero Walking Tour in New York City. I saw old news footage, at the Apartheid Museum, which transported me back in time. I came across actual 'whites only' signs and heard the stories of people deeply affected by the terrors of apartheid. I cried through most of the tour.

I felt deeply impacted and emotionally heavy leaving the museum that day, but not enough to start making a change for others. I had no idea where to begin!! It was like finding yourself in a relationship with a partner who'd suffered previous trauma and abuse – you hadn't caused the damage, but understanding what they went through meant you could be more empathetic and positively responsive to the behaviours triggered by the hurtful past.

Confucius says, "I hear and I forget. I see and I remember. I do and I understand." In 2003 the latter part of this quote came true, and it was vital for my understanding of Ubuntu:

Build perspective with compassion.

The first event was on the 22nd of February 2003.

At the time, I was working as a salesman at The Pro Shop in Woodmead, Johannesburg. South Africa's leading golf retail outlet. I'd recently 'graduated' off the tills which enabled me to earn commission from sales. On this fateful Saturday, the afternoon shift was drastically short-staffed so they asked me to help because I knew how to use the system.

Shortly after taking my post with the other two staff members, a large 'bang' sounded out to my left, near the entrance. I saw a salesman running for cover, which looked incredibly odd. Then I felt a pain in my left hip, just behind me, as though a mate had smacked me. I jokingly turned around to hit him back. It wasn't a friend. It was an armed robber hitting me with the muzzle of the gun, he yelled at me to open the smart box – a device the company used to drop cash into. The smart box, as the name suggested, had a job to do, and that was to hold the cash until the right machine was used to open it. The cash would then be collected by armoured vehicles for safe passage to the bank.

For the next two minutes, which felt like twenty, I went into autopilot. I opened cash draws to give him whatever hadn't been dropped into the smart box yet. His hand was shaking. My heart was pounding. His nerves caused his finger to pull the trigger, and that's when the first gunshot went off. It ricocheted off the floor into one of the cashier's legs while she crouched down low. I saw blood splatter onto the floor, and all I could think about was how I needed to get them to leave so I could call an ambulance. I leaned across and opened another till.

I saw his hand shake as it held the gun, then suddenly it exploded while he was barely a foot away from me. I felt the pants on my leg whip around. Instinctively I bent down and grabbed my leg, I thought I'd been shot too.

CHAPTER 2
THE INGREDIENTS THAT MADE IT ALL POSSIBLE

I hunched on the ground with my hands clasped around my leg, he yelled at me to open the smart box again. My ear was ringing from the second gunshot. Amazingly, the bullet had gone through my pants but missed my leg. I stood up to explain that I couldn't open the smart box, so he pointed the gun straight at my face. I thought this was it. Where could I be shot and still live? Maybe my shoulder? I raised my hands in submission, I dropped my head, I looked at the floor and waited for the next gunshot.

He ordered me down on the ground and demanded my cell phone. And although there were at least seven landline phones behind the counter for me to use, idiotically, I pretended not to have a phone because all I could think about was getting that ambulance. Thankfully, no calls came through on my number in that moment.

As he took his opportunity and fled, I saw something that had a profound impact on me. He dropped a R20 note but spotted it and came back to pick it up. This was when I realised how badly they needed money and that even a R20 note meant something and was worth coming back to risk it all for, it's something I still think about to this day. I'll never condone his actions, but that made me question how bad his life was that this had become his best option. It made me think about his circumstances.

Turning my attention back to the scene, I was thankful that the cashier's leg wound wasn't too serious and everyone was alive.

It's all a blur between calling the ambulance, the police arriving, and giving my statement. Eventually, after speaking to the police, I walked outside, the adrenalin faded, and I collapsed onto the curb sobbing uncontrollably. The duality of how close I came to being shot and losing my life, yet still being alive to think about it, shook me to the core. I drove home on that hot summer's day with all my windows open, singing as loud as my voice allowed me to. I was alive!

I've never taken my legs or my life for granted since that day. I didn't know it at the time, but that situation had rewired my brain to start saying yes to more opportunities I'd normally say no to in the past.

On a personal level, experiencing such a traumatic event taught me how important it was to process emotions as well as the value of talking it out. The Pro Shop was amazing, they made sure we all saw a psychiatrist and provided the necessary support for those of us who weren't coping. My biggest blessings were having my parents to talk it out with that evening and then having a stock take the next day to openly discuss what happened. At the group session the following Monday, we heard other people's perspectives on what they were going through when they heard the gunshots and how they thought they would be killed. It was a moving experience. The group session was important because I saw how quickly some people took four men's actions and blanketed an entire race with their hatred. An entire race didn't do this, it was just four men that did it.

This became a powerful layer for me to use going forward – no matter what challenges I faced, it wasn't going to be life or death.

Two months later, my good friend Jono moved to the UK and asked me to join him. I had never wanted to live in the UK. The weather was too miserable, but luckily, he pushed me because otherwise, I might never have left Johannesburg.

I finished my marketing degree in June and by August I had arrived in London, England. Not only was that where I met the lady who would pull me to Cape Town – but it was also home to Harrods, the world's leading luxury department store – a store where I found my new job. Suddenly, something came over me. I had no idea where it came from, but I got the urge to find a charity to volunteer with. The urge came with questions....

Who do I support? What would I be doing? And how would I even begin searching for options?

The next day, our department meeting shared that the Chairman's Children's Christmas Party needed volunteers for October, which was the following month. I wondered if they'd been listening to my thoughts. You couldn't ask for something, get it, and then turn it down, so I signed up and would become 'The Dancing Bear' dressed in a panda bear suit. I danced because I was nervous waiting above the escalator while the families arrived.

CHAPTER 2
THE INGREDIENTS THAT MADE IT ALL POSSIBLE

It was crazy, no one could see me, but I was petrified. The children were a mixture of terminally ill, disabled, or in hospital. This was the day I learned how such a small effort to become the dancing bear could bring so much joy to children. But perhaps there was even more joy felt by their parents, who silently mouthed 'thank you' through tears as their children enjoyed a break from a harsh reality. I may have stunk to high heaven in the 45 minute tube ride home after sweating profusely in that bear costume, but I was filled with gratitude.

Then my next pivotal year arrived; I was back in Cape Town, and it was 2015.

Our company hosted a transformational workshop in July and it was led by Professor Jackie Naude, author of *Finding the Rainbow*. This was the first time I'd been involved in a dialogue that spoke about Apartheid from every perspective with a diverse group of people from a variety of backgrounds.

She didn't start with Apartheid. She started with the Boer War in 1899 and spoke about what the British did to the women and children in the first-ever concentration camps (no – Hitler didn't invent them, the British did). She led us on a journey from their perspective of how being attacked, decimated, and treated so poorly made them defiant and made them stand together with one point in mind: that they would never be humiliated like that again.

Her narrative was not about saying 'this justifies anyone's actions', or that it was wrong; she simply went through our history (something I wished we had done at school) and explained the actions that led to future actions.

At this point, I should explain why we were having a transformational workshop to begin with and what 'transformation' in the South African context means.

After Apartheid ended, the government mandated corporations to work with them to help rectify the injustices of the past. BEE (Black Economic Empowerment) and Affirmative Action became scary words to whites and large companies. They believed it was a drastic over-correction meant to subjugate whites in the workforce.

These terms, without a full understanding, made me feel uneasy too, and disgusted that I could be rejected for a position just because of the colour of my skin. The irony! I didn't grow up wealthy. My parents didn't have it easy. For years, my dad worked harder than most people I'd ever met in my life, sacrificing weekends and his annual leave to earn more money just so we could eat and break even at the end of the month.

How dare I be discriminated against now with reverse racism! I didn't personally gain from Apartheid!

I was very opinionated on this topic prior to the workshop. Then, Jackie began to explain in detail what privilege looked like for me outside of monetary gain. I could choose where to live. My dad wasn't forced to work insane hours in a mine hundreds of kilometres away from us, and I didn't need a pass to move from one suburb to another. I also had a birth certificate, and I wasn't treated like an animal or told how little my life was worth.

Additionally, I was given top class education, not the bare minimum that non-whites were given because it was assumed they were going to be labourers anyway. The list was unfortunately longer and far more brutal than that.

I listened to colleagues share their stories of how Apartheid affected their lives. I listened to how the ANC government's BEE program wasn't about appointing black people ahead of whites – it was about creating a sustainable long-term plan to educate and move workers up the ranks over the years to significantly help change the proportions of leadership to match the country's demographics. It was supposed to be a plan to help balance the injustices of the past by creating opportunities for the future.

Corporate companies buried their heads in the sand. They didn't engage in dialogue to understand what BEE meant and continued as they were. Eventually, the government grew weary of corporate's inaction to demonstrate a willingness to execute their wishes. So they started penalising companies that didn't adhere to BEE and that didn't achieve scores in line with the diversity recommendations for the organisation and its leadership structures.

CHAPTER 2
THE INGREDIENTS THAT MADE IT ALL POSSIBLE

Unfortunately, as with any other instituted action, wealthy people saw an opportunity and started creating companies which were predominantly black, to 'invest' equity into, so they could get a higher BEE score to appease government regulations. At face value, it was great, but was it good for the people needing a hand up? Not so much. Essentially, the rich got richer and the people needing the assistance were drifting further and further behind.

My eyes started opening and seeing colour for the first time, as if I was only able to see in black and white before that.

Soon after that, 'Zuma must fall' became a hot topic. Marches and protests expressing dissatisfaction with our president Jacob Zuma's government sprouted up all over the country. Zuma's alleged corruption during his nine-year tenure as the President of South Africa seemed to know no bounds until the sudden firing of one of the state's greatest cabinet members and Finance Minister; Pravin Gordan. This irrational and suspicious act sparked outrage and 'enough is enough' dissent throughout the country.

Over time, our economy lost R250 billion rand. Billion. That's $16 billion. Marches were justified, our country was being ruined by a government that had neither the ethics nor the will to handle the job! Then, in December 2015, I attended one of the Marches in Cape Town, and something became blatantly obvious.

It was 99% white.

Where were the rest of our countrymen and women?! This glaring absence got me asking why. It made me engage where I'd been absent before. I asked the question, 'why don't you march against a president clearly damaging the country?' My righteous aura of self-proclaimed protector of the country and its desire for 'all' to live equally was dealt its first sobering blow.

'Where were you when the Marikana massacre happened? 34 unarmed civilians disputing wage issues on a platinum mine were gunned down – where were you when we marched then?'

25

This question struck me hard, I'd never been this embarrassed by a lack of behaviour before. I had no answer. I was stumped by my own inaction while 'trying to do the right thing' now. I was instantly educated on the perspective fellow South Africans held. I was enlightened to what was endured every day by many people who never enjoyed the same enthusiastic level of support.

This reinforced my realisation that while I knew about the horrors of Apartheid, I'd never asked people to share their experiences. Like "don't ask, don't tell," kind of thing, and let's just move on. It was easier to pretend.

Just like my earlier analogy – if you dated someone and loved them, doesn't that encompass meeting them at their level of trauma to listen and understand them? No matter what? After all, how can you understand someone's behaviour today if you don't have all the information on their past experiences?

It made me realise that for all the research and 'understanding' of Apartheid I'd done – I'd never taken the time to ask my friends and colleagues what their lived experiences were. After a couple of months of grappling internally with this dilemma I finally faced up to what I needed to do! I needed to ask them if they'd be comfortable sharing what their life had been like through Apartheid.

Feeling more nervous than the first time I asked a woman out on a date – I approached them one by one with the single intent to listen to their stories. If they wanted to tell me, that is. Gratefully, they all agreed. One by one, I sat across from them. Not to atone, not to reply with 'yeah but...', and not to justify my tolerance. Just to listen with the purpose of gaining a better understanding. Within five seconds, every single one of their eyes glazed over while recounting stories of their experiences during Apartheid.

I began to hear how Police drove into their neighbourhoods, fired at will, and sent children as young as eight diving for cover behind walls. Another story detailed how the Police broke through the front door late at night for no reason and ran over children laying on the floor of their tiny shack. Families were dragged out in handcuffs, beaten and bloodied. And now that the door had

CHAPTER 2
THE INGREDIENTS THAT MADE IT ALL POSSIBLE

been smashed down, they had no protection against criminals prowling the township for the rest of the night.

I was told how scared to death they were just walking down the street as white people passed them by. They feared the terrible acts that could be carried out against them without any consequences and how easy it was for them to be jailed even if they'd done nothing wrong.

I was being transported to a very different country from the one I'd grown up in. One of unimaginable pain, fear, and trauma. A multi-generational experience. Those who suffered weren't only parents or grandparents, they were people my age too. For the first time, I connected on a human level with what Apartheid did, and the effects still being felt to this day.

Privilege conversations usually make people think of money and wealth. They were never about being free from police harassment, having access to equal education, or getting the opportunity to pursue your dreams. Before this, the conversations had never been about having the ability to just be yourself freely, but now they were.

I'd never condone people burning tyres on the N2 highway from Somerset West into Cape Town – but I suddenly understood why it was done. What would I have done if my parents had been treated like this? How would I handle it if, post 1994, they were still living in a shack with unfulfilled promises of jobs and safe homes to live in? I'd also feel ignored, neglected, and abandoned.

I developed an important understanding; **while I may not have been personally responsible for the suffering of others – it didn't mean I couldn't be part of the solution to empower them .**

Putting a name and a logo to my idea to Climb Table Mountain every day.

Ok, so this didn't start off well. Firstly, I was introduced to someone coined as a 'whizz', which created high expectations. He promised to work with me on the name and to help me create a logo. I kept pushing to meet up with him, but

I just ended up waiting, waiting, waiting, and then nothing. I'd already gotten requests for interviews on the radio just as a friend got me onto the second show of 'The Honest Truth' with Smile FM's Benito Vergotine, so I needed to come up with a name for the challenge, and I needed one quickly!

I threw some ideas around; '365 Table climbs', '365 ways to love', 'Table Love', 'Mountain of Hope', and even worse, 'Love in a mountain' — but none of these resonated. The word 'ubuntu' popped up in the back of my mind and hummed with my body like a tuning fork. Most importantly, it conveyed the essence of what the climbs were all about.

Ubuntu is an African word that encompasses the spirit of humanity. It's an understanding that I am because of you. "Umuntu Ngumuntu Ngabantu," which can be translated as, "a person is a person because of or through others." In certain regions of South Africa, when someone did something wrong, they were taken to the centre of the village and surrounded by the tribe for two days while they spoke only of the good things they'd done. They believed each person was good, yet sometimes made mistakes, which was really a cry for help. They united in this ritual to encourage the person to reconnect with their true nature. The belief was that unity and affirmation had more power to change behaviour than shame and punishment.

Ubuntu is humanity towards others.

This may be why things like jails didn't exist in African culture.

Honestly, I was a little worried about using it in case it was offensive in some way. That was until I posed the question to Sizwe! The way his eyes lit up when I asked, 'what do you think of 365 Ubuntu Climbs?', made me realise how misplaced my thoughts were. I'd made another assumption and was happily proven wrong this time. Anyway, I was ecstatic that this crazy white guy was able to use it.

CHAPTER 2
THE INGREDIENTS THAT MADE IT ALL POSSIBLE

It's interesting how my brain, clouded by fear, tried to rationalise a thought which came from a place of pure love and tried to create reasons for me not to carry through with it. Ubuntu was in the middle of the name; it was at the heart of the project, and as the year progressed, I became schooled on its true meaning in a way that went beyond my original intentions to understand and teach its essence to others.

Now that I had a name, I seriously needed a logo. I knew I wanted the logo to somehow reflect the period of a single day while having a mountain in it, too. I started experimenting with websites that offered free logo designs.

Thankfully, Stefan came to my rescue. I knew him from a party we connected at on 01.02.'03, it was impossible to forget that date. Even then, I was impressed by his impeccable eye and his design skills, he was definitely in the right field. Truthfully, I'm not sure why I didn't go straight to him to begin with. I remember when he first moved to Cape Town in 2009, he found a gorgeous two-bedroom spot with the most incredible views. Besides building our friendship, I witnessed the magic of his work and constantly saw the fruits of his labour, so he was certainly the man for the job.

Once I had a basic design that I thought would work, I sent it to him.

'Give me a few days bru – lemme sort something out for you'

True to his word I got a beautiful, simple, and elegant design back. It was a jagged mountain with four wavy lines at the bottom that represented the sea, and twelve triangles neatly placed around the circle like points on a clock. A perfect representation of the daily challenge, which also included twelve points representing each month of the year.

I LOVED IT!!! My only feedback, which was backed up by my Family, was how we could get the mountain to look more like Table Mountain. Stefan made the simple adjustment and BOOM! 365 Ubuntu Climbs had a logo! His explanation about why he chose orange was beautiful and purposeful:

"I really went with orange because to me it represents the sunrise after a dark night. It represents cycles and the promise that even the darkest nights are always followed by the rising sun. Hence why the background and images are predominantly a dark shade of black and white. It's the sun that breathes life into the sea, the mountain and nature."

This was incredible because orange also represented enthusiasm, determination, success, and encouragement!! Everything I needed to keep me going! Thanks to his help, I went into December feeling far happier than I was in November after being so badly let down. Stefan's logo became the focal point for the year to come.

Gareth, another friend of mine, was recommended to me to help create a T-shirt design. I thought about printing T-shirts for those wanting a memento, and I also thought about having caps made.

With the logo done, phase two for the T-shirt design kicked in. December was pretty chaotic at the best of times, so I chatted with Gareth and gave him an outline of what I was looking for.

"I'd like an outline of Table Mountain on the front, with a silhouette of a climber and the logo. I'd like a space for two different options – one where just the month, like January 2018, is visible; and another for someone wanting a limited-edition shirt which would have the specific date and associated climb number on it. An example, if they joined on a specific date their shirt would have '22 February 2018 – 53 / 365' underneath the climber"

"No problem Andrew, I'll send you something tomorrow"

It was a very simple design, and I chose grey T-shirts to highlight the Orange in the logo. The grey also represented the colour of the mountain. I also had the idea to print T-shirts for the milestones, like day 100 and 200. When the time would come, I'd choose a light shade called 'petrol blue' – all from a local producer called Fittees. The simple design made it easy for me to supply Gareth

CHAPTER 2
THE INGREDIENTS THAT MADE IT ALL POSSIBLE

with a date and climb number for people that wanted them – he also gave me the option of sending 12 designs, one for each month and ready for the printers.

The T-shirts were done and I designed some caps too. With my expertise in building business trackers, I'd be keeping a record of the days people joined, their names, the data around the kilometres travelled, time spent on the mountain and the elevation gain. Anyone buying a cap could get their individual number sewn into the side of the cap if they wanted.

The T-shirts would become my standard gear to wear for the year, and would be added to my collection as each triple-digit milestone was achieved, they would also act as marketing wherever I went. Stefan and Gareth demonstrated how people and businesses could help charitable causes and make a huge difference by donating their time and skills. I'm eternally grateful for their help with the logo that was created, and for the gear that was branded, this truly brought my idea to life.

All these things amplified the excitement building inside of me. I was pushed at every stage while developing the concept. Next, it was all about developing the mindset, the physicality, and the emotional strength to match the spiritual commitment that was driving me to succeed. I also knew exactly what the next steps needed to be.

What I didn't know was how much the next steps would ask of me and how rude of an awakening my need to prepare would be.

> "Marriage is hard. Divorce is hard. Choose your hard. Obesity is hard. Being fit is hard. Choose your hard.
>
> Being in debt is hard. Being financially disciplined is hard. Choose your hard. Communication is hard. Not communicating is hard. Choose your hard.
>
> Life will never be easy. It will always be hard. But we can choose our hard. Pick wisely." ~~ **Unknown**

CHAPTER 3
TURNING AN IDEA INTO REALITY

It's one thing to have an idea, and it's another to turn it into reality, especially when it has never been done before, and you have no template to follow.

For five years at work, I was amazed by the number of people who used the elevator from the basement to the first few floors of the building. I made it a personal commitment to use the stairs every day, no matter how many times I needed to stop on a floor to talk to someone. This experience must have been what inspired me to abstain from taking any elevator trips for the six months leading up to the start of my summiting journey.

CHAPTER 3
TURNING AN IDEA INTO REALITY

At home I lived on the eighth floor which meant no matter what, I would have to override my brain's desire to take the easy route. While eight floors had no physical impact on me, it became abundantly clear how quickly my brain defaulted to the easier, more convenient option, a worrying factor knowing there would be nothing easy about the next year. You would be amazed if you knew how quickly it played games with me. After climbing my stairs at home five times already that day, midnight came and that little voice piped up.........'No one will know'.

Oh, but I would know.

I couldn't afford thoughts like these in the upcoming year, and with 188 days until I started, I knew how important it was to build the habit of overriding that voice. I knew it would crop up, probably at the worst time, but I had the power to build the discipline that would override it.

As August came around, I heard a business coach ask if we were '212ers'. He explained that water boils at 212 degrees Fahrenheit, not at 211. So, the challenge was in digging deep for that extra degree to reach 212 degrees to 'make it boil'. I used that thought process to climb the stairs back home after realising there were nine floors. That is when I began to climb that extra flight. Mentally, it did wonders for me. Being home I would reach my goal of climbing Table Mountain for the day. One small action repeated at least 880+ times across five months reinforced a mindset to keep going and inspired me to 'do one more'.

It was important to understand all the 'negatives' associated with my plan because of how easy it was to become unrealistic and get wrapped up in only the good aspects of what I was committing to. I had to consciously face all the negative possibilities and the 'what if's.......'

- What if no one supported me and I didn't raise any money?
- What would happen when the weather was atrocious? Wind, rain, heat, and a combination of them all!

33

- What if I got sick?
- What if I got injured?

I had to confront each one of these dragons and face the harsh realities surrounding their answers. I had to deal with the idea of being tied down and bound to Cape Town for an entire year, unable to go anywhere else – including to Johannesburg to visit my 94-year-old grandmother. I calculated that by the end of 2018, just that one year would represent 2.56% of my life—a fraction that would continue to get smaller the longer I lived but would also provide exponential growth and learnings I'd never forget.

That first question was immediately put to the test as very few of those close to me supported the idea, understood it, or shared in my excitement. Then, the day after my idea was conceived, everything came to a head while attending a black-tie gala event for a charity with Martelize.

'Forget what he does – ask him what he's doing next year' she interjected.

We found ourselves sitting at a table with the charity's host, a few business owners, and Lisa Thompson-Smeddle – the founder of One Heart for Kids, which was a non-profit organisation focused on supporting under-resourced schools with materials that helped kids learn to read. Later on that evening Lisa shared some staggering statistics with me, she mentioned that the literacy rate is 34% at grade 4 level! This was completely heart-breaking, but also solvable. She burst with excitement about my idea, and with 25 years of experience in working with the United Nations (UN) and sustainability, her mind began to work quickly.

'I have so many ideas I'd love to share with you! I've been working with corporates for years so I'd like to help you put together some proposals. I'd love to support you, this is such a cool idea.'

Really? I couldn't believe that the day after my idea came to me, I had the good fortune of meeting someone excited, knowledgeable, experienced, and willing

CHAPTER 3
TURNING AN IDEA INTO REALITY

to help me!! What an amazing Friday night that was. Later on we swapped details and made plans to connect.

I was bursting with excitement but then I landed hard, back down to earth and experienced the complete opposite feeling as the entire weekend went by without a single message back from any of the excited Whatsapp messages I had sent to my family sharing this fortuitous connection. No excited whoops, no 'wow that's unreal'. Just radio silence, and it hurt. Was I delusional? Was my belief in this idea's potential to build community unrealistic? Driving to work on Monday morning was probably the worst since the first time I heard I didn't get the job, and it turned out to be one of the longest days of my life. Just five days out from leaving and no work to distract me left me feeling deflated all day.

Driving home, I decided to take a detour via Table Mountain. I wanted to stand below the mountain I'd be climbing every day so that I could become invigorated and enthused once again. I arrived just after 17:00 and parked close to Platteklip Gorge's parking area for a better view back towards the mountain so I could see it in all its majesty, like a natural temple to behold.

With my head tilted back, I took as many deep breaths as I needed. I thought about what climbing up there every day would be like. Wind. Rain. Heat. Cold. Maybe even snow. Climbing for an entire year meant there were no seasons to hide from. I would experience it all.

I started remembering my vision of asking for R1 per climb, and how quickly that would add up to something significant enough to empower those struggling on the back foot or just hoping for an opportunity. I watched as the sun was about to go behind the west face of the mountain, then I turned to sit on the bench behind me that overlooked the city. I took another deep breath. I could feel the mountain's presence behind me, like a protective guardian. It was a still day, not a breath of wind and just a sliver of cloud on the horizon over the ocean. The late golden sunshine trickled over the mountain revealing all its cracks, crevices, and undulations. I started to cry. My world had been turned upside down and there was nothing certain in my future. I felt isolated, and alone. Then that first question came back and hit me; it was as loud as can be.

What if no one else supports this idea??

With that thought in my mind, I remained there on the right-hand side of the bench, occasionally glancing over my left shoulder at the sunset, slowly descending in the valley between Table Mountain and Lion's Head. Fifteen minutes passed; it felt like an eternity. Then, I noticed something that blew me away.

ANDREW

My name was carved into the wooden backrest of the bench. I had to come to the bench to find myself. I had to take a picture because I was sure no one would believe me. Hell, I was sitting right there, and I didn't even believe it! As if that wasn't enough – a mongoose appeared barely two metres away. I'd never seen one here before, and now it happened at the exact moment that I saw my name. Something about this timing felt crucial. It could've happened when I arrived, or when I'd left, but it didn't, it happened at the same time I saw my name carved in front of me. I don't believe anything happens by accident, so I quickly googled 'Mongoose spirit animals'. Whether you believe in things like this or not – the words I read on my phone are exactly what I needed to hear:

Mongoose is a sign of courage; it teaches us to defend ourselves with pure integrity and righteousness to experience a result that will benefit both sides. This is a special skill of mongoose people; they can settle an issue with someone without exerting too much effort and without resorting to other conflicts. It's a reminder that we should pursue our goals and passions and acquire desirable outcomes. It is telling us that if we love what we do, then we will see it as a hobby, and we'll continue to find joy in doing it.

It was a reminder to pursue our goals. Something profound happened inside me. In that moment I found an unshakeable strength, together with the internal

CHAPTER 3
TURNING AN IDEA INTO REALITY

fortitude that had always existed. Those attributes supported my ability to make a clear decision:

Even if nobody supported me – I was doing this.

For the first time in my life, I wasn't looking for outside validation or permission to go after what I wanted. It's amazing how a quote can suddenly appear and its meaning can resonate even more deeply because of the moment we find ourselves in. This one from Dr John Demartini struck a chord with me:

'When the voice and vision on the inside is more profound than all the opinions on the outside. Then you've begun to master your life.'

Learning was nothing without application. This was my opportunity to take the first step to build the mental fortitude to complete the challenge. It made me think about how I've treated people who shared their hopes, dreams, and desires with me in the past. What questions did I ask them? Did I project my insecurities and experiences onto what they wanted to do? Did I support them in the way that they needed? Probably not. But lately I'd become more aware of my own behaviour and the impact it had on others. I now ask better questions and I ask how things relate to people's lives instead of projecting my own point of view.

I was incredibly grateful for this experience and the lessons that came with it. Judging the responses of others through my eyes was the same as them looking at my idea from their angle. I was forced to look deeper to cultivate a stronger understanding about why most of the time we understand or meet others from our own limited experience and understanding. The process of understanding this made me resilient, and best of all – it reinforced my ability to listen to my own intuition. This was the first test that would gauge how much I believed in this. Just because I made a brave choice, it didn't mean the rest would be easy. I was about to embark on the toughest challenge of my life and something no one in history had ever done before. Why would I expect any part of this to be easy? More importantly – why would I want it to be easy?

There was no one to ask for advice; no set plan to follow. No one was watching over me being my 'boss'. My determination, discipline, commitment, and persistence were going to be pushed to the absolute limit. My time for talking was over. It was time to put my beliefs to the test and act!

A big idea was like going to a seminar or workshop where I'd learned new tools and the energy swept me up as I felt invincible. The real test came when day to day life 'got in the way' and that shine started to fade. The value came in understanding what my goal was and being honest about my current situation, I'd need to make sure that I was able to plot the route and clearly mark out the timelines. I would support that thinking by making small adjustments every day instead of doing something big once off.

This 'setback' while my idea wasn't even a week old, helped me entrench an unbreakable spirit into my being so that nothing or no one could deflate me again. Well, at least I thought so. I left the mountain rejuvenated in my commitment to see the idea through. I was reaffirmed of the power my plan had to build a community and bring people together to tackle tough challenges instead of complaining about them. I knew there was a lot of work to be done before 2018 even started. First off, I had to build a training program that would progressively increase the physical overload to create an on-ramp and get my body up to speed. This meant climbing Table Mountain once a week in July; twice a week in August and September; three times in October, culminating with five back-to-back climbs up Table Mountain before my conference in Los Angeles.

While I never doubted my physical capability to accomplish this, I knew having no breaks for an entire year was going to be gruelling and would take its toll on my legs and body. The physical on-ramp would teach me that the mental challenge was going to be as tough – if not tougher – than the physical one. Maintaining enthusiasm and drive with no days off was rapidly becoming my ultimate challenge to overcome.

CHAPTER 3
TURNING AN IDEA INTO REALITY

Although my challenge had the luxury of catching the cable car down, there were still going to be some instances when my legs would have to work a double shift. Bad weather as well as a two week yearly shut down for cable car maintenance meant I would need to climb down too. In my head I made it easy and convinced myself that it would be 100 days – a third of the year. I decided to make all my training climbs up and down to mimic those days. It's often said that your training should be more challenging than the actual event, but simulating half a year's worth of fatigue was impossible. I tried by doing an early leg workout at the gym and then climbing up and down the mountain straight afterwards, but I knew that even that wasn't anywhere near what the reality was going to be. Still, every time I successfully did these mini challenges, I was building my ability to override the 'snooze' button.

Thankfully, the second question about wondering what to do about windy days, rainy days, and heat waves was answered while still training. The hot days taught me that I needed to start at the latest 8am to be off the mountain before 10am or else there'd be nowhere to hide as the sun baked the exposed gorge. At certain times of the year if I failed an early morning climb and made it for a mid-afternoon climb then I'd be in the shade as the roasting African sun would move behind the mountain.

I had some opportunities to climb in wet conditions too. This gave me the chance to evaluate question four – getting injured. Intuitively I knew by creating an onramp with my training, my body would be ready by January 1st. Poor preparation was what ended my trail running days in 2012 when I overestimated my abilities and underestimated the challenge. I started as an instructor for *British Military Fitness* (BMF) in 2010 to earn some extra money. An outdoor body weight class designed from the British Army basic training regime and the original 'bootcamp' training. It was huge in the UK even with their poor weather conditions. Here in Cape Town on the Sea Point Promenade, classes took place at 6pm on Monday & Wednesday and at 8am on Saturday mornings. It was a wonderful group of people from various backgrounds and fitness levels, who kept me on my toes to produce enjoyable classes that not only built functional fitness but also provided some extremely challenging workouts.

This is how I heard about the *Platteklip Charity Challenge* in 2012, which saw mountain enthusiasts climb Table Mountain, via Platteklip Gorge, as many times as possible between sunrise and sunset to raise money for an under-resourced school. The proceeds went towards buying supplies and computers so children didn't get left behind. The route started at the Lower cable station with a 2km walk along Tafelberg road roughly 300m above sea level. To the left the city nestled in the bowl as Lions Head and Signal Hill created a lip while Devils Peak to the right completed the bowl. Then onwards up Platteklip Gorge and across the top table back to the upper cable station. That was one lap which was roughly 5 km in total and over 720m in vertical gain. I had no clue what two laps was like but my ego pledged six climbs which seemed like a good number. This was during some of my fittest years so my confidence reigned supreme. Perhaps too confident.

I remember cockily driving to Platteklip after work one afternoon to get up and back down the mountain as fast as I could just as a test. But just once. Then, on the day of the challenge the mountain brought my ego back down to earth. By the time I started lap five, my right hip was in serious pain. I learned why you don't train for a marathon by sprinting. I wasn't even halfway up, and then began doubting how I was going to finish my fifth lap, let alone six.

Around halfway a group of us all on lap five tried to spur each other on. We needed it, we were all suffering and taking serious strain. Eventually our conversations turned to what number we'd pledged to do. Funnily enough, we'd all pledged six.

Three quarters of the way up, between the towering cliffs either side of the fault line Platteklip ran through, we were done. It was abundantly clear to me that if I had attempted lap six, I'd have ended up taking a ride in a mountain rescue helicopter because of my ego. After 7 hours and 33 minutes on the mountain, I bowed out. I'd never look at Table Mountain the same way again.

CHAPTER 3
TURNING AN IDEA INTO REALITY

That day during the car ride home my ego reared its ugly head. Feeling no pain while seated I started cursing myself for not mustering up the spirit to at least attempt lap six. My girlfriend at the time dropped me off at home, so I decided to test my idiotic notion by taking the two flights of stairs up to my flat. Those baby steps were a joke compared to the 2 579 step climb up Platteklip Gorge, yet it felt like a twenty-minute mission just to do that small section. I hardly managed one step at a time, never mind attempting two steps at a time. There was no way I'd have made it without doing serious, maybe even permanent damage.

Five months later, and I hadn't even attempted a run, then I finally took the plunge on a business trip to Durban that September. My attempted run ended up with me walking after just one kilometre. That closed the book on my trail running for good. Weighing over 100 kg, I wasn't exactly built for running. The damage must've been caused by unconsciously preferring my stronger dominant right side when climbing up over bigger gaps on the mountain. But the lesson was learned.

I drew some wisdom from that experience which helped educate and prepare me for the summiting journey I was about to attempt. After all – I didn't just want to complete the challenge, I wanted to come out of it as unscathed as possible. There was another type of injury though that I realised was a risk especially with the lapses of concentration that happen when undertaking long and intense missions on the mountain. Broken legs, twisted ankles and broken wrists were all results I wanted to avoid. This made every climb up a reconnaissance mission to see which rocks had come loose, had moved, or were too dangerous to step on coming down. Each climb became an opportunity to practise complete attention and focus on the task at hand. Why twist an ankle on the 500 000th step versus any other? I was learning what was within my control and making sure I didn't take that responsibility for granted.

That led me to question 3 – what would happen if I got sick? Notice I said 'if' and not when. It was both intentional and an honest audit of the past 20 years of my life. I couldn't remember the last time I had the flu, and most of my colds had been from partying hard and running my body & immune system down. Based on history I was confident my body would stack up health-wise, but on the off chance I got the flu? I committed mentally to make up any days I was unable to climb by doing doubles in proceeding days. Flu would most likely put me out for a week, and I wouldn't climb until my heart was ready to handle the stress without having a heart attack.

This was another story that made me grateful for my healthy body. As a child, I'd visited the hospital more than my age. Ear issues needed grommet's, there was whooping cough, tonsillitis, mumps, and chicken pox, that all assaulted my immune system before the age of 6. I didn't have any scientific proof, but I believed this was the best training my immune system received that helped it become what it is today. As an adult I contributed positively to this by always being active, sleeping extremely well, learning to deal with stress, never smoking and I've always enjoyed eating loads of fruits & vegetables. All those factors made me feel confident I wouldn't get any serious infections.

Even though I was born partially deaf in my left ear, it was actually the mumps that took the rest of the hearing away completely. That was important because from an early age I was forced to tell teachers and children I'd met that I was deaf just in case I missed something they said and they wondered why. Of course, there were many times I used this to my advantage claiming 'I never heard you' which of course, they had no recourse for. But of course, it only revolved around things I didn't want to do.

The curious thing though was the responses I always got: *'Oh shame that's terrible that you can't hear in your left ear.'*

But I always focused on being able to hear in my right ear.

What a gift to constantly be reminded from a young age that I get to choose what I can focus on. This single-handedly embedded an unshakeable positivity that has served me through some rough days. Even in my 'bad' I've been shown the good, and it was up to me to look for it – no matter how painful that might have been.

CHAPTER 3
TURNING AN IDEA INTO REALITY

Lastly, that left question 5 - What if I didn't make any money?

The nature of what I was doing, the way it stirred my soul, showed me just how important this journey was. Looking at all my finances, I made a calculated decision with the package I got paid out, knowing it would keep me afloat for 10 months. I also needed to absorb my living costs for an additional 8 months while I completed the challenge, keeping in mind that new opportunities would arise from that.

I was able to drastically reduce my standard of living as my expenses became food, my monthly medical aid, rent, and petrol to get to and from the mountain. Now only a 16 km round trip, a weeks' worth of driving to Table Mountain was the equivalent of just one day trip to my old work - a huge saving.

I kept feeling a little fear around not earning steady money and felt myself defaulting to wanting to get a part time job that would create some financial flexibility. But every time I thought that, a voice inside told me that my entire focus needed to be on this challenge to extract all the juice that I needed for success. I knew there was a serious amount of work on the way that included data capturing, writing a journal, and co-ordinating with companies & individuals that would want to climb with me. There was also going to be PR, social media, public talks, organising events, working with the charities to use the funds, networking and so much more that would feel like I was doing an MBA.

I had mental blocks regarding money all my life and this was the first time I felt released from the weight of all the years it consumed me. I realised my opportunity to do something that's never been done before required 100% attention, I was able to commit myself completely largely due to my discipline which helped me save and create a nest egg. That discipline was instilled by my parents, which is why I am forever indebted to them for everything great in my life.

November 2017

Training was starting to take shape; I'd completed five consecutive climbs up Table Mountain which culminated on my birthday. I felt satisfied as I prepared to jet off to the US for my business trip which was aimed at garnering international support. I'd finished four and a half months of training and felt fantastic, but more importantly I was injury free. I was in a strong position now and it had me wondering if I'd be training this hard and purposefully had I not sustained such a major injury back in 2012.

Now I'd be gone for three weeks, but upon return I'd have an excellent opportunity to climb while fatigued because of the intensity of my flight schedule. I'd be flying out of Miami at 21:30 November the 27th, and then I'd arrive in London midday (8 hours 40 minutes flying time). The flight back to Cape Town left at 21:40 giving me about 10 hours of layover followed by an 11-hour 30-minute flight which arrived back in Cape Town at 10 am. This was a total journey of around 30 hours, so I'd lose 6 hours coming back east across time zones.

November the 29th hit and I was just 33 sleeps away from the challenge. In Cape Town, November is the start of summer and there's no way I'd be climbing up the mountain during the peak heat at midday. I got home and unpacked but seriously struggled to keep my eyes open before heading for my first climb in 24 days. Luckily it was in the late afternoon shade.

I pretended I was a year into the future and that this was how my legs and body would feel on climb 333. A while back before that I started tricking myself, I'd repeat the day's number of the year over and over on each step up the mountain. I also played games telling myself, 'Wow Andrew – your legs are holding up so well for 333 days of climbing'. I made the climb! It was a struggle, but it was also a huge boost of confidence after such a big break and long trip back. When I got back home, what happened was more than just the most intense sleep ever, it was more like a mini coma.

CHAPTER 3
TURNING AN IDEA INTO REALITY

But there would be no rest for the wicked as I had to jump start myself before shutting down too much. My friends of 20 years, Paul, and Quintin arrived from Johannesburg the next day and we headed up for their first ever summit which they thoroughly enjoyed. I felt strong, and that was a bonus! The climb with Paul and Quintin was a mini triumph and felt even more important after the calamity I experienced in Florida during my trip.

My purpose after the business conference was to join others for a three-day mastermind retreat at our coach's home. I was pumped! I had great conversations with people from around the world. I was doing my best to muster up support and it led me to finding Huni - my crowdfunding page's first donor all the way from Iceland. Not only was Huni the first donor, he would go on to become a huge financial supporter of my mission.

Then I was presented with my second biggest test of will, commitment, and belief in my project. I got that Mike Tyson punch right to the face. Imagine spending a shit ton of money on an international coach and then getting excited about learning to boost business opportunities that would help ramp up the international potential for crowdfunding... But instead, when the time arrives to have a one-on-one session with the coach, he tells you to *'get this saving the world bullshit out of your head.'*

That's exactly what happened and my world collapsed!

While my self-belief about my physical capability to tackle this was unshakeable – my mental self-doubt issues about whether I should be doing this were exposed and I was completely rattled. I thought I knew devastation before, but boy was I wrong! All that training. All those interviews I'd done. The commitment I'd already shared with my three chosen organisations was all just flippantly waved off and disregarded as I was told 'they'll move on.' I felt like I was lost in a maze covered in fog in a foreign country that didn't speak English. Early in July I'd thought about taking this global and in less than a week, I had the opportunity to speak in front of an international audience of 2000 people! I'd asked the universe and the opportunity was delivered almost immediately – so how could this be happening? Everything was supposed to go smoothly, right? He was supposed to love the idea and rally his network of people behind it to attract loads of support. THAT was what was supposed to happen. What happened was the complete opposite, my nightmare had materialised.

It was almost as though everything I'd learned the previous time I felt unsupported evaporated. What I realised now was that I had started shifting back towards my limiting beliefs, I thought I wasn't good enough to raise the money on my own with the climbs. I placed all my bets on this 'cosmically aligned introduction', as I saw it. I thought this was the perfect piece of the puzzle to kick start the challenge with a great partnership which would have donations rolling in from January the 1st. I had given all my power away to someone else.

Thankfully, this interaction was a far deeper experience that gave me more than one amazing gift. Firstly, another one of his students based in Cape Town was Karel Vermeulen, he'd interviewed John Travolta at the business conference. His story was an incredible one, which transformed his life and pushed him from broke to a seven-figure income in two years. I was feeling as low as I'd ever known, but in my depths of despair Karel's name came to me, I put some thought into it and decided that I wanted him to coach me. After all, he'd be coaching from experience.

Our partnership began less than a week after I arrived home and our first session was 6 hours. He carefully dismantled the absurdity of the experience I'd had and then he reignited the fire in my soul with even more gusto than I thought possible. Not with fake bravado or pandering motivation, but simply by asking me questions that reminded me why I got so excited in the first place, he also helped me reaffirm my belief in the potential of this project. I was grateful to have his entrepreneurial experience in my corner.

The second benefit of being told to 'forget about it', was the gift of it being a perfect final test before starting my climbs. A colossal year awaited and there was no room in my head for self-doubt and I couldn't let outside criticism break me down. I needed laser focus, and this was the perfect test. I also recognised my fault in mentally relying on someone else to help me hit my monetary targets. What would I have learned if some knight in shining armour had swooped in to do all the work? I was focussed on trying to control the outcomes (money raised) instead of the input (the journey).

I've found value in asking the right people my most pressing questions. Just as I wouldn't ask a plumber how to build a house; so too was I silly to expect a guy totally fixated on money to guide me on my pilgrimage and to counsel me on matters of the heart. I've never enjoyed these negative experiences, but I certainly enjoyed the benefits I reaped from them, in the same way that the view at the top of Table Mountain was sweeter after climbing. I believed this dreadful experience was one of the main reasons I was able to develop the mindset needed to attempt my project with such enjoyment and gratitude.

The icing on top of this trip was that it enabled me to visit a woman I'd recently met a month earlier while she travelled to Cape Town. A mutual friend, Rochelle, introduced us virtually. Jessie was the polar opposite of this painful experience. She was a rock in my support group, one of my biggest cheerleaders and she was an amazing teacher. I think most people had 'given up' on me finding that someone special, they thought I was too fussy, and I didn't believe in settling. Every woman I'd been blessed to get to know and spend time with was an amazing human being; but we simply weren't the best fit for each other.

You hear about having a feeling and a deeper knowing when you meet someone. Jessie instilled a sense of peace I'd never experienced before, and I felt wonderfully fortunate and blessed for her to be part of my life. She never doubted for a second that I had the abilities or the will to tackle such a huge task. When we 'blame' people for our bad experiences, they should immediately get the credit for the good too. Technically speaking, the coach that initially broke my spirit also gave me a week with Jessie in San Francisco, somewhere I'd never been before.

I didn't feel it at the time, but I was being shown what real support looked like and most importantly what it felt like from a partner. I was also learning why it was so important to choose who I shared my dreams with and who I allowed to become part of my inner circle. If I sought advice, I'd ask someone with experience, compassion, and a genuine interest in my growth.

With my final mental test done and dusted, all that was left to do was to push my physical capabilities to the brink before heading to Johannesburg to spend a week with my family for Christmas in the African bush. I decided to climb Table Mountain Wednesday, Thursday, Friday, then Devils Peak on Saturday, Table Mountain again on Sunday, Monday, Tuesday, Lions head on Wednesday followed immediately by Table Mountain. Ending on December the 20th. These eight days and nine consecutive climbs would be my final test.

Everything was going great until I woke up Saturday early with the wind howling. Where I lived in Sea Point was protected, so if it was getting rattled by a gale force, then I shudder to think what the constantly blowing Devils Peak was going to be like. One by one messages popped up on my phone as people cancelled. I stayed in bed dying to remain in the cocoon of warmth and sanctuary for my battered legs after enduring three consecutive summits. I remember looking at the ceiling while the wind slammed into the windows, then I fast forwarded 365 days....

You won't have this luxury next year, get up!

And so I did.

The powerful gusts were relentless, so much so that I could lean into the wind as though I was Michael Jackson in his 'Criminal' video. I had a chuckle at what would happen if the wind just suddenly stopped and I landed on my face. I watched cars pull up only for people to get out, pause, and then get back in to drive away. I was the only 'fool' on the mountain, but it was good practice for what was to come. I must admit, the hardest part was always just getting out of bed. Once that happened the rest flowed easily for me.

CHAPTER 3
TURNING AN IDEA INTO REALITY

It's crazy to think how small that first step was in comparison to the rest and yet, was by far the hardest!

The climb was such fun. Alone on the mountain I cruised up, pausing when I first managed a glimpse over the saddle with False Bay in the distance. Climbing further gave me the opportunity to take another break to admire the best view of Platteklip Gorge. I could make out every twist and turn snaking its way up the gorge. I took a moment to focus on one section which enabled me to watch colourful dots moving up. The sky was littered with clouds in a hurry to pass across. It created the most beautiful blue textures. It wasn't even 7:30 yet, but I was getting close to the top and feeling grateful that I hadn't let the cancellations, warm bed and wind deter me.

I sat up at the top like I was sitting behind a Boeing 747 before take-off, with gusts ripping behind the steady stream as though nature's engine was being revved. I laughed out loud at the insanity of being there but felt at peace in the solitude. Alone at the top I felt compelled to take photos of the sun's rays beaming down through the clouds, as though someone in heaven was pulling the curtains back. Focusing my gaze, the rays danced across the cape flats creating a peaceful sight.

I climbed down on a high and decided to turn right on to the saddle instead of left. It was a route down the northern side of Devils Peak I'd never done before. I couldn't help but think that if it were any other circumstance, I would've cancelled this hike too and missed out on a tremendously fun experience. I made sure to water that seed every day for the next fifteen days.

My last training day was superb. We started at 5am to finish my 24th training climb up Lions Head where we'd watch the sunrise up top. Lisa joined to make it a perfect start. She's another phenomenal human being who became a rock of support in every way imaginable. Lisa's magic unfolded in the way that she donated, followed through with her climbing commitments and spread my messages all over social media as well as in person.

Dashing off to her first meeting of the day, we said goodbye and exclaimed how the next time we saw each other it would be a mere day or so away from starting. The day that felt so far away was now almost upon me.

After watching her drive away, I headed up to Platteklip for the last time in 2017, starting at 7:33am – the sun was already over the eastern part of the mountain and bathed the route in sunshine. This would be my 49th time up Table Mountain and my 87th training session in total across all routes. It felt surreal to climb knowing how close I was, but I was more interested in the way my legs and body were holding up. After this final push, they felt the strongest they'd ever been. Even without professional help to monitor my progress I felt that my training had been spot on. The excitement built up with each step I took. I'd become accustomed to the challenges that the start of the climb presented; my mind shouted out in horror for me to turn back – but my body found a natural rhythm by the time I reached the first waterfall. My breathing became meditative. The 'pain' in my legs was a non-issue because I knew it wouldn't last forever.

Listen to your body. Find the pace it's comfortable with. Maintain that pace. Focus on every step. One step at a time.

I reached the contour path in great spirits. After a quick flat interlude, there was a signpost that let you know it was time to turn up the mountain. One, two, three bends, were reminders of the majestic cliffs and the upper path that was now in plain sight. It was a sight that always filled me with a deep sense of connection. It's a space that became my spiritual home. Others thought I should stay away from this route seeing as I'd be doing it every day, but for me it was important to start day one with a deeper understanding of what I was in for instead of waiting until the 49th climb on the 18th of February.

After the steep corner I arrived at a route called 'Left Face Mystery B', with a very sharp bend before the path's steepness petered out. This disheartens many by dipping down for a good 30m before one of the longest and toughest steep sections hits you. Next, I headed past a boulder the size of a small house precariously perched on the mountain side of the path with a steep drop off to the right, millions of years of erosion carved an ever-deeper gorge below. One could easily be lulled into a false sense of security as the path flattens out, only to become the steepest and most direct part of the section going straight up. Usually, bodies litter the steps here as people try finding shade to catch their breath from sky high heart rates while others around them try to defy gravity and climb up.

Finally, after an eternity of going straight up I arrived at a gentler section before another steep corner that brought me to halfway rock - a section the same height as Lions Head. Here you find a boulder half buried that allows its northern side to slope enough to provide a cool backrest for those needing an extra minute or two to recharge. From here, it's just two more corners to get to one of my favourite spots on the mountain which is the first up close and personal opportunity to stand under the majestic cliffs. I'd always take a minute to stop here, I'd always felt a deep sense of awe in the size of the mountain, the sheer scale of how small we really were in the grand scheme of things, and I'd appreciate the unexplainable natural beauty that's existed for aeons that was also here to provide me with an incredible challenge. This is where the gap between the west cliffs and East cliffs were at their greatest. As I wind my way up, the gap becomes narrower, the steepness increases, and it almost feels like the tiny gap at the top keeps moving away from you and getting smaller.

It's nature's gallery with gorgeous works of art at every view, faces in the mountain, flowers gracefully reaching for the sun out of cliff cracks, birds navigating the fynbos for nectar, a stream of colour contrasting against the earthy rocks and grasses. Maybe even some water droplets waiting for their turn to bungee jump off the cuddle grass.

With every turn there was another wonder, every step brought a new perspective of the height I was taking on. Climbing quickly meant the cliff face I stared up at was suddenly the bottom of another cliff, and a boulder I called 'the Guardian' which was sitting atop a cliff as though it was protecting the entrance to this sacred place. I wanted to call it the character Idris Elba played in Thor – but I could never remember it to tell people! Even now I had to google it to see that it was Heimdall. I thought of him because his character was all-seeing and all-hearing for everyone in the universe and stood at the entrance to Asgard on the Bifrost Bridge. The 'Guardian' had a flat face which faced Cape Town. It reminded me of the old TV's that had that bulge behind the screen. I'll stick my neck out here and say the 'Guardian' was the size of 22 men.

From here there were just 18 corners left, which included a path decimated by a rockfall, then there was a waterfall corner and the second longest steep section. Soon I'd be at Ubuntu Rock. I gave it this name because on my training climbs back down, I would stop and sit on it to visualise the year challenge. It became a beacon of how close to the end I was getting. Then onwards it would be 6 corners and 6 minutes away from the top of Platteklip Gorge.

The top section, usually bathed in clouds, is green and lush from the abundance of water. I always feel like I'm in another world here as bonsai-ish trees twist their bark in artistic designs, and car sized boulders litter the ground too lazy to roll all the way down the mountainside. Massive rocks lay on their side ushering you up the final stretch to a point when you ask how on earth do we get to the top without ropes?!

Then, rounding the final corner reveals the stairway to heaven. A tiny passageway about 6 feet wide is the final staircase with rock covered in lichen and scars that rise above you on each side. An oasis of trees and shade awaits you, the perfect spot to turn around and gaze back between the tiniest of gaps allowing Devils Peak to sneakily photo bomb its way into view.

This time I didn't have to go all the way to the cable station, so I took a moment to enjoy my last 'non challenge' climb view before making my way down. It was a vastly different experience climbing down and a complete feast for the eyes with its wide expanse and open landscape snapshot. It's such a contrast because on your way up your view is mainly just the next few stairs to climb, but now you're fighting gravity down and feeling the impact of the large gaps that resemble box jumps at the gym more than normal stairs. There was no need to rush down, my legs were definitely feeling the load they'd been put under the past 9 summits which meant I could take it easy through the danger zones while pushing it on the easier bits - which I took advantage of because of my excitement to see my family.

Off the mountain and spending a week at Zebula game lodge was the perfect soul nourishing breakaway with my special people which gave me the absolute maximum amount of relaxation that only the African bush could deliver. Having lived away from my family while I was in London and Cape Town for a combined fifteen years, we learned to maximise our time together; it was always quality time.

I was blessed to have my parents come visit for at least a week every year, so back in September they had the opportunity to climb the route and saw what it entailed. For years, as long as my memory goes back, my mom battled with her thyroid and heart so joining her on a summit attempt was amazing. Slowly but surely, together, we made it up, and that gave a special edge to our excited conversations three months later over Christmas.

My brother-in-law, Terence, is a machine, and back in 2016 completed The Cape Epic - the toughest mountain bike race in the world. His dedication and commitment to training was a shining example of what it took to tackle something so gruelling. It was wonderful to have people in my inner circle that had a wealth of knowledge and experience to learn from. My sister also has thyroid issues and adrenal fatigue - seeing these effects first hand coupled with my mom's years of struggle reminded me how important it was to be grateful for my healthy body. This helped me appreciate how blessed I was to even contemplate taking on this challenge; but more importantly it helped me see the strength in people that struggle with their health but never complain and never use it as an excuse to become bitter.

There was a bit of fun to be had too, my youngest niece, Katie, had the honour of shaving off all my hair. I'd never grown my hair long before and as this year was my own pilgrimage of sorts, I decided to shave it off and grow it all year. We'd go on a journey together and come December the 31st, I could look at the January the 1st climb, (the tip) and the final climb, (the root) all together. I did this knowing I didn't have the best shaped head for a shave (I did it in grade 11's summer holiday vacation) and warned everyone beforehand. *'I Do not. Look good!'*

On December the 29th with just two days remaining I landed back in Cape Town – the break had done its job and I was ready to go home. I was itching to start and was comforted to realise that had my gran still been alive today, it would've been her 100th birthday. Everything felt aligned, I was mentally strong, I was physically rested, and my heart was full. All that awaited me was to climb Table Mountain once a day for an entire year. I was ready to face whatever tests got thrown my way and I knew they were all going to be part of my growth journey.

I just had no idea how quickly the very first test would arrive.

"When we can believe without seeing, our heart opens, and the path becomes a pilgrimage. Our eyes light up, seeing everything through the empowering lens of love – and gratitude" ~~ **Andrew Patterson**

CHAPTER 4

JANUARY – TAKING THE FIRST STEP INTO THE UNKNOWN

December the 31st brought with it two birthday celebrations to attend. First, it was Tiff's breakfast in Vredehoek, a suburb nestled just below my new teacher & business partner – Table Mountain. Incredibly the person that was sitting next to me had a shirt that said, 'the best view comes after the hardest climb'. Really? The day before I start?! You couldn't make this stuff up! It made me smile all sparkly-eyed. I now had less than 14 hours until midnight, and I was chomping at the bit to get cracking. I was restless, and while everyone else spoke excitedly about their plans for the party that night – I was like a grandpa hoping to be in bed by 22:00.

I wasn't 100% sure when I got this idea, but the plan was to create the perfect bookends in 2018 by watching the sunrise on top of the mountain after the first climb, which meant a 4:30 am start, and then catching the sunset after the final climb on December the 31st. It felt like the perfect way to start and finish a truly epic journey.

With the early start, I'd miss seeing the New Year in, instead I'd be waking up at 3:30 am while everyone else was still madly celebrating the start of 2018. Just before I bid the birthday girl farewell, we agreed on a chat at the top to celebrate the first successful climb. 'Deal!' She said excitedly, 'Let's FaceTime when you're at the top – I'll still be awake – I promise!'

The second birthday was Nicola's 50th celebration, it was just ten minutes up the road from Tiff's venue. My plan was to 'pop in' and wish her before heading to Dave – another friend I'd promised to visit on my way home. Nicola started her day with a champagne brunch as a warm-up before the later arrivals were due to turn a mellow day into a fully-fledged sunset house party. Her beautiful home sat high up on the slopes of Table Mountain overlooking Cape Town below. It felt like Table Mountain was eager to get going by pulling me closer every chance she got. Gazing back after ringing the doorbell, the mountain seemed to loom larger with a slightly ominous presence. The top section was hidden behind a veil of clouds on what turned out to be an unseasonably grey day, but a welcome sight for our drought-stricken city, which was rapidly running out of water at the peak of our summer.

At peace, I waited for the door to open, but little did I know, I was about to be given my first major test.

In and out to wish her Andrew...........That was the plan!

I felt like a bit of an intruder as Nicola celebrated with four of her closest girlfriends. She waved it off, and with a 'cheers' handed me a glass of champagne and immediately asked how I was feeling.

CHAPTER 4
JANUARY - TAKING THE FIRST STEP INTO THE UNKNOWN

'I'm excited, itching to get started. I've done all I could to train and prepare. Eager for the wait to be over now!'

'Are you staying for the party?! I have an extra room too if you need.'

I hadn't even set a foot on the mountain yet, and test #1 arrived unannounced. It was extremely tempting. I mean, I didn't have to start at 4:30 am to watch the sunrise, right? I could easily stay, celebrate, sleep late, and do an afternoon climb. After all, we were celebrating a special milestone. At least that's what the sneaky voice of temptation was whispering to me. No one who knew would even judge this. The reality was that no one even cared. It had no real bearing on the significance or on the outcome of the challenge.

Or did it?

If I folded now and compromised the very first climb - what else would I compromise later in the year? Worse - what cracks would it create in my psyche? This little moment would define me because I knew. And that mattered.

A beautiful saying from Marie Forleo gave it a powerful perspective: *"To be responsible, keep your promise to others. To be successful, keep your promises to yourself"*

What started off as a small brunch with six of us, rapidly grew as more friends arrived. It didn't take long for the conversation to detour back to what I'd be doing all year. Very coincidentally, my deeper explanations resulted in a sneaky refill - lifting my temptation as though it was a buoy in my glass. Making this decision harder still was the fact that I wasn't guaranteed a view of the sunrise. The current overcast conditions were forecast until mid-morning, and added to that was the potential for light rain at my scheduled start. Staying could save me from being rained on or, I could be diligent; leave, get up early, do my climb, and easily be surrounded by grey mist on climb #1. It was quite anticlimactic, really, unlike other massive events, there were no camera crews, media, and hordes of people congregating to witness the start. It was just me. Alone in the pitch-black night - **Starting the journey of a million stairs.**

I had promised Tiff a phone call though...

That's it!

Well, that and the fact that my inner circle knew about my idea for a sunrise start. That instantly snapped my mind back on track! And the resolve to overcome the negative thoughts came from the same place the idea originally did - a place that knew how important this was to me. There'd always be another party and many more New Year's celebrations. But only one opportunity to watch a sunrise on the very first climb and start the year in the best possible way.

Later, as more friends arrived, it got harder to leave, and then it hit home that nothing about what I was about to do was going to be easy. I'd mentally prepared myself for this, and now I was getting an early taste of the mental questions that were going to be asked of me. Admittedly, I stayed an hour or so longer than I wanted to, but something amazing happened on my way home that warmed my heart with the deepest gratitude, a feeling I still hold to this day. My dear friend, David (no - not the one I was on my way to see, another one!) knew my ridiculous plan to start early and messaged me to check in......

'How are you doing my buddy? You ready? You still starting at 4:30?'

'Man, I'm more ready than EVER to get started! Yep - that's the plan'

'Awesome - glad to hear that. I know you want to do your first climb alone. Checking if it's okay to come and meet you at the start to wish you on your way. Totally understand if you don't my friend'...

I was floored that he would sacrifice his own evening to wake up at 3:00 am to meet me. To give me a massive high five, hug, and maybe a little pep talk before watching the darkness envelop me. It never occurred that someone would do this for me. Ever.

'WHAAAT?!! Are you kidding me?? That's incredible! Of COURSE you can come bru.'

CHAPTER 4
JANUARY - TAKING THE FIRST STEP INTO THE UNKNOWN

It was one of the most thoughtful, impactful, and meaningful things a friend had ever done for me. I was about to undertake the most challenging year of my life, and now knowing that someone would be there at the start ramped up my excitement, changing the dynamic from an 'anti-climactic start' to something far more exciting. It felt like I was being 'rewarded' for sticking to my guns and leaving the party. It gave me the perfect start to my year and became a precursor to the generosity of the time, money, and spirit I'd experience. Instead of starting late, on the back foot, and not at my best – I'd start fresh, empowered, and energised – a huge difference.

But still, I was there later than I should've been, Dave had dinner for us and was waiting for me to join him and some friends who were down from London. He was also going to play a pivotal emotional support role throughout my year of climbing – a fact I wasn't aware of yet. After dinner, I was restless, unable to focus on anything but the following day. I soaked in my last hugs, and good luck wishes for 2018, and then I left.

Finally, I arrived back home after leaving at 8 am! It had been a long day, but thankfully a full one. I was grateful I didn't have to sit at home waiting. With nervous energy peaking, I set my clothes out and packed my backpack. Alone with my thoughts, I was worried I wouldn't fall asleep. I chose my Platteklip charity challenge shirt from 2012 to start off with - a reminder of the five summits I managed in one day. There was also my old warm British Military Fitness Jacket, another bright red waterproof jacket I got from my parents in case it rained, two litres of water, my Adidas Terrex boots with ankle support, and lastly, a torch. Everything was ready.

Six hours to go! The clock was ticking, and morning was on its way!

A 10 pm bedtime wish ended up being closer to eleven. If I'd known what I know now – I would've used breathing techniques to calm down. Thankfully though, my eyes closed on one of the most eventful years of my life - and they stayed closed.

All the turmoil. All the training. All the planning.

All the tribulations.
It all evaporated.
It was time for the next step.

Suddenly I was awake, the moment of truth had arrived. I was grateful my alarm clock did its job because I was meeting David at 4:15 am. This gave me enough of a window for a 4:35 am start at the latest and meant I had 63 minutes to reach the top. All my training gave me confidence and reassured me I'd make it up in time for the 5:38 am sunrise.

I was blessed with my proximity to Table Mountain. Living at the bottom end of Sea Point across the road from the swimming pool meant my route up to work had minimal traffic and was fairly pain-free. Around the corner from where I stayed was Kloof road, which meandered through Fresnaye and around the base of Lions Head, with Clifton neatly tucked down below to my right. The route provided a winding road with gorgeous scenery - a passenger's dream road, encouraging you to stare out and soak it all in. Just before reaching Camps Bay High School, you'd come across a slip road to the left taking you up Kloofnek. It's a steep 2km (1,24 miles) stretch which I'd previously cycled up for hill training. At the top, there's a second stop street that intersects with Camps Bay Drive. Hout Bay residents use this to reach the city; while tour companies use it to access Signal Hill Road – another beautiful route past the start of Lions Head climb. As you snake along the 4km road to a lookout above Greenpoint, you reach the paragliding take-off point (north); and lastly Tafelberg road – the only road up to Table Mountain (southeast).

Fortunately, crossing this intersection was the only time I would experience traffic on the twenty-minute journey. This time I was pumping soul-lifting music, singing, and allowing all the excitement to flow through me. It was the start of one of the greatest days of my life. My headlights illuminated the road ahead while I passed massive Stone Pines (or Umbrella Pines known for their canopy shapes) on each side of me. It was quiet. No cars. The nerves intensified as I crossed the intersection and began the steep climb up Tafelberg Road to reach the lower cable station.

CHAPTER 4
JANUARY – TAKING THE FIRST STEP INTO THE UNKNOWN

It was as exciting as the moment my bum hit the seat on an international flight. All the anxiety of getting through customs was done, the waiting was over, and at the other end of the flight, I'd find new experiences.

Pitch black, I pulled over at my first predetermined photo point. It was an unseasonably cold morning. My first official photo of the year was a shot of the darkness and an oncoming car lit up ahead. The lower cable station sat with Table Mountain as its backdrop while its ridges created a bridge between the heaven of clear blue sky and ancient rock earth. The summit line traced across almost unbroken from the bottom left corner of the photo to the top right corner where the upper cable station was perched. In the darkness, though, there were just four lights from the lower cable station and a car 20m ahead with late-night partygoers. One was walking towards my car in the photo - perhaps annoyed by my lights. But onwards I went with just 2 km of road left to reach the start of Platteklip gorge.

I decided that every day as part of documenting my journey, four photos were guaranteed – this was a way to share how different the views could be from one day to the next. It was a small choice with grand lessons: I now know that this process was teaching me to search for and appreciate the uniqueness that each day brought.

Moving along, I reached a point on Tafelberg Road just above the suburb that was probably in line with Nicola's raging party. Two points that were separated by open mountainside, yet thanks to different choices, were worlds apart. I tooted the horn a couple times as if they could hear me, but I probably just annoyed the local wildlife.

As I drove on, another batch of partygoers came into view with drinks in hand, parked with the city lights sparkling below. But soon I arrived, and spotted the legend Mr Thompson, waiting in the solitary car. Unless someone else had decided to climb Platteklip this early on January 1st??

What a pleasure it was seeing and embracing him. It's also crazy how different the experience became as soon as I had the company of one. I'll treasure our selfie till I die. It will always serve as a beautiful reminder - never underestimate the impact a kind deed makes in someone else's life. No words could convey my gratitude for his sacrifice, an hour drive round trip plus a ten-minute intermission to break up his sleep. He'd be back in bed when I'm about halfway up.

'You better send me a picture from the top buddy' 'For you? The world bro.'

Dave shook his head at how mad I was to take on such an incredibly Herculean task. He wondered if I knew what I'd really gotten myself into and if I'd successfully complete it knowing the high risk of bad weather, illness, or injury. In fairness, that was most people's worry. But time would tell. Then he got into his car and sped off. I was alone again, in the darkness, so I jumped straight into my routine created in training. First, I messaged 'Safety Mountain Tracking Group 6' - a specialised safety WhatsApp group created to track the routes and progress of mountain users.

1 pax / Up Platteklip Gorge to the Top Cable Station down same way/ ETA:

08:30 The person on duty (and yes there was someone) acknowledged receipt of my message. *Copy Andrew, be safe and good luck!*

The poor people in my group would be getting two messages every day, all year, from yours truly, and I knew that if ever I saw 'John has left the group', I was going to have a chuckle. Next up was my gratitude ritual aimed at connecting with the climb:

I'm grateful for my healthy body. I'm grateful for my legs that work, that are strong enough to do this every day. I'm grateful for my five senses that enable me to experience the beauty the mountain offers me. I'm grateful to be so close to home. I'm grateful to my family, my friends and Jessie that support me and make this journey possible. Thank you for always watching over me, protecting me, loving me, teaching me. I'm ready and open to learn whatever today brings me.

CHAPTER 4
JANUARY - TAKING THE FIRST STEP INTO THE UNKNOWN

The wait was officially over.

I stood up, and instinctively took a photo of my left foot on the first step. I'd probably heard this saying a million times, but today I felt it....

The longest journey starts with the first step.

I calculated that I'd be climbing just under one million stairs - 973 560 to be precise. I took a deep breath, pressed play on Endomondo - my tracking app, and put the phone away as I started climbing. The beauty of technology meant I could accurately tell you it was 4:34 am. Another special feature of the app made it possible to connect with others and allowed them to send a message of support while training, like a pep talk, if you will. The phone would read the message out loud and robotically; comically, it started with:

Babes you're on golfing mode not climbing. You must change it.

I told you golf was usually one of the only reasons I'd be this excited so early in the morning! Thanks mom - a constant source of power and support throughout my life, she was up to 'watch' and track me on Endomondo from the beginning. I changed it to hiking and put it back into my pocket. It was incredible how quickly my eyes adapted to the darkness. I chose not to use my torch, and the city lights below helped me see more than you'd think. I knew that at a steady pace, I could climb in under an hour, but I preferred pausing briefly on each step to ensure it was secure instead of using the torch. It felt like a beautiful metaphor for the year ahead - I knew the route, I just couldn't see it.

I was grateful it wasn't raining, but the darkness lingered, leaving me clueless as to what weather was waiting for me at the top. My body felt great, my legs charged onwards like an excited dog that had just been taken off the leash. It was hard to believe I was last here 12 days prior. It's a bizarre feeling going from pent-up excitement and adrenaline to finally doing my first climb. I'd love to be running up here to match the build-up, but this wasn't that kind of challenge.

Attrition, mental fortitude, stamina, perseverance, commitment, appreciation. This wasn't a glitzy fast paced sexy challenge, but I knew with every day that passed, the intensity would build, as would the trust I was nurturing with donors. A surge of energy pulsed through my body as excitement and purpose collided with another successful step. For the first time in my life, I felt aligned. Mind, body, emotions, and spirit 100% in unison. It didn't take long to understand the intensity needed. With each step, my heart rate climbed just as rapidly, and on average doubled in the first five minutes from about 60 beats per minute to 126. I'm sure the added excitement of being the first and only person on the mountain made it even higher.

One day at a time, step by step.... This was my mantra for the year ahead, and I repeated it with every step.

I reached the first mini-milestone - the contour path, which ran below the sheer rock cliffs above the lower cable station in the west. From there, it moved across the front face, around Devil's Peak and across the entire eastern slopes of the reserve above Newlands and Kirstenbosch Gardens before reaching Constantia Nek. It's the first section of the climb that's flat(ish), offering some relief for the lungs and legs. Usually, the road was visible, which allowed me to see how quickly I'd climbed in such a short space of time.

The history of this mountain is phenomenal, as the second oldest mountain range in the world after the Andes, it supports one of the richest plant species on the planet: fynbos (fine bush), found only in the Western Cape of South Africa. One of six plant kingdoms, it covers the smallest surface area in the world - not even 1%. Per square metre, it's more diverse than the Amazon jungle and has more plant species than the entire island of Great Britain. I was excited to experience the many incredible faces fynbos presented throughout the year, as various flowers bloomed, splashing colour on the canvas of my journey.

It wasn't until Ascension Corner that the darkness started dissipating. The birds came alive, and I pretended their chirps were shouts of encouragement.

CHAPTER 4
JANUARY - TAKING THE FIRST STEP INTO THE UNKNOWN

I decided to pick my first stone of the year (photo number two of the day) as this transition from night into day began. Each stone would represent the days climbed (#1), the climbers joining me (none), the donations received, and ultimately the people the donations aimed to empower. Choosing a stone wasn't just a mark of respect, but also a way to keep myself engaged throughout the climb and a wonderful way to observe the three distinct rock layers Table Mountain was made up of. Eventually, I'd have a memorial of stones collected from all over the mountain – including the top.

As I moved upwards, the light began to creep in, but a bank of clouds still covered the top sections. My heart sank a little, I really hoped a clear sunrise would christen 365 Ubuntu Climbs. Considering our drought though, the unseasonable rain trumped any personal desires I had for a picturesque setting. Most questions at the party focussed on what happened when it rained. Thankfully – I wasn't the wicked witch of the West.

'If it rains, I get wet! The weather isn't an excuse this year. Truthfully – I hope I have to do 200 climbs in the rain so our dams can fill up!'

At the time of this climb, the collective dam capacity was 26% - with at least four months until the rainy season began; it wasn't looking good. After three years of minimal rain, we were all praying for a wet winter. Running out of water was a very real threat. These clouds brought a blessing and an individual 'curse', that reminded me about one of the things completely outside my control - the weather. When the gorge is shrouded in mist, it has a mythical appearance to it. Like entering a forgotten sacred land.

I was halfway now, and the greyness was lit up like a 100-watt globe behind a pane of frosted glass, and my luminescent green shirt was the brightest thing around. That was, until I saw my first Orange-breasted sunbird. Possibly one of the smallest and most gorgeous birds on the mountain. Their tiny 9-15cm (3-6 inches) body was yellow with an orange breast, its green head was separated by a blue collar. It was my first experience on the mountain alone, I wondered....

How many climbs would I do in this kind of solitude?

Zig-zagging between the cliffs, I reached Ubuntu Rock, where I'd decided to place each day's stone. This was where I always stopped in training as I made my way back down. The purpose was to stay grounded and ensure each climb wasn't about speed, taking it slow gave me a chance to sit and appreciate the view. I used my time to visualise 2018 being safe and successful.

It was just 336 steps to the top of the gorge from Ubuntu Rock – a special place that would become a beacon of hope for many tired legs and souls over the year to come. I knew how many steps it was because I counted! I searched online for Platteklip's total number of steps, but never found an accurate tally, so on August the 10th, I decided to count using a finger to represent one hundred. Thankfully, I didn't lose count! My findings were that the climb had 2579 steps of vertical gain from the road to the top of the gorge.

With impeccable timing, the silence was cut by the robotic voice reading another of Mom's messages...... *'You must be near your rock'.*

It made me smile, I remembered bringing my parents up here back in September. She climbed victoriously onto the rock to get a picture. Thankfully she was feeling good enough health-wise to make it all the way up. Not only could she visualise exactly where I was, but she could understand what the climb entailed. I kissed my first rock and put it down. Rock number 1: Placed.

I was still about six minutes from the top of the gorge and 15 minutes from the top of Table Mountain. I didn't pause for too long because I'd be damned if I missed sunrise after everything else I did to get there. Clouds or no clouds – I was going to make it!

When I made the summit, I let out a 'WOOOOOHOOOO' of excitement and snapped a selfie (photo number three of each day). I felt slightly dejected as the grey surrounded me, so I headed along the plateau to my 'end point' – a manmade balcony that extended over a cliff. It was the perfect place to take my daily top picture (photo number 4) because it showed the upper cable station, Lions Head below, and the Atlantic Ocean. It would perfectly show the contrast in weather from day to day and an epic change from the start of the climb to the finish!

I was ecstatic that 1/365 was under my belt, but my focus quickly shifted to getting back down safely. Then something extraordinary happened, and thankfully I have pictures of it because even after typing this, I had to go back and check! The grey seemed to disappear through a wormhole, and the path in front of me got lighter. It forced me to look up, where I saw blue sky and was then spun around to face east. The clouds parted, and I was granted another reward for not giving in to temptation.

I was blessed with a delayed sunrise on top of Table Mountain on Day 1 of 365!

It was gorgeous. The glowing ball of life peeked over the flat mountain, illuminating the surrounding clouds bright orange, the only visible blue was through a tiny rectangle that opened just perfectly. After just over an hour of climbing in the cold and dark, the rays felt especially warm on my face. Filled with gratitude – I closed my eyes. It was every bit as awe-inspiring and meaningful as I had envisioned.

This was the perfect start, thank you.

I tried a video call with Tiff, but the signal was poor, so I had to make do with a voice call as her birthday raged on in the background. It was amazing to think I had the company of David at the bottom, my mom during the climb, and then Tiff and her party cheering me on at the top over the phone. These acts of support taught me the essence of Ubuntu.

After soaking in the beauty of day one next to the cable station, I began my climb back down. A little overzealous, I yelled *Only 364 to go*!! I immediately regretted this, but it reminded me to embrace my new mantra: One day at a time, step by step. I had no interest in waiting in the cold for two hours for the first cable car, so I turned around and headed east across the top back to Platteklip. The clouds rolled in again, like a curtain closing the show while the sun retired to the green room. I was back inside a cloud now, but witnessing 2018's first sunrise at the top made that first ascent so much more special.

I came across climber number two for the day at the 'Stairway to Heaven' - the final section where the cliffs close in on you until they're arm's length apart.

'How's the view?'

'I'm afraid the clouds just closed in again. Sorry.'

It was wonderful to witness so many people beginning their New Year on their best foot. I was almost halfway down when Achmat - my mountain brother, greeted me with a beaming smile. The day before, he'd completed his 131st climb for 2017 and was wasting no time in getting #1 for 2018 done and dusted. Seeing him on my way down made me feel blessed.

Achmat is part of a handful of people I see regularly on the mountain - the locals, if you will - like Jack, Wayne, Lisa, Susanne, Dixie, Don, and of course, all the mountain guides; Hendre, Kathy, Stuart, Lynette, Cliff and Muki.

Achmat's friend took a proper snap of us using an actual camera and not a phone. He shared my excitement about how my year would progress. He laughed, because people thought he was nuts for doing this three days a week. If anyone understood the toll this route took on the body, it was him. He'd been a tremendous mentor. His constant words of support and the care my mountain brother showed every time I saw him were invaluable and meant so much. I knew I'd be leaning on him as the year entered the business end for sure.

Climbing down was the opposite of the solitude experienced on the way up, the mountain seemed to wake up and come alive with eager people pushing their capabilities on Cape Town's iconic rock. In my opinion, it's a fantastic way to start a new year.

CHAPTER 4
JANUARY – TAKING THE FIRST STEP INTO THE UNKNOWN

Reaching the bottom was my first chance to celebrate a successful climb without injury or problems. Job done! I'd planned early climbs all week but realised before starting this challenge that I need to be flexible and remain focused on today, experiencing it for whatever it may bring. There was no good, no bad, there was just an experience to be had. If I thought about the number of climbs left or how many months lay ahead, I'd get overwhelmed. I wasn't climbing the mountain 365 times – I was climbing it once, for 365 days.

After 3 hours, 19 minutes, and 38 seconds on the mountain, I was feeling far happier than what I believed I would have felt if I'd stayed at the party.

'Safely off the mountain! Thank you for tracking – and wishing everyone a fabulous start to their new year.'

With five hours of sleep and no more adrenalin left, I felt alive but knackered. All I could think about was getting some serious shut-eye, so I quickly sent David the pictures I promised him, then slipped into the greatest snooze of my life.

First climb: check

First solo climb: check

First up and down climb: check First sunrise: check

Next: climb #2

On day two, I bought a yearly cable car pass. It was an incentive for locals to save money while still being able to enjoy the mountain frequently. Some hikers enjoyed catching a lift down after the tough climb up, while others took a ride up, giving them more time to explore the vast network of paths that spread across the top and back table. A one-way trip was R150 compared to the R640 for a yearly pass. But my guesstimate was that I'd be climbing up and down about 100 days due to severe storms and wind, which meant that without a yearly pass, it would cost R39 750?! Instead, my R640 card would become the most used (and economical!) of all time.

I genuinely felt love and warmth from all the staff, and they quickly made me feel at home. Nandipha was the first. She worked at the gift shop inside the upper cable station, her radiant smile was the perfect tonic for my legs and spirit. They did their best to look after me, which didn't go unnoticed.

My fourth climb started at a more respectable hour – 7 am, so I'd see staff waiting at the bus stop at the intersection just as you turn onto Tafelberg Road. It was a steep walk up to work which wasn't great if you were like me. It meant you'd be sweating profusely by the time you reached the top – especially if you were wearing work clothes. As a youngster, I remember going to golf with my grandad, and whenever he saw the caddies walking up or down, he stopped and gave the men who could fit into the car a lift.

That memory flooded my mind so I slammed on the brakes and reversed back to the bus stop. Their beaming smiles of gratitude were the perfect start to any climb. It gave me an opportunity to meet even more of the staff.

Most of my training was done alone, which made me contemplate what I'd do on days when unfit people joined. Should I apply cut-off points to help 'preserve' my legs? Do I have to turn people away? How can I leave people on the mountain? None of these questions felt representative of the Ubuntu spirit that this challenge was about.

Being alone while training naturally centred my thoughts and kept me focused on what I needed to do to be successful. It didn't feel that selfish to have cutoffs, after all, multiplying an extra hour or two by 365 added an additional month on the mountain. Not five days a week, 9-5, but a full month. If you started the clock at 00:00 on the 1st and stopped it at midnight on the 30th. That was over and above the normal time it took to climb. This wasn't a challenge about speed though. It was about pushing my capabilities in a way that gave others an opportunity to be part of something bigger than ourselves. We could have the same goal, but only I could overcome the challenge laid out by the mountain to reach the top. I now understood why 'ubuntu' kept prodding me. It was one word that perfectly expressed a social experiment to build a community of people around self-mastery, and service to others. It was impossible to understand how much better my life was because of the inventions and work of others.

The first five climbs were all solo and would give me the space to focus on myself and develop a rhythm without distraction. My first cash donation on the mountain happened on Thursday the 4th, after a tourist questioned me about how often I did this. I let him hear my story and he quickly reached for his wallet, handing me a note. For the first time, I noticed Madiba's smiling face looking up at me. I felt his presence, cheering me on. (Madiba is the name of the Thembu clan to which Mandela belonged. It gets its name from a 19th century chief. All the members of this clan can be called Madiba. Mandela was called Madiba as a sign of both respect and affection)

I was surprised at how easily I was able to wake up at 5 am to enjoy the mountain in the cool morning light. As a lifelong professional snoozer, it was a refreshing change to bounce out of bed energised and inspired for physical activity instead of rising begrudgingly.

Then Friday arrived... our beloved Cape Doctor hammered through, rattling and flinging around anything that wasn't bolted down. The Cape Doctor was the name given to the South Easter, the Western Cape's prevailing summer wind that tormented Capetonians from December to March. As I mentioned before, Sea Point was protected, so if it was pumping there – I knew it was doubly worse everywhere else. In 2017 it was so strong it closed the world's largest timed cycle race - The Cape Town Cycle Tour. Picture cyclists desperately holding onto super lightweight carbon fibre and aluminium bikes as the wind picked them up like rag dolls and flapped them around like flags. Check out this video on YouTube to see exactly what I mean: *100km/h wind throws around cyclists at Cape Town Cycle Tour.*

Thankfully, it wasn't that bad on the mountain when I got there, but it was enough to close the cable car. The tablecloth was flowing beautifully over the lip of the mountain. The Tablecloth is the name 'lovingly' bestowed on the orographic cloud formation, which normally forms during the summer months when Cape Town's south to south easterly pushes moist air against the mountain's east slopes. The air is forced to rise, and as it climbs, it cools, causing the relative humidity to increase and flow down the front north face. From a distance, it's a spectacle as Table Mountain's flat top is covered by a cloud just as a tablecloth is thrown over a table in preparation for a meal.

Days like these were a treat, close to the top between the cliffs, the cloud demonstrated exactly how the wind bounced off the walls and spiralled down, trying to flatten everything in its path, it was like being in nature's wind tunnel. The powerful ripping of the wind would roar across your face and ears, making it almost impossible to hear anything else. I find it incredible how the plants have adapted to survive such an assault. I used to think climbing down was most dangerous in wind like this, but now I realise it's far deadlier going up. The minute I performed a big box step-up, I became weightless for a second. If a severe gust suddenly blew, it could easily push me off balance, and backward with nothing to grab onto.

Walking down is tougher on the joints and muscles, and in this wind becomes a balancing act of leaning back just enough to stay upright and not get pushed down the mountain. With the wind so consistently strong, I could keep leaning backward. Being 6"4' was another advantage I had, I could step across the bigger gaps with greater ease. I always felt sorry for people walking behind me, unable to make a stride the same way I could. The more I acknowledged these smaller details, the more grateful I became.

Although it was still early days and just my second climb back down, my brain couldn't help but extrapolate the ratio; 40% of the year would mean 146 days up and down – 46 more than my guestimate. Gulp! It was an intimidating figure, and immediately I regretted crunching the numbers in my head. I swiftly swept it under the rug and reminded myself how my training was always up and down.

CHAPTER 4
JANUARY - TAKING THE FIRST STEP INTO THE UNKNOWN

The down climb was a completely different experience, the view embraced you, and your lungs weren't gasping for air. It provided space for deep thoughts and today I was focused on my excitement for tomorrow which would be my first group, thanks to Karel. Originally planned for his birthday on Sunday, the forecast of rain shifted it a day early, making my first group of six people on the 6th. It would be my sixth early start, and I made that choice because weekends had additional factors to consider. Timing was everything. Firstly, once the sun rose above Devils Peak to the east – Platteklip gorge got roasted by the sun. From 8 am it got unbearably hot in the gorge, and on days with hardly any wind, the rising hot air had a suffocating effect. Many unsuspecting tourists were caught out hearing & believing you could 'walk up' and arrive unprepared with little to no water. I suggested two litres per person as the minimum.

Secondly, Platteklip was fast becoming a popular outing, causing traffic jams on the narrow sections with higher volumes of people choosing to start their weekend on the mountain. With sections dropping off steeply there was no room for error, especially when people were on their way back down. The infamous 'red chopper' was often seen hovering over Lions Head and Table Mountain to rescue injured climbers, or in worse cases – recover the bodies of those who had lost their lives.

Table Mountain's proximity to the city was a blessing and a curse. Blessing because of the easy access everyone had to enjoy the beautiful views high above the Atlantic Ocean. Curse because people took that proximity for granted. It's a national park. It's wild, and often creates its own weather that can change in minutes. From searing heat to icy cold winds, clear skies to thick mist disorientating people. The mountain is big, scrap that, huge! You only realise this when you get up top and see the vast space between Constantia (east), Camps Bay and Llandudno (west), the city (north), and Hout Bay (south).

As a boy scout in my teen years, I'd been dropped off in the middle of nowhere with nothing but a compass to find my way back. The motto was 'always be prepared,' and it stuck with me. That's why I carried extra water, a warm jacket, and two space blankets to assist unprepared climbers. The earlier the start, the more time I had to ascend in cooler conditions and the quieter the route would be.

One of my biggest supporters, Lisa, surprised me as she walked towards us and joined the first group. I should've known she'd be here for this. The first of what would become a record number of climbs with me.

Karel generously asked his group to make a financial contribution to 365 Ubuntu Climbs instead of 'gifts'. It was also his first time up the mountain. In fact, only Lisa had been up before, so this meant we had five first-timers. Seeing the mountain through their eyes was magical.

Conquering Platteklip created a vastly different kind of fitness. While I was extremely fit from climbing, it didn't mean it would automatically translate into a stellar performance on a bike, running, or swimming. The reverse was also true and left many 'athletes' feeling the strain on their first ascent. The relentless assault on your legs was brutal.

Karel got an early present; a bank of clouds slowly rolled in below us when we were about halfway up, and it looked as though we were above the surface of a white lake which was now lapping the lower edges of the mountains. It took reaching the top to reveal just how expansive and beautiful this new canvas was. Only the tip of Devil's Peak stuck out and joined the top of Table Mountain, creating an island effect in this heaven created on earth.

Enjoying the view and basking in our accomplishment of summiting, Karel sprang a surprise on me. Not only did he voice his pride at seeing my growth in reaching this point from the lowly devastated figure that walked into his office a month ago; but he pledged one of biggest donations ever by an individual. The fundraising was now well on its way, with this R5 000 being the 27th donation of the week – a contribution which brought us to a total of **R12 704.84**.

I chose a public crowdfunding platform called *Backabuddy* for people to donate because it allowed international donations too, I loved the transparency of being

CHAPTER 4
JANUARY - TAKING THE FIRST STEP INTO THE UNKNOWN

able to see everyone donate and the running total that came with that. One of the aims was to distribute the funds as they accumulated, this would give donors a level of transparency and would build trust. One of the unintended benefits was the opportunity to read the comments from friends and strangers alike – the Ubuntu family.

Adele, a friend of 18 years, wrote, *'Looking forward to 365 days of your incredible inspiration. Supporting you all the way to the top.'*

Rob Coutts wrote, *'Amazing idea and I hope to join you a few times if possible!'*

Another friend Verity wrote, *'So inspired by what you're doing! Let the magic unfold xxx'*

These twenty-seven donations warmed my soul and had a profound impact on my heart. It helped douse the first fire of doubt that had me wondering whether this project would be supported or not. Karel's generosity capped things off beautifully and reminded me how inspired the thought was to seek him out for coaching.

Six climbs down – 359 to go.

TO DATE:

Time on Mountain | Distance | Vertical Climb Equivalent | Alone | Up & Down

14 hours 46 minutes / 43 km / 1 equivalent Everest Summit / 5 solo / 2

At this early stage I was eternally grateful for such a positive steady start. But I was under no illusions and knew that all it would take was one misstep to jeopardise all the work that had been done so far. What was the difference between thousands of safe steps and one bad foot placement? The right measure of concentration and focus!

This was about to be tested far sooner than I'd hoped for.

We must embrace pain and use it as fuel for our journey
~~ Kenji Miyazawa

CHAPTER 5
JANUARY - HELL WEEK

Backabuddy was terrific, they made sure I had a couple of weeks of climbing under my belt before reaching out to their network of journalists and media contacts with a January 16th press release. With my challenge being unique and because of the lengthy duration, 365 Ubuntu Climbs was chosen as one of Backabuddy's focus points for 2018. I wouldn't be able to donate 100% of the donations because of the 5% Backabuddy admin fee, but the charge was worth every penny in this case.

Overnight, the story exploded across TV, Radio, newspapers, and a variety of online platforms. There was no onramp for this freeway! Suddenly, an intense spotlight was thrust onto me and the journey I'd started, but as daunting as it was, I was grateful for the publicity so early on. People wanted to know how to follow my journey; how to contribute, and, if based in the Western Cape - how to join me on a climb. DKMS Africa tracked and noted every instance their name appeared in the media because of its association with 365 Ubuntu Climbs, One Heart, and Habitat for Humanity. This is how we tracked the Rand value of the publicity that was generated, just as it's done with paid advertising. My

CHAPTER 5
JANUARY - HELL WEEK

story became amplified by a factor of four - another reason I was happy that I listened to my gut and stuck with three charities to support.

Speaking as a master of ceremonies at weddings or delivering work presentations is one thing, but being interviewed live on air is a whole new kettle of fish and something I was forced to learn - quickly! Thankfully, my talk in Johannesburg last year in front of 2000 people taught me the benefits of sharing a message as opposed to talking about myself. That focus helped channel my nerves and fear as the days quickly filled up with interviews from across the country. I was thrown into the deep end, but my vision became my armbands and kept me afloat.

I find radio interviews are easier to do, and I get them more frequently because they have less restrictions. Producers would phone me and ask, *'are you available in the next twenty minutes?'* to chat. My funniest moment was with 5fm, one of the largest national stations. I managed to spread the word in time for family and friends to tune in and listen to give me feedback. Thankfully, Zane prepped me with great questions for the press release to formulate my answers before the pressure of a live interview.

My timing was a bit off for this interview, though, so I had a laugh replying to everyone's messages......*'They caught me off-guard, I'd just got out of the shower - I was in my underwear the whole time!'*

There was a negative side to all of this though. I made the mistake of reading comments online under articles posted on social media. An avalanche of online warriors gave their negative two cents worth on the challenge. It made me wonder if they'd even read the article. I was baffled trying to understand the connection between what I was doing and their views.

It stung, so I instantly decided I'd stay off the comments section in the future. I've always lived with the understanding that what happens to me is out of my control, but how I choose to move forward is within my control. Easy, of course, when things are going well. Pretty different when I'm in the middle of it. I had to sit down with myself and have a stern talking to. Did it really matter what someone else typed about the challenge, good or bad? It didn't matter. Their opinions weren't the ones climbing every day – I was.

Hindsight made it easy to see I wasn't expressing myself completely. The intense week I was having kept playing tricks with my mind and made me question myself again and again. Back in December, I wanted to have a fundraising launch party, but I postponed it because I worried about attendance. Self-doubt had spoken up – 'do it in January when you've got some days behind you!'

The good old *'I'll be ready when'* scenario that never arrived. You guessed it, with those negative comments hiding behind door #5 in my mind, I decided it was 'probably best' to do it when I had a serious chunk of climbs behind me. How ironic, not a shred of doubt behind my ability to do the challenge, but a mountain of doubt piling up behind whether it would be supported.

Truthfully, I could understand the scepticism behind this challenge. Every day? The whole year? What about winter? What about the wind? Injury? What happens when you get sick? I almost predicted what the next questions would be. There was only one way to prove any detractor wrong – my actions had to match my words. Maybe that was exactly what I needed to finally overcome, the worst critic of all – me!

As the exposure exploded, most of my climbs were still being done alone, giving me the flexibility to juggle start times with the interviews that had been booked. The interesting aspect of my interviews was that, in other instances, they usually took place before or after the extreme event – not during. This meant I was constantly updating my interview answers with new experiences. For example, my first international cash donation happened on Climb 12 and came from Philip – a Belgian who was here to make use of the notorious South Easter to kitesurf. We connected after he'd been out to dinner with his Belgian friends and a mate of mine named Beth. After seeing his eagerness to climb Table Mountain, she told him to contact me. I laughed at our opposite desires; he wanted the wind to gust early all day every day – and I wanted it

CHAPTER 5
JANUARY – HELL WEEK

calm! He was a fascinating man, and I got to hear about his hiking travels in Patagonia – a magnificent location high on my list of places to visit. Time with Philip was the first experience that reminded me about my travel restrictions for the year, and although I was nailed down to the Cape, my challenge gave me the opportunity to meet others and hear about their travels. It also put into perspective how lucky I was to be living in Cape Town. Most people had to spend thousands to experience it for just a few days or weeks at best, but all this beauty was in my backyard.

As we said our goodbyes, he dashed off to his car, then came walking back with a wide grin and handed me €100 (about R1500), *'That was absolutely fantastic Andrew! Thanks for taking me up the mountain today – here's a little something towards your challenge. Best of luck for the rest of the year'.*

It certainly wasn't little in my eyes at all! It had been a real pleasure taking him up, and I appreciated his contribution. After that, I was flying high, especially now that my body was four days into uncharted territory. Before this, the most consecutive days I had in training was eight, and my climb with Philip was the 12th consecutive climb.

As the publicity increased, a woman by the name of Margolite made contact with me and requested to join in on a climb that was scheduled for Wednesday, the 24th. Meeting her was a treat because she'd completed 100 climbs in 2017 up the same route! Although still early in the year, she missed her life-changing experience. Her eyes shone as she recounted the stories. Learning from someone else with such enthusiasm and passion for climbing was special! She raised money for 'Life Child' - a safe house for children in Philippi. As a woman alone on the mountain, safety was a concern. She'd see other climbers and make sure she was just behind them to appear as part of the group. On one such occasion, she asked a couple if they'd mind her walking behind them – they turned out to be the owners of 'Life Child'! She fell in love with their work, so all the money she raised for them went towards protecting vulnerable children. I loved hearing stories like this.

It was also interesting hearing how her body had more niggles now that she wasn't climbing compared to last year when she was so much more active. Her appreciation for the mountain grew with each climb she took on. She showed the same uplifting energy towards what I was doing, and it completely lifted my spirits, especially after hearing what she did to maintain her enthusiasm all year. Between her and Achmat, I had pioneers to call on in times of need. The timing of our climb couldn't have been better because I was rapidly descending into the week from hell.

Karel joined me for his second climb. Again, living up to his promise, his intention was to join on multiple climbs so he could experience an array of weather, seasons, and times of day. He got all three in one day! Firstly, we started in the dark with the aim of experiencing a 6 am sunrise up top. Next, we got extreme wind, and then it was bitterly cold at the summit. Many visitors are surprised by the stark contrast between the summer heat at the bottom compared to a huge drop in temperature of at least ten degrees (18° Fahrenheit) at the top. Today's wind guaranteed my sixth climb back down for the year and Karel's first.

It's a tough job trying to explain the wind strength, mostly because, unlike other places, it's consistently strong (hence why Kite Surfers love it), but now and again there's a surge, a violent gust so powerful it feels like someone's grabbing you and pushing you around. With wind now playing such an important part in my life, the weather app Windguru became my best friend. This nugget came from the staff at the cable car company, and the app offered me the most accurate readings for weather patterns and wind, which was particularly helpful with its data relating to Table Mountain.

'Search Windguru Table Mountain – that'll give you the forecasts we use'

Typical summers are calm in the morning, with gale-force winds building up throughout the afternoon. This explains my first week's climbs, which were all morning sessions. I did, however, decide that at least once a week, I'd do an afternoon climb. This would give my legs a 'mini break' with an extra twelve hours added to the rest period, but most enjoyably – I wouldn't have to wake up to an alarm.

Of course, the opposite applied when I switched back to mornings, this would have me climbing Table Mountain twice in twelve hours, so careful analysis of these different scenarios before starting was critical. Proper planning and some forethought allowed me to incorporate this into my training, intentionally doing an afternoon climb immediately followed by an early climb. I'd gone through every situation and combination to test the impact, to mentally prepare, and to trial a plan B. This was not a year for excuses, and my mindset needed to be solutions-oriented.

There were potential situations I couldn't plan for, though; the very nature of the challenge with all of its unknowns, and the impact of doing a climb every day. Some things had to be taken on the chin. For instance, one windy day on its own wasn't that bad, but string a few together and I'd have another level of intensity to deal with - that would be a vastly different story.

Karel and I tried desperately to shelter out of the icy wind and settled on the floor behind the stairs leading up to the café - a welcomed relief out of the relentless wind. He came prepared with coffee and sandwiches, which instantly kicked the mood up a bit. While we sat talking, I showed him the app that explained the unlikely odds of the cable car running while the mountain was being battered by the southeaster.

On the app, there were two rows with wind speed; one was for average speed while the second was for the gusts. They were colour coded which allowed you to quickly spot the dangerous times beforehand - the days were also broken down into three-hour slots. What you wanted to see was white or blue blocks - that was excellent and meant minimal wind. Next was green and yellow which signified a breeze - these conditions were helpful on hotter days. Then there was orange - this was where the darker shades became a cause for concern. Next, there was red, pink, and purple - these were no ordinary days.

Karel and I were in the red, so we had a better chance of growing wings than seeing the cable car come up. It was time for us to head down, so I shared some mountain safety tips. On the way up, we both looked like Golam from Lord of the Rings – hunched over and staying as close to the ground as possible to avoid sneaky gusts that were waiting to catch us. They were powerful, and one mistake at the wrong time would have meant a catastrophic fall backwards.

Coming down was an entirely different ball game – we paid close attention to any changes in the wind, leaning backwards and adjusting ourselves accordingly. I didn't want to get myself into a situation where the wind was controlling me and forcing me to move faster than I was comfortable with. It was like driving a car – knowing your breaks would help maintain that feeling of control. I made sure I was always on the side of the path closest to the mountain so if a gust pushed me off balance, it wouldn't pose a risk because I was away from the edge. And anytime I needed a break, I sat down, focussed my concentration, and continued onwards with a fresh mind. On the larger drops down, I climbed down sideways. Slow and steady was the motto for days like these.

The heat we generated on the ascent was a much-needed advantage, but sadly it was lost again climbing down because of the wind that turned us into icicles, making our hands numb in the process. As we fought our way down, it intensified, it became intimidating, like a drill sergeant hammering us about our pace and wildly hurrying us down the mountain. *'Oi! Get a move on! You're dawdling!'*

Finally, we made it down safely in 3 hours and 40 minutes. My brain was exhausted and drained from the intense focus and concentration given to every single step, my body was feeling the effects of the constant physical exertion, and my joints were crying out for rest after the impact of each step.

Windguru provided a 10-day forecast, I was in for another two days of this.

Ah, I'm so grateful for my longer legs!

CHAPTER 5
JANUARY - HELL WEEK

The interviews with the press the past week had been nonstop; this was my first clear day, and it was rush-free. All I needed to do was head home and rest up for the next climb. That night, I had a dinner party with friends. Even with all the hum & chatter, my body was able to attract my attention and get a message through to me, I felt a tickle of sparks in my throat. I tried ignoring it, I thought I just needed a good night's rest....

I'd soon find out just how wrong I was.

Friday – January the 26th

With an afternoon climb scheduled, I enjoyed waking up later, but alas, the tickle was still present, and more aggressive. It wasn't that bad, but it was enough to create doubt. To add some fuel to that fire, the weekend had some serious plans in store. My friend Greg had organised for a group of us to stay on top of the mountain at the Scout Hut. I'd never been before. At 16:30, we were going to meet at Platteklip to split the supplies load and set off. This would give us enough time to reach the hut before dark. I spent half the day going backward and forward on whether to go or not. I was torn. Half of me said it was a once-in-a-lifetime opportunity – go! The other half said there'll be another time – rather sleep at home and manage the throat. Time was running out, I had to make a call, so I impulsively decided to give it a bash.

While I would've loved to stay there the whole weekend, my plan was to sleep there just one night, then early the next morning, I'd catch the cable car back down – later that Saturday afternoon, I'd do climb number 27. That was the plan, the wind had other ideas though.

My memory of the hut's proximity to Platteklip was way off. I was about to be reminded of an extra two-kilometre trek that I'd conveniently forgotten about, a trek that felt like double the distance in the wind.

The wind was completely INSANE. I'd never been skydiving in my life before, but I imagined with the blasting gust in my face, I was pretty much experiencing it already. When I arrived to meet Greg and his friend, the tablecloth had reached the road. THE ROAD?!? A seven-hundred-and-twenty-metre wall of cloud flowing at up to 100 km/h (62mph) was violently lashing the base of the mountain where we were due to start our climb. That's when I realised the size of the tablecloth illustrates the strength of the wind – we were in for a rough time.

Ironically, our original weekend last year in November was cancelled due to wind. Greg and I still climbed that day because I saw it as an opportunity to train. THAT – had nothing on today. I've never experienced anything like this in my life. Standing on the road, we all had a look of disbelief on our faces, 'Are we really doing this?? Yup...'. Not surprisingly, ours were the only cars there! We were on our way, and nature wasted no time; grim evidence of the wind's power greeted us just past the first waterfall. A massive branch from a mighty oak tree had snapped off and was flung 20m down the gorge like a piece of plywood. We're talking about a branch at least 8 feet long (2.4 metres) and as thick as an athlete's thigh.

Staying the night was going to be a blessing; it also meant our bags, which were crammed with food and extra warm things, provided additional weight, which doubled as some extra defence against the power of the wind. We had bags of wood for heat and cooking together with other packets which acted as stabilises in each hand. My mind tried to stay focused on each step while trying to ignore the pain of the extra weight and the onslaught of wind. It was a struggle. Slow and methodical, with frequent stops to refocus our efforts against the relentless onslaught of the southeaster that was funnelling down the gorge. My concentration levels were at DEFCON 5.

Achmat caught up to us, and our faces screamed 'WTF'!! I say screamed because that's what I had to do to be heard. It was a full-on assault on the senses. I stopped climbing for a moment but was still working against the wind. I watched the plants getting smashed around, it honestly felt like the wind was trying to uproot everything. I now understood how one of the gorge's plants got nicknamed the 'hikers' friend' – it was known to support the weight of anyone who fell and grabbed onto it. Their incredible root system went deep into the rocks thanks to millennia of adaptation and trying to survive the vicious wind.

CHAPTER 5
JANUARY - HELL WEEK

Every foot was planted with laser focus, as though we were climbing a ridge high up in the Himalayas with nothing on either side but tragedy. No thought was given to the discomfort of the climb, no thought was given to the madness of the mission, no thought was given to the growing fire in my throat – there were just no thoughts at all. All focus went towards putting one foot in front of the other and maintaining my balance just enough to achieve one solitary objective – summit number 26.

As we reached the top of Platteklip, we took a well-deserved break and celebrated a mini victory for a job half done. Achmat had to climb back down while Greg and his friend headed straight for the hut. I made my way up the last section that took me to the top table. I navigated through the dense mist that enveloped me as the tablecloth covered everything in its path. I still managed to take a photo without my phone being ripped from my grasp. Trying to hold it still for a moment was a challenge; it felt like I was holding onto an invisible kite that was thrashing around somewhere above me. A blurry snap was all I could muster, the roaring wind made it impossible to shoot a video! In my frustration, I shouted eight words.......... *'This is ridiculous! No video today too windy!'*. Those words stoked the vicious fire that had been raging in my throat. I could no longer ignore it.

My walk to the hut was painful. Besides misjudging the distance, I'd also forgotten how dramatically the terrain dropped and rose again – a far cry from the gentle flat stroll I 'remembered'. I was tired, annoyed, frustrated, and I just wanted to get out of the wind. Was this a treadmill I was on? I had no bearings, and I was totally wrapped up in the grey clouds that were whizzing past my head. I'd lost my sense of humour and in pure frustration after reaching boiling point, (and just to make my throat better), I dropped the packets, tilted my head back, and, like an erupting volcano, let out a blood-curdling cry of emotion.

Idiot! That aggravated my throat, and as the light started fading, I got fed up. Suddenly, I had the patience of a three-year-old with a milkshake in front of him. To top it off, I couldn't see the sun, just thick dark clouds slamming into me and stealing the last of the day's light.

We left at 16:42, so the journey was five minutes shy of three hours, and I arrived 19 minutes before sunset. Out of the mist, the wind, and the hell of the climb, the four huts appeared – I made it! Well, so I thought. I wasn't sure which one was the scout hut, I also wasn't sure who was joining us, so I walked up to the first one, which had a group of people comfortably enjoying coffee outside the front. As I glanced around for a measure of familiarity, I got nothing but blank stares in return – wrong hut, I thought! Luckily, they pointed me to the next spot, which they believed had 'Greg' in it. I casually strolled through the door.............. still no Greg!

Crazy though, I'd found someone else instead, it was Blake – the founder of Love our Trails and orphanage owner. Another quality human being focused on using his skills and resources to make the planet a better place and raise awareness to create lasting change. We'd been introduced at a PechaKucha event in July 2017, and after exchanging details, I'd met up with him for a coffee to learn and ask questions.

'What are you doing here?' he says bewildered.
'I didn't know you knew Greg'
'Greg Who?' 'Hillyard'

'How do you know Greg??? He's not in this hut though'

'Wait, What? You just happen to know him and I'm at the wrong hut?! Isn't this the scout hut?'

'No that's further down'

By this point, I was over it. I was done! I wasn't having fun at all and just thought of my couch, which would've felt like a dream destination. I was also craving something to soothe my throat. I made my way back outside and continued the search. I should never have agreed to come here. Well done, Andrew, you chose the harder, crazier, and more stupid option.

CHAPTER 5
JANUARY – HELL WEEK

The sun disappeared as I arrived at door number three. Disheartened by the eery lack of human movement inside, I remained cautious as I burst through the door – 'I'm home'. Please let this be home! I'm exhausted......PLEASE!!! I was greeted by Greg's frame sitting at the table, with another group of climbers that had trekked up from the east via Kirstenbosch Botanical Gardens. Instantly, I weighed up my options, considering how rotten I felt. I had zero desire to eat, so after a brief chat about our epic journey up, I decided to lie down for a bit. I apologised to everyone and excused myself. It felt so good to lay down on a free bunk. Perhaps my eyes would gently shut, and I'd drift off for a bit......

Wrong!! I was not on a good streak.

I had no idea what time it was, but the candles had been blown out, and everyone had gone to bed. Rather than enjoying a warm, rejuvenating sleep, I felt like I was travelling on a plane enduring the 'sitting upright sleep'. It was pitch black. Just the wind was partying late into the night, and I couldn't get comfortable. Eventually, the cold became unbearable, so I stumbled around in the dark, searching for my bag.

I'd decided clothes would be fine and left blankets at home. Mistake! My rain jacket was all I had as a 'blanket'. It was better than nothing, but the minute a piece fell off, I woke up to 'tuck in' and then went back to laying in the foetal position while battling to swallow with the fire in my throat. I had no idea how long this went on for, all I could think of was...... *How the hell am I going to climb tomorrow?*

Saturday – January the 27th

My nightmare was real! As I woke up, the sound of the wind still rattled the hut and reminded me of what lay ahead. Forget climb 27 – I still had to climb down to my car, and I knew there was no way the cable car was working. The big question was.... Do I take the longer but flatter route? Or the direct & more physically intense route back to my car?

Greg's friends must have thought I was the most unsociable person alive, I barely stayed half an hour after waking up. I just wanted to get home. So, I set off and took Kasteelspoort, a gorge that cuts down through the Twelve Apostles. I decided this longer, flatter option was best for me because I'd be more protected from the wind and I'd be out of the sun. This side of the mountains rose majestically out of the ocean, flanking Table Mountain on its west. Climbing down, I finally reached the pipe track. Another flattish contour path which ran above Camps Bay. It was an old route carved out to create space for a pipe that sent water from Hout Bay to Cape Town. There were still sections where you could see the old, rusted pipe sticking through the rock. I was grateful for the flatter section and happy that I finally made a good decision. I was deep in thought about why I had this sore throat. I knew it wasn't by accident.

After 8km and a little over two hours later, the sight of my car almost made me weep. I could almost feel my couch.

Finally, I got home around midday, and knowing the wind wasn't going to improve, there was little time to rest. I had four hours of downtime before heading back out. This was not a position I wanted to be in so early on. As I drifted off to sleep, the first pinprick of worry crept in. Besides telling Greg at the scout hut, I'd kept this predicament to myself. I didn't want the decision of potentially missing a day to be on anyone else's shoulders but mine.

As 15:00 rolled around, I was dejected but found comfort and some comic relief as Lisa visited before joining me on her third climb. She shared a recent idea she had about shaving her hair off.

'I have clippers you know. We can do it now,' I said with a devilish grin.

I'd never shaved anyone's hair off, especially not a woman. Nevertheless, she took the plunge and went for it, which was a welcome distraction from the business end of the day that lurked like a test I hadn't studied for. She felt like a change and hoped this would shed some negative elements of her self-belief in the process. Hmmmm... this was something I could relate to. The experience was liberating for her and a real laugh for us both.

As I stared out my window at the vista of Lion's Head, I realised the bank of clouds I could see flowing was actually the tablecloth visible from my flat. Any remaining hope I had that the cable car would operate was now gone. Lisa shrugged it off and said she was still coming. If she could plug into my brain and see what I saw the day before, I believe she'd have chosen otherwise. But her support truly meant more than she realised.

While not as bad as yesterday, it was still howling around the 60km/h (37mph) as we started. Talking was out of the question, so we receded into the silent crevasses of our minds. My two windy climbs during training – while good practice – were nothing like this. I was forced to recon with the reality of knowing that many challenges like this were still awaiting me. It was impossible to know the extreme end until it happened. This was an early exercise to prepare me for what winter had lined up when wind, rain, and cold would combine.

I pointed out the snapped branch and Lisa's eyes widened. She was shocked when she saw the tree it was ripped from. It was a very sober reminder early on. That was one of the benefits of being on the path every day, I got to watch life in action, and I got to experience the subtle mountain changes in real time. Previously I'd just walk past thinking nothing of it. Imagine being here the moment it snapped off!

Each climb became a reconnaissance mission for the next day's climb. Paying close attention to the path was essential; especially on days like this when I climbed back down. Knowing which rocks were becoming loose from human erosion meant the difference between a terrible accident and a safe foot placement.

My legs were feeling it. I tried desperately to stay focused on the climb, but the fatigue kept dragging my mind into the future. My throat was still screaming at me, and it didn't feel like I'd had any rest. It all just felt like a complete shit show – there wouldn't be any screaming out loud today.

Climbing back down for a third time and second in one day was taking its toll. I kept thinking about the idiotic decision I made the day before, I felt like chastising myself, but honestly, not only would it do me no good, but it would just deflect my attention away from where it was needed. I was excited about my bed. It's crazy how my mind jumped from the insanity of the current climb, to being home in bed, and to the fact that I hadn't even finished a month of climbing yet. I was struggling to hold back the feeling of intimidation that the weight of what lay ahead was causing – I needed to focus on the steps right in front of me. I got it right for a while with some meditation, but inevitably my thoughts kept bulldozing their way in.

Finally, we made it down just before sunset, the sanctuary of the car was a welcome relief. It's incredible how quiet it was inside after almost three hours of being battered by the wind. Both our faces were pictures of gratitude. Lisa broke the silence,

'Bru, that – was – INSANE! I've never experienced anything like it before.'

After three days of this, I wasn't sure I could handle another one. The sore throat wasn't hindering the climbs physically, it was just painful to swallow. Which wasn't great at each water break. Had I bitten off more than I could chew?

Sunday – January the 28th

I never thought waking up to the sound of silence would spark such joy – No wind! Just a beautiful stillness for weary legs that had covered 22.1 km (13.8 mi) in gale force winds in 7 hours and 32 minutes on the back of 25 days on the mountain – this brought me to a cumulative total of:

66 hours 29 minutes / 192.1km / 5 equivalent Everest Summit / 18 solo / 8 up & down

My legs and brain felt equally tapped out. Swallowing was accompanied by razor blades.

CHAPTER 5
JANUARY - HELL WEEK

Eating anything was out of the question. I finally staggered from my bed to the couch around mid-morning, going backwards and forwards in my mind about whether to climb. The mind games were in full swing. Was I just trying to be a hero, or was this part of what I signed up for? Was I using this as an excuse? If I took one day off now and made it up again – would that become a habit? These were pretty damaging thoughts I had consuming me on day 27 of a year-long challenge. To make matters worse, a fire broke out below the start of Platteklip Gorge, I could see the smoke billowing above Lion's rump, and a friend from across the bay sent me some pictures.

Was this a sign to skip today's climb? Or was I just looking for an excuse??

Fires during summer were an unfortunate reality in the Western Cape. With no rain, the ground and vegetation are kindling. Throw in high winds, and a flame quickly turns into a raging fire. We've had some horrific fires in recent years; the most notable was a tragedy when 2000 shacks were destroyed in Hout Bay. The year before that, another devastating blaze ripped through half the Cape Peninsula and burned for a week.

Luckily Platteklip isn't the only way up, it's just the most direct. I've decided each milestone (50/100/150/200/250/300/350) would be a different route as my 'reward'. I may have to do one earlier than expected.

My mom joked how only I could do other routes that were longer and harder, calling them 'rewards'. Besides language being important and a powerful influencer for motivation, I genuinely believed they were rewards. They acted as little beacons breaking up the year with a change of scenery. It also gave me an opportunity to explore new parts of the mountain I'd never seen before. Choosing new alternative ways of defining these events with language certainly helped boost my ability to remain spirited. I was far from high-spirited though.

I checked in with the Safety Mountain tracking volunteers and learned that the fire was under control, so I didn't need to use another route. Then some news broke that left me with the heaviest of hearts...

> *"The City of Cape Town's Fire and Rescue Service is saddened by the passing of 33-year-old firefighter, Candice Kruger (also known as Ashley)," the City of Cape Town said in a statement.*
>
> *"Kruger passed away in hospital yesterday after collapsing on the fire line on the lower slopes of Table Mountain. She received medical attention, but efforts to resuscitate her were unsuccessful. The cause of death has not yet been established."*

While I was grateful the fire started on a windless day, the news of Candice's tragic passing overshadowed my gratitude. My deepest condolences to those close to her, she gave her all and will remain a hero.

I was deeply moved, and my mind felt scattered..... I had to shift my thinking! What about my climb? I still hadn't decided - my throat wasn't getting better after mixtures of hot water, honey, ginger, and lemon, and the warm salt-water gargling wasn't helping either. My conflicted thoughts battled it out and eventually came to an agreement... I'll go, but much slower than usual. If, at any point before halfway, my body takes flack or I start struggling, I'll turn back. It's a deal!

I set off from the lower cable station at 17:17, focusing on slow measured steps. The joy of the calm conditions was tainted by the ever-burning furnace in my throat. Seeing the cable car running again was a huge boost too. It felt much slower than normal but 2 hours and 4 minutes later I was up at the cable station. I hadn't eaten all day, and drinking water on the way up was limited to emergencies only.

Had I ever experienced such excruciating pain while swallowing? Maybe when I had tonsillitis as a 5-year-old – but nothing in my memory banks compared to this. Gratitude was the overwhelming feeling after achieving another successful summit AND for the cable car ride down. Problems always seem like the end of the world, and this felt no different, so I dosed up on Echinacea Force, applying it directly to my throat, then some more hot water, lemon, and ginger, as well as salty warm water gargle. Then Rest!

CHAPTER 5
JANUARY – HELL WEEK

I wasn't even contemplating an early start for my next day's climb, but my heart sank. Thinking about the days ahead overwhelmed me. Tired, frustrated, and somewhat defeated – that was the end of week 4.

Please.... Please let me wake up feeling better and able to swallow again.

Monday – January the 29th

Is it even possible to feel worse? Am I ever going to be able to swallow anything but liquids ever again? It certainly didn't feel like it, as this was rapidly becoming the longest four days of my life. I was starting to feel weaker because I hadn't had a decent meal in two days. My body and heart told me this was a localised throat infection. But why now? What's caused it?

The past few years, I'd paid close attention to the few injuries and illnesses that had come my way, and with further studying, I developed an understanding that injuries and sickness were related to our emotional issues. Every time something happened, like when I injured my back at gym and now this sore throat, I knew it was related to an emotional block.

The pain in my throat was linked to my inability or willingness to express myself regarding the challenge. I could do without the attention, but the two were inseparable – and I'd to come to terms with that. I was having an internal battle that pitted the promotion of my climbs far and wide up against the fear that I'd be judged as an attention seeker. I was struggling to articulate my message to the world. Consciously I knew that I couldn't separate myself from what I was doing. I struggled to accept that people's interpretation of this initiative was about them – and not me. Clearly though, the battle was worse than I realised.

Coming off the back of a few weeks of media interviews, my body was sending me a message on how I was handling it all. This challenge was an expression of myself and my desire to push my boundaries while adding value to society. Deep down, my childhood insecurities and fears that tortured me were boiling up as a reminder that they were still there - unresolved.

I didn't know this at the time, but the throat is the gateway that connects the head and heart. Looking back now, I can see that what was being highlighted to me was a release of the fear related to the sharing of my journey and speaking from the heart. I needed to stop allowing my head to censor and redact what my heart wanted to spread. The morning was spent thinking about why I wasn't standing up for my truth and what I needed from myself to make this project a success. It was my focus all day as I admitted my fears out loud, putting them on the table....

I fear being ridiculed

I fear not being supported

I fear being misunderstood

I fear being unsuccessful

This was the first time I'd voiced these fears out loud. I started repeating how I accepted the challenge of 365 Ubuntu Climbs, and with it, the responsibility of communicating what it aims to achieve.

Trying to find some way to soothe my throat, I bought some ice-cream – which apparently is the worst thing for sore throats! I was smart enough to check that, but dumb enough to do it after I'd already started eating it. Anyway, while I ate it, my throat's fire seemed to ease. As I drove to the mountain for a 17:09 start, I felt deflated. For the first time, I felt physically in trouble. No motivational quotes and no amount of positive thinking was going to get me through this.

Take it slow, slow, slow.

I found parking under the trees just past the lower cable station. I must have looked like a dejected child walking home after being bullied at school. Reaching Platteklip Gorge for my gratitude ceremony, the words 'I'm grateful for my healthy body' carried new meaning. How was I going to finish? Would I wake up in pain again tomorrow? I still had 336 days left. I couldn't focus. Please just let me get to the halfway point unscathed. One more step. One more. After a

CHAPTER 5
JANUARY - HELL WEEK

thousand of those and feeling a bit woozy, I collapsed onto halfway rock and forced some water down. I lingered, staring through the view in front of me, I was faced with a big decision.

Knowing Safety Tracking was 'watching over me' gave me comfort and a gentle push to go on. I had support. Still. Thoughts about whether this was all ego kept weaselling their way into my head. During the break, my heart rate quickly dropped. This was the light I used in a very dark cave to keep my motivation in check because I know an elevated heart rate - anything over 80 while resting, is an alarm to take note of. Whether at home, in the car, or resting on the mountain, mine was consistently dropping under 60 and that's good.

Usually on my solo days, I put my head down and listened to some music for a boost. On this climb though, I listened to sessions created by Huni at Focus Gym - my new friend from Iceland and the first investor of 365 Ubuntu Climbs. His 'Walk the Talk' audio sessions were designed to be listened to while walking, there was also another session meant for laying down and relaxing at home - these were powerful tools.

Huni's a purpose alignment coach, and his audio sessions are created to inspire happiness, joy, purpose, and to motivate action needed for better physical and mental health. How incredible that this came to me as my internal battles of 'unworthiness' and doubt manifested physically as a sore throat. His voice reminded me of my true purpose and the inner voice that was guiding me perfectly every time. His words were exactly what I needed and pushed me to start practising more self-love, and acceptance for what I was doing, and for the purpose behind this mission.

How often have I done something for a specific result, only to learn something completely unexpected? More times than I'd like to admit! Perhaps the purpose of this daily climb would bring a completely unexpected consequence for me - maybe a message only comprehensible once I'd fulfilled this 'prophecy'.

I listened to it on repeat. My slow, steady, and measured steps got me to the top in the same amount of time as yesterday's climb, which felt impossible knowing how slowly I'd just climbed. This gave me a jolt of confidence, a much-needed boost. Clearly my body and legs were coping, and my decision to keep going was justified – autopilot must've taken over.

My lack of food though was taking its toll, and I had a dizzy spell at the top. The sunset was gorgeous, but I only enjoyed it from the cable car as I rushed straight to Simply Asia to force some food down. Forget the pain of eating creamed spinach as a child, this was now my most painful meal.

I wasn't defeated, just dejected. It was my fourth night in a row of wishing for relief the next day – any relief! It had been a day of deep reflection, facing my fears and grappling with my inability to handle them head-on. Huni's audios were a blessing. They offered the lifeline I needed to liberate myself from pity.

Retiring early, I couldn't wait to escape the torture – even if only for a few hours.

30th January

I learned the hard way that when something feels extreme in life, EVERYTHING becomes extreme. My thoughts, my relationships, my eating, my recovery, my fatigue, my moods, the weather – all seemed to veer away from the healthy middle ground. This week gave me an early glimpse into what was waiting for me in a year full of climbs and no days off.

'I'm not sure you know what you've gotten yourself into' was a sentence regularly launched my way. Do we ever know what we're getting ourselves into though? This had never been done before, but I was changing that! So far this battle had been gruelling, but I was still standing.

A good night's rest, coupled with day three of being alone on the mountain, meant doing what I needed most – more horizontal couch time. I was clinging to a thin rope as my throat showed a slight improvement. I was no longer

CHAPTER 5
JANUARY - HELL WEEK

swallowing thousands of razor blades, now it was just hundreds. I forced another meal down, but three days of poor eating had already done the damage. My climbs took an extra quarter of an hour. It doesn't sound like much – but with burning legs and lungs begging me to stop, it felt like an hour.

Time on the mountain was becoming a fluid concept, especially when I was on my own and ignoring my phone. Perhaps if I'd made time another yardstick, then things would've been different. It was only when I paused the app at the top that I could gauge the performance. On a day like today? I'd never have guessed it took 2 hours and 16 minutes to summit – It could easily have read three hours. Whether lost in my own thoughts, engaged in intriguing conversations, or fatigued from the endless steps over the course of the day; time seems to have a different meaning on the mountain.

Thankfully this time, there was no dizzy spell, and I was excited to enjoy the sunset. The opportunity to relax and enjoy what I'd missed over the past few days pulled me up the final section, but the weather had other ideas as thick clouds rolled in and wrapped us up. Thank you mist! I empathise with what it must have felt like as a tourist to fly all this way and see nothing but mist. Luckily I'd be gifted with another opportunity again tomorrow, this sadly wasn't the case for the throngs of tourists clambering to snap a semblance of a view through gaps in the passing cloud before it was too late.

Then suddenly it hit me.... Tomorrow's successful climb would bring me the first month's trophy! A worthy milestone, and some much-needed proof to help me acknowledge the progress that had been made. THAT – pumped me up and made coming back in 24 hours an exciting prospect. And how about some extra sprinkles of joy to add to the occasion? Yes please! It was the second full moon of the month – a blue moon to kick the year off with. The last blue moon was in 2015 – July the 2nd and 31st, so this was going to be a treat.

Watching it rise at the top would be the perfect way to celebrate climb 31, and one full month of climbs completed. What a finish to a week from hell!

January the 31st

While overjoyed at waking up with a healthy throat again, nature seemed to take pleasure in throwing my plans out the window. Or maybe it was just teaching me not to place emphasis on outcomes and to embrace the uniqueness of whatever was flowing my way. It could have been worse – my sore throat could've persisted, or I could've had an overcast evening with no view of the second full moon at all. Or even both!

Instead, it was another savage windy day that closed the cable car – had this happened over the last few days, I'm not sure I would've been able to climb down. My climb was an opportunity to reflect on my overall progress and how I'd handled everything that was thrown my way. I was also blessed with a lesson on how to tweak my mindset for coming back the following day simply by seeing how the tourists missed their sunset opportunity. With 334 climbs ahead, I forced myself to feel sad on the third last corner near the top. I felt as though this was the last time I was ever going to see the beauty of the mountain. I let that permeate throughout my body until I reached the top and let out a loud celebratory 'whoop' (now that my throat had healed!) for a successful summit, this immediately made me feel excited about coming back the following day to do it all over again. I did this until it became second nature, and I wasn't even pretending anymore: **I was just excited to come back!**

I practised the same excitement for the down climbs too. It was the perfect opportunity to do so because the wind-swept days provided something I love – solitude, and that meant peace to contemplate. I had the top of the mountain all to my lonesome. 1 in 7.7 billion people on this planet, and I was the only one on top of this majestic rock. In the peace and quiet of the howling wind, I decided to make my way down the path to watch the full moon rise up into the sky. I desperately wanted to watch the full moon rise at the top, and maybe if I didn't have 334 climbs left, I'd stay.

CHAPTER 5
JANUARY – HELL WEEK

It was all about managing the risks while still finding ways to enjoy new experiences in the process – I'd have many more full moons throughout the year to try again and watch it rise from the summit.

It's impossible to convey what a relief it is to feel healthy again – to swallow water with ease, complete bliss. It was my ninth climb back down already for the year, and as the last person off the mountain, it was exhilarating.

It was my first time between the cliffs this late, with the sun moments away from setting. I got to see the softest shadows hugging the mountainside. Sunset was at 19:52, with the full moon due to rise at 19:45. I panicked, I'd gone too far down to see it rise in front of me, so I stopped in my tracks and opened my SkyView App (it shows the stars, moon & sun positions) to gauge where it would make its grand entrance into the now lilac sky. It was just below the horizon, but it was on its way, soon it would pop up in the kink on Devils Peak's outline. Perfect. I sat down quietly in the presence of my teacher and her striking cliffs, waiting patiently for the moon. After everything it took to get to this point, I was filled with a deep sense of accomplishment. One month down – eleven to go.

I sat in marvelled silence as the blue moon peaked above the distant Drakenstein mountains, which were perfectly nestled above Devil Peak's northern spine. The sky was alive with celestial blues, lilacs, pinks, oranges, and yellows – a magnificent canvas for a rare occasion. A blue moon happens every 2.7 years, but *two blue moons* in one year, that last happened in 1999, and the next instalment after this year would be in 2037. I don't remember 1999; but one thing's for sure – I'll never forget this year and the show the moon put on.

With the city lights glittering below, I was beaming as endless gratitude welled up in my heart; for this sight, for my now completely healthy body, for the donations pouring in, and for 365 Ubuntu Climbs being one month old. This had been a huge test, but I knew the real challenges were coming. There'd also be many more beautiful moments like this. And after those? There'd be more challenging days. **Just like life.**

I still had a hurdle to overcome - the delayed project 'launch'! First, it was December, then January – each time, self-doubt stopped me because 'the time wasn't right' and it wasn't 'important' enough. I'd been projecting my own insecurities, saying, 'people would support me when....', and 'when' never arrived. The work I'd done over the past two days in understanding the root cause of my throat infection helped me finally choose a date to host it - Climb 100 on the 10th of April. It would be a celebration of hitting three figures of summiting and an opportunity to share how we'd started using the money raised for DKMS Africa, Habitat for Humanity, and One Heart.

I was learning that no matter what I did in life, obstacles were consistent, and forced me to evaluate how much I really wanted what I was pursuing. It challenged the implementation process and tested my resolve. It gave me the opportunity to feel what the end result would be like and allowed me to use that feeling every day to drive me forward.

I get to put that to practise with 334 days left, searching for, and appreciating each day's uniqueness in pursuit of creating as much joy each day as I would at the end.

January Stats:

3 days 6 hours 19 minutes 27 seconds / 225,89km / 6,03 equivalent Everest Summits / 22 solo

climbs (70,9%) / 9 Up & Down

(29%) TOTAL DONATIONS: R55 393.17

Greg: 'Good luck, Andrew! Therese, Clara, and I enjoyed meeting you on the mountain on Jan 4 and will be cheering you on from Denver!'

Michelle: 'I battle with procrastination. Thank you for the inspiration.'

Stefan & Ally: 'That's R365 from both of us because we know you'll make it to the end. So proud.'

> "In Africa there is a concept known as 'ubuntu' – the profound sense that we are human only through the humanity of others; that if we are to accomplish anything in this world it will in equal measure be due to the work and achievement of others."
>
> — Nelson Mandela

CHAPTER 6
FEBRUARY – BUILDING ON SOLID FOUNDATIONS

Is it possible to climb Platteklip barefoot?

This question popped up on one of my training climbs. I'd just read an article on earthing and the benefits of being barefoot in nature. The article centred around reducing inflammation. As a young boy, I adored running around on the grass barefoot in our garden, and to this day, the feeling is still complete heaven. With a full year ahead on the mountain, my curiosity went beyond just reading the article. A few days later, my question of whether it was possible or not was answered, on my way down, a man, whose name I'd later learn was Jack, climbed past me with no shoes. Every time he machined up and down Platteklip I was in awe. Shirtless, in red shorts, dripping sweat from every exposed part of his body, with his earphones like a drill sergeant blasting music to push him up the mountain. Seeing him today for the first time gave me the permission I needed to add another dynamic to an already difficult task. With a yearlong challenge ahead, I was conscious of preventing risks like ankle injuries - even a simple cut under my foot could fester and become something more without enough rest.

On my next training climb - I'll give it a bash. Admittedly, 'next time' wasn't the smartest decision because it happened to be a cold overcast day, and within ten minutes, my feet felt like two blocks of ice. Although successful, I learned a lesson - to ensure that I always had shoes in my bag , just in case. I decided to do a barefoot climb every month on the 11th day (weather permitting), but when February's second barefoot climb ended, I couldn't stand the thought of waiting for a full month again, so I added the 22nd to the roster. Barefoot climbs brought incredulous looks, shaking heads, and outbursts of shock.

'That's crazy! You're gonna damage your feet!' 'Have you tried it?'

'No'

'Then how do you know?'

Responding to people's outbursts by asking them how they knew if they'd never tried gave me an opportunity to challenge their perceptions. In this case, what they thought, and the reality of the experience were polar opposites. Whether it was people joining the day's climb, or passers-by on the mountain whipping their shoes off - it was equally rewarding to see them enjoy the experience as they shattered a preconceived idea. Barefoot is the way we're intended to experience our home - and it was a way for me to appreciate my new 'university' even more.

I believe this decision was the single biggest reason I never twisted an ankle or suffered any major falls all year.

Why?

Because barefoot, there was no room for error or mind wandering. Simply dragging my right foot and clipping the sharp end of a stone step was enough to snap me out of autopilot to a more mindful state. It was unclear to me then, but these mindful days of practice were exactly what I needed for the windy days and stormy rain-filled climbs looming ahead.

Being barefoot allowed me to connect deeply by feeling every change in texture and temperature. Cooler stones acted like air-conditioning for my body on warm mornings. Undulations and ground textures that my hard shoe sole usually overlooked now became a joyous experience as I felt the contoured shape of the rocks fit underneath me perfectly. One stood out, just before the first waterfall, it was a perfect fit for my toes and forefoot, cradling it as though crafted by a cobbler.

The barefoot days were great opportunities to bring me back down to earth. Not that I felt I was being arrogant with my progress – but if ever I did become complacent, then the barefoot days quickly sparked my awareness to life.

Stay focused, mindful of each step and intentional about the perils or complacency.

One day at a time, step by step, was becoming more than a mantra – it was a perspective I began to take on life.

As you read this now, I'm certain there's something in your life that feels overwhelming. I invite you to put the book down for a minute and to step outdoors with your shoes off. Ideally, if you have some grass, go stand on it and wiggle your toes. Take a few deep breaths.... Now bring this question up into your thoughts... 'What can I do today?'. Dwell on whatever enters your mind while you enjoy the experience of being completely connected to the ground. It may seem like a simple act, insignificant possibly, but just like the barefoot climb taught me mindfulness for the approaching winter storms – this today may impact your future in ways you could never dream of.

Just trust.

There are always unintended consequences to the actions we take in life. I enjoy looking back on what I thought were small decisions, only to see how they blossomed into something grander than I ever could've imagined. It's a powerful point as I try to focus my attention on increasing the momentum created from January's publicity. Even though solo climbs allowed me to establish a powerful base – the point was to get others involved.

I started by dismissing thoughts of what I didn't want to happen and focussed on what I wanted instead. I'm idealistic, so I visualised twenty people joining per day – the sweet spot to retain intimacy with everyone. This calculation forced me to create a 'me day' that would ensure I had the chance to recharge.

I'm an introvert at heart, I love it and need alone time to recharge, but having climbs with larger groups taught me more about being an extrovert. Then my analytical corporate brain began running through the sums:

20 people x R365 = R 7,300 per day,

6 days a week = R43,800 which = R189,899 a month That's R2,277 million for the entire year!

This may have been a bit optimistic. It sounds amazing, but completely impractical. Hindsight allowed me to say with certainty that I would've burned out before the first winter storm battered the mountain. Besides it being a gross exaggeration of my ability to manage 5,760 people; giving myself 52 climbs to recharge? I was being delusional.

I chose Mondays as my 'Me day'. Why? Great question! I envisioned weekends to be busier by default, which made it the perfect day to decompress. Also, Monday being the start of the week made it so much more special. Besides my birthday falling on a Monday, it was the day of the week I started this journey, the halfway mark fell on that day, and the last climb would fall on that day too.

Oh, and in case Mondays didn't have enough going on – I was born on a Monday!

Because I enjoyed being alone, the thought of no one joining all year didn't scare me off. January's quiet start gave me the freedom to focus on myself and develop a natural rhythm. I was grateful for those 21 solo days at the start, they provided a solid base to build my individuality which helped me cultivate an identity for 365 Ubuntu Climbs. January was a 'me' month, but that quickly changed, and February became the 'we' month. Ubuntu was about collaboration, and all the relationships I'd nurtured till now began to bloom. I focussed on networking to get as many individuals as possible to participate, rather than having the big organisations do the heavy lifting. I believed in the power of individuality and connecting with others to create powerful forces of change.

Future Females is an organisation that embodies this way of thinking, and it's visible in their communication with the world. Future Females: *We're a movement aimed at inspiring female entrepreneurs, and we're committed to supporting their success. We provide a platform digitally, physically, and emotionally where women can connect, inspire, and collaborate with each other, and access the resources they need to succeed.*

I started this partnership back in December and became a guest writer after attending my first event. I'd written on topics like Goal Setting, Balance & Self Care and Breaking through Self-Doubt. Lianne, my friend who introduced us and who is also their mentor, shared the progress of my project from the beginning. I explained my purpose and extended an invitation to organise a 'Future Females' climb. Wasting no time, they settled on building a group for Friday, the 9th of February. This would become the 15th day climbing in the company of others and just the third group. What a gift! It was shared with their community which is already over 5,000 strong!

Climbs like these offered people an opportunity to grasp the enormity of the task at hand and helped develop a deeper understanding of the solutions each charity was implementing. Lauren & Cerina (founders) continued to do an amazing job building a purpose-driven global organisation which was now in over twenty cities around the world. That vision extended to 365 Ubuntu Climbs.

There's an aspect of supporting others that often gets overlooked and that's the 'simple' act of sharing the idea or plans with others in your community – you never know how a spark lands and what positive knock-on effect that may have down the line. Here's a perfect example of that; it's through them that I met Raghmah Solomon – one of the seven monthly donors who would give from the heart throughout the year. Another was my friend Astrid whose actions earned her the accolade of being one of the top generators of donations. She continuously shared my project with her network in the property industry, and even invited me to speak at an event scheduled on the 28th of February. She also introduced me to Joshua and Susan Crook – another pair of amazing human beings who became champions of 365 Ubuntu Climbs. When I needed it most, my network of incredible friends rose to the occasion.

Then there's Harry and Dani, who'd built a community around their love of music. They put on private festivals for small groups to ensure an intimate family atmosphere was maintained. No surprise at all that my connection with them was thanks to Lisa. Quality begets quality. Harry and Dani's events taught me a great lesson; those who were responsible for creating an initiative set the standard for how it operated and for the people it attracted. They organised a climb through their 2,000-member strong Facebook group. They also used their October event for financial support, and donated R20 of every ticket sold, which quickly added up to R8 000!! It was incredible how quickly micro-donations like R20 stacked up into something significant when everyone contributed. Through this network, I met amazing friends like Avril and Craig. Avril joined multiple climbs, she also arranged a team building for her company to climb, and fantastically donated R10,000 in the process! Climbing with them on a muggy overcast day was a wonderful experience and really made me feel part of their team building. It brought with it so many fun moments, like watching them excitedly survey the city below to find and point out their office building to me.

CHAPTER 6
EBRUARY - BUILDING ON SOLID FOUNDATIONS

What a change February was, being joined by groups, bigger and bigger – this was the month of 'We'. It showed me that while things may appear 'quiet' – you never know what's happening in the 'background' that's contributing to the success of a project. It was humbling being on the receiving end. It felt like a supportive hand on my shoulder, acknowledging my mind's question of 'would this be supported' with a reassuring smile to say 'yes'.

Craig's climb with the Summer Camp group was particularly powerful. After four solo days on the mountain, I met with Craig, Colleen, Harry, Dani, and their young son Dylan early on a blustery Sunday morning. Now 56 days in and wiser, I knew the wind offered little hope for a cable car ride back down. This day stood out for a few reasons; being the 56th climb of the year meant I had 309 more to go. My birthday climb was going to be my 309th climb (which coincided with my 39th birthday – some serious universal alignment right there!) with only 56 days remaining. It conjured up ideas of how that day would feel compared to these 56 days. One difference that instantly raised its hand was how my legs would feel, and how loud they'd be screaming.

Craig's explanation of just being there and what he'd experienced gave me an instant boost. As an independent tour guide, his tours took him all over South Africa. He was one of the first to jump on board the minute Dani announced the date for the climb. It was tight, he was also booked for a two-week tour with a two-hour flight to KwaZulu Natal. His flight was the night before our climb, and it was delayed, he only arrived home after midnight. With a 7 am start to our climb – this was the kind of dedication that inspired me!

I lost count of the times people pledged to join and bailed at the last minute. Legitimate reasons aside, hearing people enthusiastically preach their excitement the night before, only to cancel the next morning was bizarre and disheartening. Even more baffling, though was hearing... *'I really want to support you and do a climb with you'*, only to hear nothing from them again. If they'd said nothing – there'd be zero expectation in my head.

Craig was a breath of fresh air and one of the few who genuinely went through extremes, he had a legitimate excuse, a solid reason to fold that no one could have questioned – yet instead, he told himself, *'If Andrew can get up every day and climb this mountain, I can get up today and join him!'*. Ironically, it's support like this that lives with me every time my legs are taking strain and my body's exhausted. *Remember Craig and his commitment.* Craig was among family and friends like Astrid, who consistently sent messages on windy days, checking in, and encouraging me before I headed out. Each message, a top-up of fuel.

For his birthday coming up that October, Craig planned a combined 90th party with his friend. Both requested donations to 365 Ubuntu Climbs instead of presents. There's a lot of negativity in the world, but actions like this reminded me that by focusing on what I can do instead of complaining about problems, I could attract more beauty into my life. Just like this…. I chose Ubuntu.

I was surrounded by incredible human beings who were willing to get out of bed early on their weekends to climb a mountain and empower others in the process. Again, it held up a mirror and shone a spotlight on how I'd shown up for my friends and family. I was also learning that it's better to ask questions about what they need versus assuming and going straight into solution mode. I'd spent a large portion of my life trying to please everyone – and that's impossible. I know I've let many people down in the past, but I don't look at it through the 'good or bad' lens anymore – but rather with gratitude for the lessons I've gained, and a deeper understanding of the reasons people are in our lives. It's not bad, not good – it just is. I could easily get frustrated by what I felt was a 'lack of support', or I could choose to focus on how inspired I felt by the amazing ways that people were supporting me. From New Zealand to Miami to Stuttgart – I felt very blessed. One of the greatest gifts we can give anyone is to let them know we're there for them in their darkest hour. Not as saviours, but as stewards to sit with them in their difficulty and shine a spotlight on the road back to possibility. There'll certainly come a time when we ourselves need it.

CHAPTER 6
EBRUARY - BUILDING ON SOLID FOUNDATIONS

On the 19th, my first significant milestone arrived; it was my 50th consecutive summit. Part of the excitement for my 'betrothal' to Table Mountain was to use milestones as an opportunity to do different routes, like a reward. Most of the routes up the mountain are longer and more technically challenging than Platteklip. Nothing requires ropes, but your upper body strength will be called on to handle sections of scrambling and to pull your full body weight up - you're also going to need a stomach for hanging onto cliff faces. Today, I chose India Venster, a route snaking its way underneath the cable car before traversing the cliffs above Camps Bay. It then brings you around the back side of the mountain and connects you to the top of Platteklip. Being more exposed, the majestic views of the city and Lions Head to the west can easily become a distraction.

It was an absolute peach of a day; I chose an afternoon climb since I'd be on my own. About an hour up, I reached the most direct section that ended up on a beautiful outlook spot. To make it safer, the National Park inserted giant staples into the rock face giving you something to hold on to with your hands and use as steps for your feet. Above this section is one of my favourite views in Cape Town - a sweeping 270-degree vista. My eyes start with the 12 Apostles above Llandudno before reaching Camps Bay. Lions Head, with Clifton's beaches below, grab my attention next and then cascades down into Signal Hill with Robben Island floating distantly in the Atlantic. That gives way to the Waterfront, the city, and the harbour with Milnerton and the rest of the coastline snaking its way north. Lastly, Devils Peak completes the amphitheatre with the Cape Fold Mountains taking guard on the horizon behind it. On clear days like this, the Hottentots Mountains behind Devils Peak are alive in the afternoon light, Simonsberg Mountain prominently sitting alone, rising high above the vineyards of Stellenbosch below. Paarl Rock and Drakenstein Mountains offer contrasting formations to admire, the former being a smaller rounded dome of exposed rock, while the latter sits majestically on guard with its towering cliffs reaching 1,590m above sea level.

It's an unusual feeling to be so close to the city and yet so high, especially with the harbour and beaches below. 1,085m (3,559 ft) above sea level is the highest point on the mountain, with the upper cable station perched on what feels like a 30-storey cliff at 1,072m (3,517 ft) above me.

I never get tired of this view, but my 49 days up Platteklip provide added appreciation.

Reflecting on the first 50 days, I was grateful with how well my fitness and legs were holding up. As soon as I reached climb ten, I entered unchartered territory, which at 40 climbs ago, already felt like a distant memory. Ha - my year and my language have already shifted into climbs and not days! I've already experienced dramatic changes from day to day. Today I had a glorious view, while yesterday started perfectly, only for a bank of clouds to swallow the summit in thick mist.

My poor guests. Thankfully, by snapping pictures every day, I was able to erase the gloomy summit with previous pictures. This provided an incentive for overseas climbers to come back and gave locals a sense of gratitude and encouragement to do it again to experience the mountain in a completely different way.

The scorching heat of the day made Cape Town's water crisis our primary focus. Day zero was lurking too close for comfort. At this rate, Cape Town was scheduled to run dry by April. We needed the approaching winter to bring miracles, rain, and relief. I couldn't imagine the added complexity of standing in endless queues just to get water to drink and to bathe in. I was praying for rain. The alternative was something I didn't want to think about or give too much energy to. Shops were already selling out of bottled water as many stockpiled 5L drums in anticipation of bone-dry taps. It was headline news around the world as we looked to become the first major city to reach a water-related crisis point like this. Some good news was that our collective efforts to conserve water meant we became the first in the world (ever) to get the daily average per person per day down to 70L - half of what was previously achieved in places like Brazil and Australia.

All I could do was my own part in reducing water consumption to using less than 50L per day and becoming an expert at showering in under 2 minutes. 50L was the equivalent of; a load of laundry (10L), a shower (10L), 1 toilet flush (9L), brushing teeth (2L), water for pets (1L), washing the dishes (9L), drinking (3L), cooking (1L), and cleaning (5L). At the very least, our statistical average of 101 days with at least 0.1mm of rain would be a blessing. That would make almost a third of my climbs in rain while bringing with it a host of other challenges. I was pumped in anticipation of Table Mountain's cascading waterfalls after torrential downpours. While we all prayed for rain – it wasn't a blessing for everyone. For those living in the shacks on the Cape Flats, a heavy wet winter was an additional element of challenge to an already consistent nightmare.

If February became the month to understand collaboration, no day highlighted this more perfectly than Thursday the 22nd, the day after my third barefoot climb. I joined Habitat for Humanity on their latest build and finally got my chance to experience what was first set in motion for me just over four years prior when Nelson Mandela died. I must be honest; it was a weird experience to be doing something so challenging yet smile the entire time. Knowing the pain was temporary, I arrived each morning feeling ready for the test.

Having started at 06:25, I was back at my car just before 08:30, which was more than enough time to make it to Habitat's offices in Pinelands for 9 am. I'd only met one of their team members, so I was excited for the morning ahead. Idling my car, waiting for Lyndall to pop downstairs, I jumped as she came out of nowhere, knocking on my window. It took her a couple of minutes before she stopped herself....... *'Oh my word, I'm so rude! Just because we've been chatting online, I'm acting as if we've known each other for ages! I'm Lyndall'* Considering her profile picture on WhatsApp was of kids, I wasn't 100% sure this was her.

The Habitat staff piled into Lyn's car, and then we zoomed off to Wallace Dene, an informal settlement half an hour away. It wasn't my first time in the area, I'd been here before, I remember the shacks and the many ingeniously built shelters that had been made with whatever spare materials were available. I did audits on some of the stores here, and no matter what time or day of the week it was, the scale of unemployment and poverty was overwhelmingly visible. After countless visits, I finally asked myself: *'Do I believe I'm strong enough to work my way out of here??'* I'd like to think so, but I'm not so sure.

Turning into the last street, the Habitat for Humanity gazebo came into sight, it really stood out like a beacon of hope. The American company co-sponsoring the build was already there working away in the blazing sun. Our African sun is relentless, and I'm always sympathetic to international people who are met with the brutal heat even before they've started working! At 10 am, the sweat was already dripping from their brows and damp patches appeared all over their shirts.

After going around the half circle and meeting everyone, I was faced in the opposite direction, and there in the distance sat Table Mountain, quietly watching over us. It's a bit unsettling to be here, but that feeling was quickly erased when I was introduced to Masande. The warmest smile radiated in my direction as we shook hands. Almost twenty, she had already seen more challenges than most of us would in a lifetime. Her quiet disposition was cloaked by the type of strength and humility we can only strive for. She lived with her mom and two siblings – her father unfortunately died in a shack fire five years prior.

The walls of the house being built were much higher than that of the tin shack they currently shared. The shack was barely bigger than the room I sat in while writing this book. Twelve square metres (130 square feet) or roughly the size of a standard bedroom, but with no windows! That's right, no windows. I tried to understand why there weren't any. The answer is heartbreaking. Windows are access points for thieves and gangs that roam the streets at night, so it's a luxury not suited for the area.

As Masande led me into her shack, I was hit by a wall of heat more intense than a sauna. Her room is made entirely of corrugated iron sheets with no insulation and zero ventilation – it's a torture chamber – not a house. Then in winter, she has to contend with another form of hell, with temperatures dropping to 5 degrees Celsius (41 Fahrenheit), it's almost impossible to keep warm. There's the torrential rain and the bone-chilling wind that cuts through every unsealed metal-to-metal corner, leaving one exposed to the biting cold. Masande shared that without proper insulation, the first family member home in winter would start scooping water out of the shack. Just as my brain couldn't comprehend climbing in storms, so too am I unable to fathom the layer of hardship and misery storms bring to townships.

It's one thing to drive past the shacks and acknowledge at a conscious level the difficulty of the living conditions – it's an entirely different thing hearing and seeing first-hand what day-to-day life is really like there.

Masande's candid about not being in university; she failed Mathematics at school and is redoing it. Her eyes lit up in excitement as she shared her plans for when she passes, she's going to study Entrepreneurship at university. At the time we visited, her younger siblings were at school, and her mom was at work. I hope to meet her mom. Raising three children by yourself in a room that barely fits a double bed under these conditions AND producing a young woman filled with this level of gratitude is inspiring. I learned that Masande had no knowledge of the water crisis, she had no idea what it meant because she'd been living in a water-scarce environment for decades. With no toilet or running water, she was forced to walk to a central point that had rows of plastic portable toilets, usually full too, and she had to collect water in buckets from communal taps for washing, cooking, and cleaning. That's kilometres of walking just to relieve yourself and collect water. This was only during the day because any female walking at night ran the risk of being attacked and raped. I'm not saying I condone burning tyres on freeways in protest of the living conditions – but I now understand why it happens. I bet I'd be doing the same. In essence, the water crisis was showing us how most people already live, albeit without the inconvenience of living without our own bathroom.

I was getting a picture of what the new house would give to a family that's already endured so much. I couldn't imagine living a year without a bathroom – never mind twenty. It was still two months before the house would be finished and ready to move into, but there was a flicker of hope inside their hearts that burned a little stronger as the days progressed towards 'that special day'– and just in the nick of time before winter too.

I was indebted to my colleague for telling me about Habitat for Humanity 5 years ago. The drive out was a sobering reminder that for every success story like this, there are a million more to help. Today cemented my belief in the critical nature of this work, it also made me realise how important it was for it to continue, even after the climbing had been done. I had an entirely new perspective on the word 'room', and what a difference one room, or a bathroom could make in the lives of a family. Meeting Masande and all the staff was like rolling back the clock to day zero for my legs. Seeing the resilience they had moved me. I didn't think my motivation could be dialled up any further. I was wrong.

As February ended, March shaped up to be a busy month. My friend Dexter introduced me to his company DigiOutsource and took the initiative to get them involved. They decided to sponsor their staff and incentivised them to climb with me for an entire month. Another beautiful example of things that happened in the background I didn't know would bear fruit. With large groups a certainty for March, my final day in February became the practice I needed.

I met Sieglende in 2017 while attending a *Sustainable Development Networks* course called *Marketing of Your Services*. She organised a group of 10, and Lisa joined, too, making it her 6th summit. Siegie chose the 28th of February for her climb because it was known as 'Rare Disease Day'. Her organisation supports the fight against a disease called 'Congenital Melanocytic Naevus' or just Naevus – a rare skin condition that affects 1 in 500,000 newborn babies. The low rate of babies affected also meant that less funds were available for research into the condition. Her son had it, and she worked tirelessly to raise awareness, so people would treat him with empathy instead of staring.

Climbing with Siegie's group highlighted what a phenomenal bunch of people they were, they shared their stories of living around the world and how each came to be in Cape Town. Originally from Germany, she'd lived in both India and New York. I loved these opportunities to talk openly about other cultures, it gave me a chance to learn about their different experiences and ultimately helped me become more compassionate through understanding.

And just like that – February was over. A month to remind me that what I sow now, will be reaped later.

2 down – 10 to go.

February Stats:

59 / 365

People Joined: 51 / 68

6 days 00 hours 19 minutes 39 seconds / 395,76km / 11,48 equivalent Everest Summits / 37

solo climbs (62,7%) / 12 Up & Down (20,3%) TOTAL DONATIONS: R99 363.35

Richard: 'iTrack Live is proud to support Andrew in his mission to empower 1 million South Africans.'

Avril: 'SABIC is honoured to be part of this journey to ensure a sustainable future for generations to come. We challenge all corporates to equal or better.'

Sasha: 'I absolutely cannot wait to do the hike this upcoming Friday with you and the Future Females Team :D'

The cure for boredom is curiosity. There's no cure for curiosity.
~~ Dorothy Parker

CHAPTER 7

MARCH – DON'T YOU GET BORED?

It's easy to assume that going back to the same place every day to do the same thing would be boring. I'm sure many people felt that way, yet my excitement continued to grow day in and day out. It sounds crazy – but I couldn't wait to tackle each day's climb now that the number of successful summits was rising beyond the 50 mark. It took me back to my cricketing days when I wanted to finish an innings with an asterisk (*) behind my score – which meant I wasn't out. Starting each month with the 'completed climbs' bucket filling up and getting heavier wasn't just psychologically relieving – it was emotionally invigorating too, and although I was doing the same thing every day – I certainly wasn't experiencing the same thing. I was about to see that more clearly than ever.

March exploded into action with one of my favourite experiences of the year. When I was up at Zebula for Christmas, my sister and family confirmed their climb. Our lengthy discussions in December surrounded the water crisis and had us wondering whether we should delay the climb until after winter. I loved that they were taking our crisis into consideration, but tourism accounted for just 1% of Cape Town's water consumption, so delaying a climb for that reason was admirable, but unnecessary. They settled on climbing between my niece's birthdays – Saturday, March 3rd, which would be climb 62.

While they took an early flight down on Kristin's 13th birthday, I started just after sunrise. It was a crisp, warm early morning climb with Stephanie, who had come down from Johannesburg, as well as Ruta – for whom this was her second climb. I was as excited as if the following day was going to be the final climb, and I was bouncing off the rocks with the energy I had just before my first climb In January.

The weekend was jam-packed, I had a group of eight international business tycoons joining the Sunday climb after their conference in Johannesburg, and I had a Skype call into Stuttgart for a fundraiser being held by my dear friend Wes to raise funds for us. What a gift it was to be able to give Krissy and Katie birthday hugs. Having left Johannesburg fifteen years ago, those moments carried significant meaning, especially since we were living 1,400 km apart. We met at the Waterfront and had some light-hearted fun as I 'handed out jerseys' in a pre-climb ceremony. We chose to do it in front of a giant yellow frame, one of seven around the city that highlighted the different views of Table Mountain. The frames were regular attractions for locals and internationals alike, all wanting to land the perfect selfie with the iconic mountain smiling in the background. Each of the shirts I handed out (for me too) had the date and the climb number: 3rd March 2018 – 62 / 365.

It was another first for me: a climb with everyone sporting a 365 Ubuntu Shirt and cap. Achmat was first to spot the girls in their tops on our way up. Right on cue, the south easter hammered through after lunch, much to my sisters' dismay. She was already nervous about climbing, so the thought of a down climb added an additional element of stress to her shoulders. My good friend Windguru helped me calm those nerves – it showed green bars in the morning, which was perfect for a cable car ride, this however was still a contrast to the current windy reality.

Then, to my surprise, I was presented with the most amazing gift all the way from New Zealand, courtesy of Melanie and Kym, who were family friends and huge cheerleaders of my journey. It was a Pounamu toki Maori greenstone necklace – a symbol of strength and courage. Its tradition states that no one can buy it for themselves, it's bought strictly with the intent of being a gift for another. I read this all in her handwritten letter (I don't even remember the last time that happened) that shared the significance of the gift as well as its purpose for protection. It would become part of my daily ritual, as I prepared my mind for the climb, I placed the greenstone necklace over my head, allowing it to rest over my heart. It will become infused with purpose and deep gratitude over the next 303 climbs. Today I still wear it as a reminder of Ubuntu and of the commitment I developed to help others express their own strength. I am deeply grateful to Melanie for her heart-warming gesture, it meant more to me than she could ever know.

While the Brown family were at their friends in Tamboerskloof, they were welcomed by the first of March's two full moons. From the balcony, they enjoyed a thoroughly imposing view of Table Mountain, but they were also exposed and at the mercy of the wind. The stories of what the wind threw around the balcony didn't help my sister's nerves which I'm sure disrupted her sleep a little later – I hope that wasn't the case. After a fabulous evening, we bid farewell and as I closed my eyes, my excitement spilled into my dreams. Luckily, I eventually switched off and got some rest for another 5:30 am start the following day.

It was a crisp morning, a gentle reminder that autumn was creeping up on me with winter's ominous figure hiding in the shadows. No doubt, our parents were glued to their phones, watching our progress on Endomondo and waiting for pictures on our Family WhatsApp group chat as we progressed. I asked them to choose a rock along the route for me to greet every day – today, we'll add four new ones. They'd also be the first family members to pick a stone, and just as I did each day, they'd be able to place it on Ubuntu Rock to commemorate their climb. Our earlier start allowed us to experience a truly majestic sight - the full moon setting over the Atlantic Ocean, creating a magical silver trail in its wake. The other benefit of an early climb was the chance to beat the heat and crowds. My sister was understandably apprehensive. Table Mountain is an imposing sight, especially if you're standing on the road, straining your neck, and looking up at the summit. She disregarded the fact that her body shut down during exercise whenever her heart rate became elevated. This was due to adrenal fatigue and an underactive thyroid.

Walking along the road, we passed the lower cableway station and I pointed out a group of seven trees perfectly lined up that I felt represented my family – one sat higher up overlooking the others, so this was my Gran (aged 93), then about 6 feet down on the road they lined up: Dad, Mom, Terence, Caroline, Krissy, and Katie. Behind them were three tree stumps – representing my three grandparents, who are sadly no longer with us.

I was overjoyed at having my family with me as we made our way along the road for the twenty-minute warmup. Nervous smiles greeted me as I turned around at the base of Platteklip....

"We're here," I said, smiling.

I removed my cap, shared my gratitude ritual, and added what this climb meant to me – I had a supportive family who flew down to become part of this challenge, and now they owned climb number 62.

Just before setting off, I told everyone... *'This isn't a race to get up, if you need a break or water, we stop'*. I preferred calling them beauty breaks as opposed to being tired and catching my breath breaks. *'I like that,'* my sister said. As we moved along, I purposefully slowed my pace, constantly checking that I hadn't lost anybody. Terence brought up the rear making sure no one dropped off pace, and within five minutes our cheeks were red, and our breathing began to get heavier. I enjoyed sharing how the old route up until the 60s used to follow the river below to our right until increased usage and human erosion forced them to build the path we were on. We had a little breather at the first waterfall, where I showed them Dad's rock and 'that branch', which was a reminder of the windiest day I'd experienced on the mountain. The next section had a sharp incline connecting it to the contour path, so we took our first water break under a set of trees. Katie pointed next to the rock my sister was sitting on and said......

'That's my rock please'

'You sure? We still have a long way to go'

'I'm sure!'

Family rock number three was locked and loaded in the memory bank. We were rapidly leaving the road below us and passed the contour path near my mom's rock. Krissy chose hers next, and although she couldn't see it now; in winter, this spot had a beautiful waterfall that flowed over a mini cliff before hitching a ride onto the path and diving down the side of the mountain through the thick fynbos. Her rock was vastly different from the surrounding ones and easier to remember, it looked a little bit like a fossil rock with thousands of lines twisting in unison around the weathered holes. It was beautiful. The next corner was steep, with roughly three flights of stairs. They had large uneven gaps between each step, but after a serious burst of effort, it became the perfect place to rest. It was also one of my 'go to' places for water breaks, with one of the last vantage points of the city before the ridge hiding Platteklip blocked the view. We were able to appreciate how high we'd climbed, while also being closer to the sheer cliff faces above us.

First quarter: check!

Caroline declared the rock she was sitting on to be hers, while Terence pointed to an outcrop located above Krissy's rock and chose the rock to be his. It was one of those that would make an epic picture, legs dangling over the side. This meant that before I even reached halfway on future climbs, I'd see each one's rock and feel their presence. This thought made me happy because it was my way of bridging the great distance between us and bringing them closer to me in spirit. No matter what the weather did in the future, their rocks would

CHAPTER 7
MARCH – DON'T YOU GET BORED?

be a constant feature to remind me of their amazing effort and their attitude towards the climb we shared.

Devil's Peak no longer sheltered us from the sun, and the change in temperature was instant. There was hardly any wind, which was unfortunate because even the tiniest breeze usually helped ease the heat radiating off the rocks.

When I climbed alone and passed others, it was easy to feel grateful for my fitness without understanding what others were going through. Today was an education in perspective. Every step increased my pride for my sister. She was stretching her capabilities and her struggle was because of her love and support for me. Once we got past the halfway mark, the gorge got narrower keeping some sections of the zig zagging in the shade. The second half was where her pure grit and human spirit took over. For the bulk of it, she fought dizziness and nausea – two things no one wants to feel ever, especially if you're on the mountain. We took it one switchback at a time with each corner a chance to stay hydrated, refuel, and enjoy a perfect moment observing the breathtaking view behind us. It was completely different compared to seeing it from the top. The tunnel vision created by the cliffs on either side was like nothing I'd ever experienced anywhere on my travels. Each step revealed what the mountain was made of, and how the vegetation flourished in such a majestic yet hostile environment. There were endless examples of how nature defied the odds as gorgeous flowers grew out of cracks in the rock face. Usually, when I'm so focused on pushing to reach the top, I miss out on all the finer details, all the little nooks and crannies. This was an opportunity to study the building blocks that make up one of the world's most iconic mountains and it certainly wasn't lost on me. I made sure I pointed this fact out to my sister as she apologised for 'holding' us up.

'Is there somewhere I'm supposed to be? Are we in a rush?' I asked.

I continued, 'There's nothing to apologise for. I'm so proud of you! Just think of the bubbles waiting for us to celebrate.'

She eked a smile out before delivering the burning question, 'so, how much further?' I'd learned a valuable lesson; that was to calculate how much more we had left to go by knowing how long we'd taken to get to this point. I constantly heard climbers offering advice on 'how much time was left' without taking vital factors into consideration – like how long someone took to get there in the first place. It's soul crushing to believe that you're 'just a couple minutes away' only for the climb to carry on for so much longer.

It's a powerful lesson on empathy and learning to understand someone's needs, perspective, and capability before just giving advice from our own point of view.

Just before Ubuntu Rock, she sat down and melted into a massive flat boulder which the family joined her on. It became the 'Brown family rock'. It'd been a herculean effort by Caroline, one that demanded every ounce of her determination. I pointed out her empty hands – she was yet to pick her stone, then she discovered possibly the biggest loose rock on the mountain.

'I want the biggest MF rock for this effort!'

I politely replied, 'if you can pick it up, I'll carry it!'

That got her laugh going again. Eventually, I picked up the stone's more reasonably sized neighbour – still sizeable though, slightly bigger than a handbag. It became the centrepiece for all the family stones throughout the year. Thankfully, we found ourselves in the shade for the last 360 steps. Mom and dad watched on Endomondo and wildly cheered us on, knowing what an effort this was. It made all the difference hearing, *'You're doing so well, I am so impressed'*. I was seeing and feeling my sister's love and support firsthand, and I'd never been more proud and grateful that she was one of six people who'd known me my whole life. She taught me another important lesson:

The value of a result shouldn't simply be measured by the output – but by the effort generated to produce that result.

CHAPTER 7
MARCH – DON'T YOU GET BORED?

In future, if I overtake someone while climbing, I'll ask myself if it's their first time, perhaps they just beat cancer, and this is a celebration of life for them. Maybe it's a desire to start a healthier way of living. It doesn't matter – I'll make sure to always congratulate and encourage them. Being on the mountain is the real joy and celebration. I incorporated this message into future group climbs, it was important they knew it wasn't about how fast we did it – but that we did it together. This was Ubuntu's second lesson.

I was reminded of Teddy Roosevelt's quote, which helped me deal with negative people and reinforced my gratitude towards those joining:

"It's not the critic who counts; not the man who points out how the strong man stumbles, or where the doer of deeds could've done them better. The credit belongs to the man who's actually in the arena, whose face is marred by dust and sweat and blood; who strives valiantly; who errs, who comes short again and again, because there's no effort without error and shortcoming; but who does actually strive to do the deeds; who knows great enthusiasms, the great devotions; who spends himself in a worthy cause; who at the best knows in the end the triumph of high achievement, and who at the worst, if he fails, at least fails while daring greatly, so that his place shall never be with those cold and timid souls who neither know victory nor defeat."

Climbing with my sister further cemented the appreciation I had for her grit and tenacity. I'll always treasure Summit 62 as one of the moments I'm proudest to be her brother. Don't just take it from me though – here's what she said about her experience:

'When Andrew first told us that he would climb Table Mountain every day in 2018 – I instantly knew we'd join him at least once in the year. It would be one of the toughest challenges for me because of my battle with thyroid and adrenal fatigue, which also means I'm not exercising and I'm very unfit. The 3rd of March stands out for me as a highlight in my life.

At the base of Table Mountain, I really had no idea what a huge challenge climbing Table Mountain would be. It became more of a mental challenge, as my body shut down about halfway up the climb and I started working out how a helicopter could land to take me off the tortuous mountain. But I realised that couldn't happen and I would have to dig deep and put on my big girl panties. Andrew and my family were incredibly patient - we had to sit and have a break after each turn for my heart rate to calm down.

When we FINALLY reached the top - I felt completely overwhelmed with JOY and admiration for Andrew who'd be climbing every day through the rain, wind, and heat, for the remainder of the year. I am so grateful we were able to experience being part of Andrew's challenge for the year!!!'

Lunch in Hout Bay at Dunes provided Caroline with the most well-deserved GnT of all time after her 4 hours and 26 minutes of pure unadulterated grit and determination. She expanded my understanding of what it means to use the word 'ubuntu'. Creating a platform that invites climbers to push their limits in a way that sets examples for others, means holding space for them to explore that. It also means not getting upset about having to take longer than I usually do. While on the mountain I often play the role of host, a good host makes people feel welcome enough to join again and makes them feel comfortable that this is their 'home' too. This immediately stood out as a contrast for my following day's group, who were all driven, motivated, and successful individuals in the country for an event that took place in Johannesburg a week prior. It was through this event's organiser that I met them. Cape Town, understandably was a stop on their trip. They were all thrilled and excited to be part of the journey I was on and to climb for such a special cause, and I was happy to host them. Sadly, only Erik and Robin contributed, tarnishing my joy as the rest failed to live up to their donation promises. Being from Europe, that was especially disappointing because €10 was R180. Sadly, this wouldn't be the last of the empty promises I'd encounter. We've got to take the rough with the smooth, I guess. It was a lesson for me to release any fixation on my own desires and replace it with gratitude that I'm able to plant seeds in the minds of others.

CHAPTER 7
MARCH - DON'T YOU GET BORED?

I was on a rollercoaster of emotions, and my disappointment quickly faded thanks to Wes, who was now living in Germany. He'd organised a fundraiser with a buffet lunch at the hotel he managed. They had a full-on family day planned and we were hoping to dial me in via Skype. Alas, technical difficulties prevented us from achieving this - a huge pity, I really hoped to thank everyone in person for their support from so far away. Wes's efforts were immense, he tapped into his South African network and messaged as many celebrities and influential people as possible to get behind the project. To see such dedication for something I was doing energised my body even as fatigue began to set in.

I met the Brown family for a special afternoon to celebrate Katie's birthday on a cruise in the bay which allowed us to enjoy the majesty of Table Mountain from the water. Everyone appreciated the effort they put into the previous day's climb, now they really began to understand my words 'you'll never look at the mountain the same way again'. They were treated to a show as the beloved tablecloth 'flew' over the front face of the mountain. It would be our last chunk of time together until their return in December. It was the perfect way to end week 9. I treasured these three days with them, and now I'd get to feel that every time I passed their rocks and stones on the way up the mountain. With all the gifts I got, it felt more like my birthday. And with our time coming to an end, it was hard to say goodbye, but years of practice had made it easier - it's never goodbye, but.... *'Until I see you again.'*

Wednesday arrived, and the emotional rollercoaster continued. The morning's climb with Lisa brought me a warning: a cold arctic-like wind blasted us at the top, it was by far the coldest this year and only day 66! I desperately tried to hide my chin under my jacket as we climbed back down (my 15th of the year) and sensed we were in for a bitterly cold and wet winter. That was truly my wish. Today's climb meant that I'd completed 66 summits which was a massive psychological win as I now had less than 300 to go. I had an appointment to see my friend Kim Worral after the day's climb. She ran an organisation called *Amoyo Performing Arts Foundation*. It created opportunities for children with no access to after-school activities, to be included and to become part of a group learning self-discipline initiative. Their philosophy is one of gratitude. *Amoyo means "spirit of appreciation" (appreciating everything and everyone).* It's a unique approach to upskilling and empowering the children of Hout Bay that's already having a huge impact; not only on the children but on their families and the broader community, too. Kim invited me to watch their final dress rehearsal. Watching the children sing and dance up close was an immensely powerful experience as they tackled topics such as unemployment and laziness. The stories were all written by the kids themselves.

Before they started, Kim told them about what I was doing. I wish I'd recorded the priceless looks on each of their faces as their jaws hit the floor. The shocked expressions they wore was one I was getting increasingly used to as the climbs stacked up behind my name. Unexpectedly, she asked if I could share why I was doing it, as well as who I was supporting. She caught me off guard, and perhaps a little unnervingly so, as they were the very people the vision aimed to support. I sat back down, and she calmly asked, *'I think we can donate R2 to Andrew and his causes, yes? And we'll organise a climb up with him too.'*

A unanimous 'yeeeeeeeeeeeeeeeess' erupted, complete with nodding heads. Their show was on the coming Saturday at the Baxter Theatre, and I wished them all the best. After what I'd just witnessed, I had no doubt the judges and audience would be as moved as I was. I walked away uplifted by another experience that left me feeling energised, buoyant, and even more inspired about South Africa's potential. I didn't think I could feel any better, boy was I wrong about that!

Saturday rolled in and oddly I was alone. I woke up remembering my dream. I was in a race where I was coming fifth. In the dream, I remembered feeling like I had extra gas in the tank I wasn't using, so I started pushing myself and proceeded to pass each of the four in front of me. An incredible feeling flowed through my body; each stride was effortless, with every cell working in unison to power myself to the win.

CHAPTER 7
MARCH – DON'T YOU GET BORED?

Driving to the mountain I replayed the video over in my head, the way I pushed myself and how well my body responded. I couldn't shake the thought, even while I was walking along the road. After all, how often does one get the opportunity to turn a dream into reality hours apart? So, I thought about it a bit more... I'm well rested, I feel fantastic, and I'm energised after Amoyo – perhaps a speed test would be fun!

As I finished the gratitude prayer, I took a deep breath and felt my body tingling in anticipation. My thoughts kept me company and seemed to enhance my emotions, this powered me forward one solid step at a time. To this day, it was my fastest ascent up Platteklip Gorge. 43 minutes and 40 seconds, to be exact. The focus and ability to anticipate each step put me in a flow state I'm not sure I'll experience again. It was almost as if each stone ahead expectantly lit up for me. It took me twenty minutes to recover at the top before heading over to the cable station. I drove home feeling on top of the world. How much better could life get? Ask, and ye shall receive...... nothing could prepare me for the message Kym sent:

'Andrew, half of the children have arrived with R2 to donate to 365 Ubuntu Climbs – the other half said they'll bring it on Monday. Amoyo will match their donations.'

That finished me and left a massive lump in my throat. My eyes welled up as I re-read one of the greatest displays of generosity I'd ever experienced. I was truly in tears. They got it. They understood what I was doing because they were living it, and while R2 doesn't sound like a lot – for children that have next to nothing, it's a larger sum than we think. That's like most people giving thousands of Rands. The following day I tried to share the story in a video on my social media, but not even twenty-four hours could remove the lump in my throat and the tug on my heart. I battled to get the words out through the overwhelming emotion of what an incredible gesture this was. Sometimes the smallest donations came from the biggest hearts.

Do you remember the 90's song Mr Wendal by Arrested Development? It's about lessons from a homeless man – it starts:

"Here, have a dollar

in fact, no brother man here, have two.

Two dollars means a snack for me, but it means a big deal to you."

I finally understood that last line. Never again would I express different levels of appreciation based on the size of a donation. Amoyo also became the first group of people I'd spoken to where everyone donated. 22 children and 3 staff members took the donations to R50, which was doubled by Kym. Only one other group all year would join them in that accomplishment – a networking group called *'Business Matters'*. Incredibly, I met them in March too. They met every Friday for breakfast at the River Club in Observatory, Cape Town. They etched their names in history by living up to their promise of joining me on climb number 146 in May. Then, another amazing team due to join on climb 105 was Amoyo's *Young Men of Change,* known for breaking the cycles that lead youth into joining gangs. What this has consistently proven to me is how many amazing and committed human beings there are around us, more than we realise.

My idea to select a stone each day to represent the climb pushed me to look at the path with a more investigative eye. Colours, size, texture, shape, all worked together fighting for my attention. It added an intentional grounding element to each climb and prevented me from climbing on autopilot. I'd also been grappling with how to build a pyramid with these stones piling up on Ubuntu rock. I started placing them in rows of nine, but I have this 'unease' about placing stones in non-numerical order. I'd been dragging my feet about moving them to build a pyramid off the beaten path to protect it from people. And then on Monday the 19th, climb 78, I found out someone clearly didn't take kindly to my memorial. Every single stone had been thrown off!

Well, okay, I suppose that's sorted then! While mad that someone did this, I couldn't help but chuckle and think that if I didn't make a decision, the universe would do it for me. It was already 17:00, and I had peace and quiet to pick up all 77 stones that were scattered around Ubuntu Rock and the surrounding path. What was my big decision? Where to build a pyramid that would be easy to get to, but out of sight from riff-raff that were uninformed about what they represented. The area behind Ubuntu Rock was packed with huge boulders, like giant Lego blocks intricately stacked among one another on a steep slope. I needed a relatively flat surface big enough to start a base that would support 365 rocks. After spending fifteen minutes investigating the boulders, I came up empty, so I scanned the cliffs on the opposite side and spotted what looked like a platform under the east cliff to the left of the path. Clearly, others had been here before, I could see how the grass was flattened in a little footpath through the dense bush. One big step across the gap, and I was on. There were three boulders, one half the size of a dining room table, the other two smaller ones. None were 100% stable, and they were stacked on each other. Hidden behind these stacked boulders was a flattish rectangular space about 1.2 by 1 metre. JACKPOT!! It was the perfect spot, complete with a magnificent view and nicely camouflaged against the backdrop of the cliffs and boulders littering the landscape. I enjoyed carting 77 stones across in what became a new weekly ritual: transferring the past week's stones from Ubuntu Rock to the pyramid. My solo Monday missions got me excited about fitting the stones and watching the pyramid grow as they joined their brothers and sisters. I wished I was a maths wizard to have carefully calculated the exact number to build the base, but I wasn't aiming to replicate the temple at Giza. The smaller stones were nestled between the larger ones, which were placed above them. This made a solid square base with 77 rocks.

I can't remember when I got the urge, but while relaxing next to the ever-growing Ubuntu pyramid, I checked the direction each side was facing. I couldn't believe it. I must've cleared the compass app a dozen times, but each time it showed me the same thing; it was perfectly aligned to north, east, south, and west. I'd love to take credit for this, but it was all thanks to the position of the boulder they rested on. Another piece of magic I'd discover later in winter: it was directly under a waterfall which seemed to wash new life into them on rainy days.

So, to the person who threw all my stones off creating an adult 'Easter egg hunt' – Thank you, it all worked out perfectly.

Astrid's 'recruitment' drive continued with help from Joshua, spreading the news of my project as far away as Australia. Keeping it local, too, she shared it with her property network and got Warren from SA Property Network involved.

The way Astrid, Joshua, and Warren used their respective networks to build more momentum behind the project was monumental. Warren invited me to speak at networking events and personally challenged members to get behind the initiative. Leading by example, he donated and joined me on Climb 79, the day that also happened to be the only one where an investor suffered a mild 'injury'. Candace from DigiOutsource got severe calf muscle cramps just before halfway. The four of us sprang into action and massaged the spasms. Not in any mood to give up, she persevered and pushed through to make it to the top while being spurred on by Warren and Wafeeq, who showed tremendous patience on an almost four-hour climb. This was the fourth of eight climbs organised by DigiOutsource. March rapidly became the busiest month so far.

Whatever leads came my way, I pursued. Especially talks. Writing this, I'm amazed at the amount of money generated through Astrid's network engagement. A prime example was her connection with Warren; this led to opportunities that ultimately turned into money to empower others.

DigiOutsource had 56 staff members join across eight days. By far my biggest opportunity to interact with strangers. This led to an interesting phenomenon; all eight days I was asked if I was getting bored doing the same route. The first couple of times, I explained that every day was different, to support this response, I showed them pictures of previous days. But the question kept coming and made me evaluate my answer enough to think deeper. Some solo climbs provided the opportunity to reflect on the boredom aspect... *What is boredom? Why would I be bored? And when have I been bored?* I didn't grow up with smartphones or technology (I remember three TV channels, all of which started their programming in the afternoon!) but even then, I don't remember being bored. I had such a vivid imagination, which carried over into my detailed dreams. I let my thoughts run loose. I thought about being born partially deaf and how I was taught from a young age to be grateful for whatever 'little' I had. The next three times I asked the boredom question, my reply got a tad deeper. This is how it went......

Besides each day bringing different weather and ways to experience the mountain while simultaneously watching the weather shift; I have opportunities to meet new people and develop my perspectives on a range of topics. Being bored goes against everything my gratitude prayer says at the bottom. It would show a lack of appreciation for the simpler gifts I have; working legs, the physicality to climb each day, eyesight to see the beauty in nature and I can hear every sound the mountain makes. Quite simply – I'm alive.

Looking back now, I wonder whether those asking the questions were driving to work along the same route, sitting behind the same desk and working on the same computer day after day? Perhaps this question reflected the boredom they were experiencing in their own lives? I hope my answers and the experience on the mountain gave them some clarity on how I chose to move forward with a greater sense of inner peace and outward purpose. Strangely enough, once I developed this deeper understanding, I was never asked about boredom again. Not once for the rest of the year.

DigiOutsource's final climb was on Good Friday, which turned out to be a beautiful day. Both my friends Louise and Dexter, who worked at DigiOutsource, joined. Having Dexter join was extra special because he was the very man responsible for DigiOutsource's support and donations. He was responsible for going to the HR department to see how they could support 365 Ubuntu Climbs. Although temperatures had steadily started dropping since the first week in March, this was the first rainy day of the season. Not the major downpour sorely needed, but a fine mist and drizzle that soaked us ten minutes into the climb. Dexter was beaming from ear to ear. Never complaining, just revelling in the joy of being on the mountain with life flowing around us in the form of water. He wasn't letting his lack of fitness dampen his experience and certainly never let it prevent him from claiming his victory on climb 89.

Dexter later shared the profound impact 365 Ubuntu Climbs had on helping him shift towards a healthier lifestyle. Changing his eating habits and getting up earlier to start training, telling himself... *'If Andrew can climb for an entire year – I can get up a couple times a week to train.'*

Anytime someone decided to live a healthier lifestyle, I was ecstatic. It just made my journey so much sweeter, knowing that positive actions grew out of a seed planted on our climb. I couldn't seem to find the holes in Ubuntu's philosophy, I couldn't identify any weak points where a loser was created. That continued to be a hard task as the DigiOutsource's HR manager met me up top on their last day's climb with a massive Golf Tournament winning cheque. Another R10,000 would go a long way toward adding another donor to the Leukaemia registry, building a home for someone like Masande, and towards providing much-needed literacy aids for children in need.

Saturday's drier weather rolled in. I was excited to watch the fourth full moon and the year's second blue moon rise on top of the mountain. Well, this is what I'd hoped for. After yesterday's unappealing weather, the mountain was buzzing with people. With Avril on her third climb and Jaclyn on her second, Avril decided to brave the queue and headed down in the cable car. After January's experience of watching the moon rise in the gorge, I decided Platteklip would be the better option. After 90 climbs, I was still feeling great, and climbing down didn't feel that much of a problem. It was my 19th climb back down and my 7th this month. Jaclyn shared interesting tales of her travels which transported me away from this mountainous existence, even if just for a second.

Though just 59 climbs separated the two events, the sun was already setting 1 hour and 11 minutes earlier, which meant that we'd watch the full moon rise in the darkness twenty minutes after sunset. For two-thirds of the climb back

CHAPTER 7
MARCH - DON'T YOU GET BORED?

down, we were in the dark but bathed in soft silver light, putting my senses on high alert. Soon we made it back to the road, the relief was palpable when both feet touched the tarmac.

After our farewells, my eyes were treated to Lions Head's pearl necklace – a string of torchlights that hung perfectly around the mountain. Unfortunately, for every light I saw, I knew there was probably another five people unprepared walking in the dark. Seeing the endless stream of moon enthusiasts clambering down was a reminder that if I'd followed the crowd, my experience would have been very different. Perhaps it would've been more focused on people, many disrespecting the mountain, leaving all their trash up top. I made the right choice, Platteklip Gorge offered a better option that allowed me to enjoy the moon from a higher vantage point, and in stillness.

As my drive brought me closer to Lions Head, the lights sparkled, and I remembered the first and only time I went up to watch the moonrise. We left early to avoid the crazy queue to climb down. I was eternally grateful I didn't have to experience that painfully slow climb back down on Table Mountain.

90 climbs had been successfully navigated. It was hard to believe, but the first quarter of the year was officially behind me. Summer was over, and I cautiously pushed on into Autumn. What a gift it's been, it's gone so smoothly.

Of course, that 'smooth' sailing wouldn't take too long to come to a crashing halt.

March Stats:

90 / 365

People Joined: 100 / 168

9 days 2 hours 3 minutes 41 seconds / 606,42km / 17,35 equivalent Everest Summits / 47 solo

climbs (51,7%) / 19 Up & Down

(21,3%) TOTAL DONATIONS: R163 333.51

Susan: "Just sharing my wealth from a recent paycheck"

Wes and Stuttgart contributors: "Proud of you Andy keep going, here's a little hump to help the momentum. W"

Raghmah (monthly contributor): "Hi Andrew. Thanks for starting such an amazing initiative."

Doesn't expecting the unexpected, make the unexpected expected? ~~ **Bob Dylan**

CHAPTER 8
APRIL - LEARNING THE HARSH REALITY OF EXTREMES

Sunday was my 'day off', not from the mountain, just a chance to sleep in. No alarm meant absolute Bliss! Around 8 am, and after almost 10 hours of sleep, I surfaced. I glanced at my phone and saw missed calls at around 00:30 from a number I didn't recognise. Before I even listened to the voicemails, my gut twisted up, I instantly knew what had happened. My car!!

My building didn't have enough parking, so I was constantly grabbing the nearest street parking available. A tracking device kept my insurance company updated on things like speed, braking, cornering, and impact alert, which was the reason I joined in the first place. In the event of a severe accident, even if I was incapacitated, an alert would go out, and I'd get the benefit of an immediate response with medical care.

I was incapacitated alright. After a massive collision they dispatched medical assistance and tow trucks to my coordinates while frantically trying to reach me on my cell. I'm sure they buzzed my flat countless times too but I'm pretty sure I was lying on my good ear and cut off from the action of the real world.

Of course, at this stage I was still in my flat with no knowledge of what really happened, but I'm sure that was the reason for the missed calls. My heart sank. I had no idea what to expect. Whatever it was, rushing wouldn't change anything, so I gingerly made myself some coffee and dragged myself downstairs with an awful feeling in my stomach. The lift opened and as I stepped out, Sam, one of our security guards, let out a loud anguished cry.

That's not good, I thought.

'Andrew I'm so sorry man! Yoh.....'

I cut him off, 'Sam, let me go look and I'll come back and chat with you.'

His pained facial expression said it all. After my full moon climb, I found a sweet spot directly across the road from the building, next to the swimming pool. I guess it wasn't as sweet as I thought.

I strolled across the road in my pajamas to my car, which was now sitting halfway onto the sidewalk. Sunday morning is prime time on the promenade with walkers, runners, and cyclists who were all staring in amazement. During the night, someone had hit my car on the back right wheel with enough force shunting me into the car in front pushing my front left half onto the pavement. The worst damage seemed to be the wheel's axle, the back panel, and a hideous mangling of the right passenger door. As I sipped my coffee wishing I'd parked one spot back, a police van pulled up next to me.

'We got the guy. He's at the police station. We took him late last night and they already have a case open with the number waiting for you.'

'Do I need to come into the station?' I asked

CHAPTER 8
APRIL – LEARNING THE HARSH REALITY OF EXTREMES

'No, you can just call us.'

Well, at least I didn't have to file a police report. What are the odds of the police driving up next to me while I survey the damage? Honestly, all I could think about was that it was April the 1st. Seriously???? In the past, I'd come up with some harmless ways to catch my family out with a well-timed April fool's joke. This time, it was on me. My insurance cover included a rental car, which ended up being a little Datsun GO. The wonderful timing of this being Easter Sunday meant that nothing would happen until Tuesday. Being just 8km from the mountain, suddenly took me to a new level of gratitude.

I felt like crying, yelling, screaming, laughing, cursing... none of which would help. Was this really happening? Was I still dreaming? Why did my most important possession at this time become the unlucky one? I called back the tow truck company and before I'd crossed the road and made my way into the lobby, we'd organised a time to come collect my mangled car. I was also about to get a front-row seat to the recording as Sam eagerly replayed the video. The parking was in clear view of one of the security cameras monitoring the entrance. After smashing into me, the driver tried to reverse and drive away. His steering column was clearly busted, and only succeeded in driving into me again! At least this made it a clear-cut case.

It hadn't been an easy road with my car, with three years of recurring water leakage issues and a variety of other problems, I was beginning to think it was cursed. No wonder my dear friend Donald hoped they would write it off! He was with me the day something exploded in the engine, and understandably he'd grown tired of hearing stories of car problems at our gym sessions.

This, however, was the start of a stressful four-month period in tackling issues with my car. I wish they'd written it off. It must've been a close call with all the repairs. Adding insult to injury, poor service delayed the whole process by a month and kept me in my noddy car. Getting my car back should've been a blessing, but water leaks started plaguing me again and had me carrying five

137

water bottles in my boot when driving to the mountain so that I was prepared for when that warning light came on. It was exhausting.

Donald was a godsend. In my extreme year, which still had three quarters to go, he calmly reassured me that if the worst-case scenario were to unfold, then we could share his car.

I still had my 91st climb to think about. I was supposed to climb with Dave and Sam this afternoon, so Dave immediately offered to pick me up with the condition that I give him a full rundown of the incident with my car. The look on his face was priceless as I showed him the photos and the video. The more I spoke about it the weirder it got. It was such a bizarre place to get hit, no matter how drunk the guy was. The road bent to the left, so he must've over-steered. I'd understand if he under-steered and hit me because he didn't follow the road, but in all the years I'd been parking outside and in a sea of cars he missed them all, including the one behind me, and smashes into mine. What are the odds? Apparently 1/1.

With 275 climbs remaining, I appreciated having Sam and Dave with me today to talk it out. I love Dave's dry sense of humour. Of all my friends, I think he's led the way when it comes to car pains. Having lent me his second car at a stage, he joked...

'Is this just an elaborate ploy to drive my car again buddy?'

How I needed that laugh. Dave and Sam showed how there was no substitute for human interaction in times like these. Especially after long chats with my family in Johannesburg; Jessie doing her best all the way from San Francisco, to Josh in Melbourne Australia whose birthday it was, everyone played a wonderful part in lifting my spirits. Josh was the surprise of the lot. Even though we'd only been 'introduced' online thanks to Astrid back in March, talking to him really grounded me. Having suffered one of the worst tragedies himself in January, he empathised in a natural and genuine way.

CHAPTER 8
APRIL – LEARNING THE HARSH REALITY OF EXTREMES

His wife and soulmate died in his arms due to complications with her medication, she was 32 at the time. Astrid met Josh through a mutual friend when he brought Roxy to be buried at home In Cape Town, which was the city she was originally from. Astrid bonded with him, and knowing we were 9 hours behind, made a commitment to reach out to him when darkness descended, and he had difficulty coping.

She shared one of my videos with him on Facebook and added that perhaps it could give him a project worthy of focusing his energy on, something to encourage and motivate him. He took that advice and immediately reached out to learn more about my journey straight from the horse's mouth. That same day he donated and shared my story on his platforms to garner as much support as possible. Every donation we received from Australia (barring my friends from school) was a direct result of his relentless support.

It took him a while to believe the story about my car, but eventually he was laughing as much as I was. It was our first proper chat where I got to hear his voice and see him. I enjoyed connecting with him. His ideas seemed to flow out at a rate of knots even as he pushed through his grief. He seemed to be handling it okay, but after my ordeal at gunpoint and knowing how the distress could linger, I couldn't help but continue to check-in. Unfortunately, I couldn't sit across from him and give energetic support just like Dave, Sam, and Donald did for me.

Tuesday's climb with DKMS Africa provided some much-needed perspective. We started just before 7 am and as we were about to reach Ascension Corner, Shelley shared an epiphany:

'You know – as tough and as difficult as this is, it will be over. Then we get to go home and get on with our lives. The people we help would LOVE to have this opportunity. For three months they're stuck inside a hospital room away from family and friends, and that's just the start of years of recuperation'.

This was a deep and powerful perspective that added even more purpose to the 93rd climb.

It didn't diminish what we were going through, and it wasn't an attempt to make light of our experience, it was a beautiful reminder that sometimes what feels like the 'worst' or most challenging thing in that moment, isn't the worst. That resonated deeply, especially after Sunday's car fiasco. What if it had happened just after parking? I could've been in the car and injured my legs. These experiences and conversations helped cement gratitude in my mind as the challenge of winter loomed. For those living in shacks, every day, all day, is a struggle. A cold and wet climb, although treacherous and unpleasant, was just a few hour's glimpse into the lives of others.

This deeper perspective encouraged me to shed the smaller things I'd allowed to consume me in the past. Would this *really* matter in 5 years' time? The answer was generally no. In fact, it may just build me in ways I'd never imagined.

This simple exercise was given to me during an *Understanding* EQ Course. The purpose is for everyone to record their earliest happy memory, and then record an unhappy/sad/horrible memory after that. Then a happy memory again and continue on.

No matter what the frequency or length of time between each dot – everyone's curve does exactly the same thing.

Two simple yet powerful insights are:

1. There's going to be a dip after experiencing a high – so appreciate the highs while they last.
2. No matter how bad the dip is – it's always followed by another high – don't get bogged down when the dip comes. Find its lesson.

Another beautiful arrow added to my quiver of gratitude back in 2014 was this; It's easier to swim *with life's* current, than against it.

Understanding life's principles, I could use them, instead of believing they were against me.

CHAPTER 8
APRIL – LEARNING THE HARSH REALITY OF EXTREMES

Image1

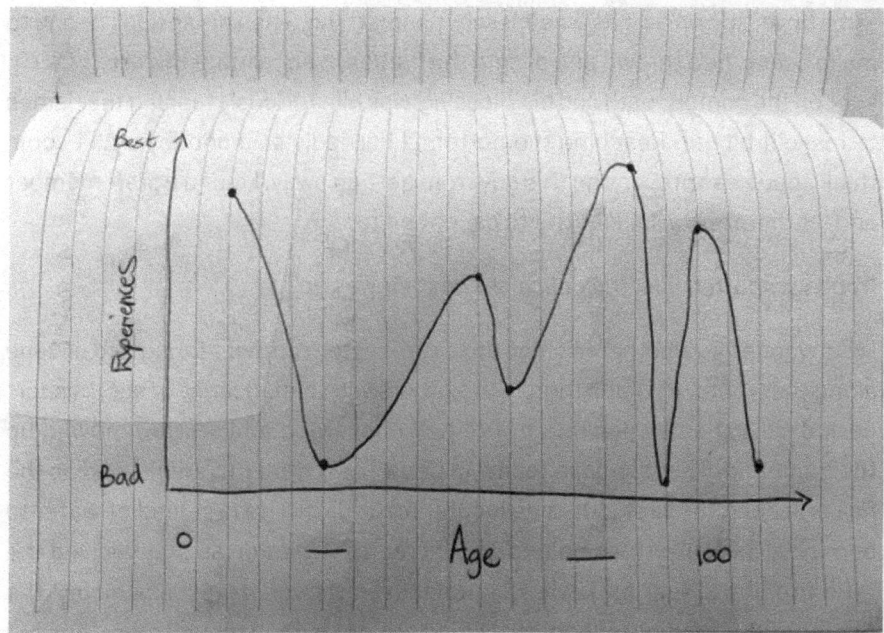

Spending four hours on the mountain today, I could feel the light changing. I watched the sun begin its journey later and farther north while tracking lower in the sky. The temperature was changing too. This same climb with Caroline exactly a month ago was an hour earlier, and yet we still had a cooler finish without mad dashes for shade at the corners between the cliffs. Our celebratory smiles were cut short as we waited to board the cable car. A thin wisp of smoke started rising into the clear midday air. Fire! We weren't the only ones to notice as the staff frantically contacted operations at the lower cableway station. They'd seen it too.

Then a second fire started sending plumes of smoke up into the air. How could it be? It had to be an arsonist, there's no way fire jumps this kind of distance and magically starts in another spot, especially on a windless day. While I contemplated that, a third fire started. As I came down in the cable car, I saw a man in a smart white shirt, and long trousers, clearly not a hiker, throwing his arms up and down as if he was 'blessing' something. Then his actions began to make sense, he'd thrown petrol onto the fynbos to accelerate the fire, a fourth spot on the contour path and his 'blessing' was him furiously fanning the flames to make it bigger. Reaching the bottom, I hurriedly said goodbye. All I could think about was preventing this guy from getting away. I found a staff member and let them know, luckily, they'd caught on too.

'Yeah we spotted him, the police are on their way up'

I was wondering whether to climb up to the western corner fearing he'd escape along that route. Perhaps there were others with him. Scarily, in such a short period, all the small pockets of fire had converged and started moving up the mountain. The response teams in Cape Town were incredible, and as the fire breached the first cliff, a helicopter arrived with its first load of water to bomb it. The skill of these pilots was incredible to watch as they tackled the third fire of the year on Table Mountain. Even though it was a calm day, the fire grew at incredible speed, searching out dry fynbos to consume. Finally, I saw the rangers and policeman drag the perpetrator off the mountain before taking him to jail.

Information came to light revealing a motive for the offender, he was apparently a disgruntled car guard who felt that starting a fire would be the best way to 'get back' at the society he felt abandoned by. His actions made him a criminal and incurred some serious costs. One of the staff I adore – Siyabonga (meaning thank you in English) – shared an African Proverb I'd never heard before: *You cannot hear a baby cry in the mother's womb*. This was the most succinct way of describing this man's actions complaining about things that he'd never shared.

The fires reminded me how quickly my chosen route could be ruled out as an option. Hopefully, this was the last fire for the year. It's certainly added to the many exciting developments the week lined up for me.

CHAPTER 8
APRIL – LEARNING THE HARSH REALITY OF EXTREMES

Mark arrived from London and fulfilled his promise by donating and climbing with me on the 4th of January. Thursday was our first climb together, and I got to meet his sister. He loved the mission and thoroughly enjoyed the English breakfast at the top, claiming it was 'the most hard-earned meal ever'. Even though he almost passed out fifteen minutes into the climb from over-exertion, he laughed about it and slowed down for the rest of the route to make it more enjoyable. I loved his outlook on life and his explanation about how special it was to do it for the first time and with such purpose.

Friday, I had my second family climb. Terence's sister and her two daughters; Michaela and Abby joined after donating and taking me up on my offer to climb. Everyone who donated received a 'Thank You' email which expressed my gratitude and invited them to join in on a climb. Even though they lived in the midlands of Kwazulu-Natal, a two-hour flight away, they made a plan.

Bronwyn, another tremendous supporter, and regular donor, joined us for her first climb. She'd often send me pictures of the mountain covered in thick clouds, letting me know she was thinking about me climbing.

Three more stones were added to the family pile and took the tally up to seven. While slower climbs were a 'rest' for my lungs, my legs still did the same hard work. I was starting to feel the impact of no rest days now, the honeymoon was over, and the eerie awareness of the upcoming 269 climbs began to live in my thoughts. After celebrating more successful first summits, we headed down to Red Sofa Café where Beth worked, and we sat outside under the watchful eye of the mountain. My excitement was boiling over too, because my parents were already on the road down to Cape Town and were due to arrive later that afternoon while Jessie was on her way flying from San Francisco. Everything was coming together in preparation for my 100th climb on the coming Tuesday and my illusive event that evening to raise more funds. Ah yes – THAT event. Gulp.

I finally settled on 'believing' that triple digits would suffice as a mark to host the fundraiser. I just hadn't quite overcome the hurdle of asking others to join the cause and to help me, help others. Three figures. It didn't quite compute. Especially when I stacked the consecutive climbs of Table Mountain up against the vertical equivalent of Mt Everest: 19 summits. It's what blew my mind the most and powerfully demonstrated how quickly 'small' daily actions added up to something significant.

It would be the first time my parents got the chance to meet Jessie, and with everyone staying for a week, there was a wonderful opportunity to build deep connections. Jessie was a huge hit with my parents. And as the year unfolded, her character was on full display time after time, leaving a trail of happy hearts in her wake. My two Endomondo pep talkers were now in the same city. My heart was overflowing. Mom and Dad wanted to join the 100th climb, but with terrible winds forecast, I used my now pro-Windguru skills and suggested the day after so they could catch the cable car down.

It was Jessie and JP's second climb, and Lisa's eleventh, which made it a perfect group to commemorate climb 100. Alone on 99, I used the solitude to take stock of the enormity of what had been accomplished, and more importantly to pay respect to what lay ahead: 265 more summits. The contrast from yesterday's perfect day to today's icy wind at the top was an indication of what was to come. It also meant it was just Jessie and I scuttling along to get my top picture, while Lisa and JP sheltered out of the wind at the top of Platteklip.

This was supposed to be my second reward climb on a different route called 'Left Face Arrow Face', but the gale force winds and poor visibility made any attempt foolhardy. I decided against it. When I eventually saw the route on Climb 111, I realised just how wise that decision was. Reaching the bottom, I was transported to my childhood when my parents surprised us with the warmest welcome. Recording us on video and cheering in the background, I felt like I was a teenager scoring my second hundred in cricket all over again. I really am blessed with amazing parents.

It was an emotional moment for me to be able to share this with them. Again, the distance between us added additional layers to my gratitude. They'd been

CHAPTER 8
APRIL – LEARNING THE HARSH REALITY OF EXTREMES

'there' online from step #1 after Dave wished me well on my first climb. Their support was constant for the next 257 900 steps climbed.

Climb 101 was a hot one, but saw my dad and my mom deliver a monumental effort in the unseasonably toasty conditions. My dad carried mom's snacks and we assisted her to the top. It was also my sixth barefoot climb, and my three special people took my tally of joining climbers up to 190.

The special family climb enabled me to point out the Brown's rocks, while adding three more stones to the family pile. Jessie got to choose her rock too, and it became the largest of the lot sitting high in the gorge just two corners above Ubuntu Rock. It was an emotional chat at the top with my parents, who were now part of 365 Ubuntu Climbs family. We reflected on the journey to reach 100 consecutive climbs, and they shared their perspective on what I was doing. Part of our conversation was inspired by the event the night before, and the opportunity my parents got to meet the very people these climbs aimed to help.

My never-ending spiral of 'not feeling good enough' didn't end because I'd finally hosted the event. It simply became part of my journey to stand in my own power and gave me the belief that my response and feelings to how others viewed this challenge or anything else I did was a 'work in progress'.

I managed to create a self-fulfilling prophecy, by not advertising my fundraiser as I should've, there were few people at the event. One of the upsides was that it gave people, my parents included, the opportunity to have all three charities in the room at the same time and gave a broader perspective of all the work that was being done. Possibly the most impactful of the three was Habitat for Humanity. Not only did Patrick (the CEO) share his personal story about receiving a home and how it changed the trajectory of his life, but Masande came too. I couldn't believe it was 47 climbs ago that we paid her a visit. She, too, agreed to chat to everyone about the progress of the family home being built. Seeing and hearing someone speak about being on the receiving end of our work and the impact it's had, lives with you forever.

The saying, *"To the world you may be one person, but to one person you may be the world" (author unknown)* – reflected the love that could be felt for you and was a powerful reminder to everyone in the room what upliftment meant to the person on the receiving end.

It forced me to take a deeper look at my corporate mindset, constantly analysing donations and whether I was 'on target'. It was draining because I was constantly obsessing over the money, and even in my personal capacity, I failed to look up and enjoy the experience and the beauty of everyday life. I remember thinking about falling short of the target and being asked later in interviews whether it was a 'success' or not. It took meeting Masande and experiencing her current living conditions to reevaluate my definition of success. Listening to her speak about not having to share a bed anymore, and now having her own kitchen, and toilet too, was powerful as it was told with a smile of the purest joy and appreciation I'd ever witnessed. Violence in townships where unemployment is rife, and poverty is at every turn has become a 'norm' for so many. Now her family could visit a toilet in peace without fear of being raped.

This is why they say the more you give; the more you get. It's a reminder to stay committed to that two-thousand-year-old challenge 'if not now, when', and keep creating opportunities for others to experience the very best of being human.

The success of any project isn't measured by the amount raised. It's measured by the impact it has on those on the receiving end.

Masande was just days away from moving in, her joy radiated through her eyes without even speaking.

More stories came from One Heart and DKMS Africa that demonstrated what Ubuntu achieves when our hearts are open. I was extremely grateful to the companies that opened their hearts and supported the event. Thanks to Roanne, Sir Fruit provided fresh fruit juice for the guests, while Helen at Graham Beck and Njongo at Distell provided some bubbles and Bains whiskey as raffle prizes.

CHAPTER 8
APRIL – LEARNING THE HARSH REALITY OF EXTREMES

Conrad put me in touch with his marketing manager at The Last Word hotel, and they donated a night's stay in Franschhoek, while Beth gave me a voucher for Breakfast for two at Red Sofa Café. These fabulous prizes were available in a lucky draw, with each ticket costing R100.

Our amazing guest speaker was an introduction from Patrick. He interviewed me for his platform called 'Awesome South Africans', which publicly acknowledges, highlights, and celebrates the awesome things South Africans are doing to positively affect change in the country. It's about conquering adversity and encourages patriotism through inspirational stories that prove anybody can achieve anything if they really set their mind to it.

Patrick introduced me to Jamie Marais, once known as South Africa's fittest man and the creator of the 'Four Giants' Challenge. You should check out his book 'Determination'. His chosen cause is the Sabrina Love Foundation - set up to care for children with special needs and their families, providing them with medical and professional support. The Foundation is responsible for providing a holistic program for every child under its care.

One of his 4 Giants initiatives was climbing Table Mountain via Platteklip Gorge 22 times in 28 hours. My head couldn't compute this, having personally been destroyed at 5. Jamie met with me over lunch in February to chat about being a speaker at my event. He agreed and gave me some of the best advice....

'Use the first half of the year as training for the second half.'

The second half was still 83 days away.

This wasn't a sexy challenge requiring speed and intensity, or a race against the clock. It was a war of attrition, a battle to stay motivated, healthy, and injury-free. I had to get up and be motivated one day at a time. His talk was fascinating. He shared the horror of injuring himself just one week before his 22 climbs, which caused severe pain on most of his summits and made him limp along the top of the mountain as early as three summits in.

What would I do if I got injured like this?

It was hard not to let thoughts like these creep in and destroy my mindset. It's one thing to think about potential problems and how you'll deal with them beforehand. It's another thing focusing on what you don't want while deep in it. Was my training enough to keep me healthy? Would I be able to stay focused on what I DO want? While I have no control over the weather, I know how strong my focus is – and for that very reason, I believed.

The week with my family evaporated like dew in the morning sun, and it was time to say goodbye to my folks and Jessie. She was showing what a machine she was, a run of six consecutive summits and a cumulative time of 17 hours and 11 minutes. Think about that. She travelled across ten time zones on two long-haul flights culminating in about 32 hours of travelling and then did six days in a row?!?! If you look up support in the dictionary, you'll see her smiling face there. Her support was rewarded over the weekend. On Saturday, we saw tahrs, very shy mountain goats indigenous to the Himalayas. They broke out of the old Zoo on the foothills of Devils Peak decades prior – taking to the mountains with aplomb and breeding like wildfire but, unfortunately, damaging the ecosystem in the process.

Sunday, *the Young men of Change* from Amoyo joined and were escorted by Kim's husband Allan and his two work friends, while Raghma, our committed monthly investor, joined us on a magnificent Autumn Day.

We started bang on sunrise at 7:11, with Allan's massive black rottweiler, my first four-legged Ubuntu Climber. Alas, the baking sun took our first victim as the pooch started too big too soon. Bounding up ahead of us and rushing back to see what was taking us so long didn't help. Allan took him back down. He was seriously concerned his dog might've had a heart attack.

It was hard to believe it had already been 39 climbs since I had the privilege of meeting and watching Bulelani, Zosuliwe, Asiphe, Athule, Siphumle, and Sakhile in that dance rehearsal. I shared my gratitude with them at the bottom

CHAPTER 8
APRIL - LEARNING THE HARSH REALITY OF EXTREMES

and let them know how they were the first group I'd spoken to where everyone donated. I made sure to look each of them in the eye as I thanked them. None of them had climbed before, and again I shared my gratitude to them for living up to their promise to join.

As we passed the halfway mark, Sakhile chatted away with Jessie a few steps behind. I could just make out their conversation and ended up hearing one of the most heart-warming exchanges all year. Now two-thirds up, between the cliffs, and over two hours into the climb – he realised what I'd committed to.

'He's doing this all year??'

'Still 260 days left for him to climb yeah', responds Jessie.

There's a pause

'He can't even leave Cape Town?!'

'Nope – the only way we can see each other is when I can make it back'

A longer pause this time before a melodic combination of sixteen words:

'I want to do something like this to help my community too when I get older.'

Only the mountain saw how much that made me smile. Thankfully though, Kim showed him he was already making a difference. By using the discipline and commitment that Amoyo was teaching him, he was turning his back on drugs and gangs, he was transforming his life with his school marks. So much so that he'd become a leader in his community, and through his example, he was showing other boys what was possible. I have no doubt I'll be reading about him many times in the future.

This week became my second longest streak of climbs where others had joined, my longest was still holding strong at 8 days back in March. Truthfully though, I needed and wanted some quiet time on the mountain.

It was an emotional goodbye with Jessie, watching her walk out of sight at the airport was tough. I collapsed into bed at home with no alarm. My heart may have been heavier than usual, but the longer sleep meant I was refreshed and invigorated to move week 15's rocks over to the pyramid. Sunsets were now at 18:22, with the last cable car down at 19:30, so a start at 16:30 gave me ample time to enjoy a solo climb.

Oh, but how wrong I was again. The climb started off beautifully, especially after running into Achmat, who was getting his bag out of the boot as I arrived. I love my high fives from him. His positive influence always elevates my mood and energises me, he's always deeply concerned with how my body's holding up. He should know! He had over 1500 summits since he started recording back in 2009, averaging about 3 climbs a week going up and down. This year he'd finish on 134.

And then, our joyous mood to start week 16 got vaporised. Barely 50 steps up and a massive flat rock, the size of half a decent coffee table, had been completely spray painted. It looked wet, as if it had just been done. The top of the rock had a red and black stripe sprayed across it, with a yellow logo of some sort, below that was a green stripe, and right at the bottom the word 'BIAFRA' in red. It was the kind of ridiculously out-of-place scene that made you want to pinch yourself. *Who on earth would do this?! Is this even real??* Unfortunately, on the mountains, graffiti was becoming worse by the day. Halfway rock used to be a majestic slab of white rock the size of a single mattress, angled perfectly enough to rest on. Struggling climbers always took advantage of its cool exterior as they built up the will to push on. It was no longer that pristine slab. We took pictures to share with both SANParks and my friend Blake from Love Our Trails, and then we composed ourselves and set off, trying not to let this ruin our climb.

We moved on, and just as the blood pressure levels dropped, smack bang on the left was sprayed rock #2 with the words *BIAFRA IS NOT DEAD* splashed in bright red on the 260-million-year-old grey granite rock. This one was about the size of a standard single-seater couch. I was dumbfounded. I also had no idea what the hell 'Biafra' was, and why it would compel someone to ruin rocks with it. I was grateful Achmat was with me because I don't know what I would have done if I'd run into whoever was doing this. Before we hit the waterfall, another small piece had been sprayed in green, about the size of two open palms placed together. Shaking our heads, we glanced up the path and found #4...BIAFRA (yellow) THE (red) RISING (green) written on the steep section next to the waterfall. This was the equivalent of covering a truck door with each word painted under the other. I was livid! Fuming! I no longer wondered if there'd be more, it was now a matter of how many. Before we reached the contour path there were another two. Achmat suddenly expressed that he was taking strain and let me know he probably wasn't going to go all the way up to the top and said I should push on without him.

The higher I got, the more my heart was racing from the climb, and boiling from walking past graffiti pieces numbers 7...... 8...... 9...... 10......

Unsure of how high Achmat would still go to take pictures, I took my phone out to capture a life-size flag plastered over a rock adjacent to the steepest section of Platteklip Gorge. As I looked at my screen, I saw two missed calls from a number I didn't recognize. It was Michael from Safety Mountain Tracking...

'Hey Andrew,

Its Michael from Safety Mountain tracking'

'Yes?'

I suddenly got a very uneasy feeling in my stomach.

'We have a hiker in distress on Smuts track and you're the closest, are you able to assist?'

'Uh, sure – I can do my best. What do you need?'

'We have a SANParks ranger already on the scene providing medical assistance.

Our emergency guys aren't even at Table Mountain yet and you're the closest we have. If you can head over and help with any crowd control needed for the helicopter on the way to assist, we'd appreciate it.'

'Sure – I'm almost halfway up Platteklip but I'll push it to reach them.'

Just then, I realised another benefit of the tracking service and being kept safe; it was always known who was where, and in this case, who was closest to help. Then just as I was about to hang up the call, a decision I made earlier came back to haunt me.

'Oh shit! I took my torch out of my bag! Do you still want me to go?? Won't I just become another hazard?'

By this time, it was around 17:15 – and sunset was in an hour.

'Yes, if you can help us, we'd greatly appreciate it.' 'Okay I'm on my way.'

'Thank you – I'm sending you a pin with their location.'

Even after 108 climbs, I wasn't feeling too fatigued yet, I'd slept late and had more than 24 hours rest after yesterday's early climb. Besides my silly decision to take out my torch, everything else was in my favour, and I was confident I would get to them before sunset. The pin came through and showed me I was more than an hour away. An hour?! You've got to love technology! But still, time was against us. Smuts track is on the eastern slopes of Table Mountain – named after Jan Smuts, who spent many hours every week walking on the mountain. It connects Maclears Beacon (the highest point on the west table) with Skeleton Gorge, one of the routes up the east slopes, as well as the Overseers huts above Kirstenbosch Gardens and the reservoirs.

I continued up once more, and before halfway I was greeted by more graffiti, numbers 11........ 12... but I couldn't stop for photos now, I was on a mission, and I was moving as if I was doing a speed test.

Once again, numbers 13...... 14....., they just kept appearing.

CHAPTER 8
APRIL - LEARNING THE HARSH REALITY OF EXTREMES

I channelled my anger, using it as fuel for the furnaces in my legs. Finally, I passed the last of the graffiti, roughly two-thirds up the climb just below The Guardian. Even though the paint seemed fresh, I didn't run into the perpetrators, something I'm extremely grateful for. My lungs were burning, and my legs were pumping. I wondered what the emergency was. I counted the corners down like a tick box exercise, straining over the steeper top section with my legs screaming at me as the steps became wider and further apart. I barely stopped to place rock number 106 on Ubuntu Rock, knowing how close to the top I was. I decided on some trail running along the flat top to reach them a bit quicker. It felt bizarre to be running and going in the opposite direction. The mountain's big, and after misjudging the distance of the scout hut, I couldn't afford to rely on my memory's version of how far they were. It had been a year and two days since my epic solo climb to Maclears Beacon from sea level, and none of my climbs this year headed along the east side of the mountain. Maclears Beacon felt like it should take me 15 minutes, but I wasn't fully trusting of that idea. It's crazy how my mind condensed distance and time.

Running for twenty minutes and still not at Maclears got the butterflies going. I periodically checked the pin, which was telling me I was still 30 minutes away. I started getting nervous. I'd never been down that side of Smuts track towards Skeleton Gorge, and I was worried there might be more than one path. As I ran, the most majestic sunset, quite possibly the best of the year, unfolded next to me, bathing the mountains in beautiful soft golden light and creating the most exquisite tapestry of colour across the clouds high above the reservoirs. Every intricate contour of the mountain below was revealed, it looked like heaven.

Checking the pin again, I paused to get a picture, it was 18:03, and my battery power was dropping rapidly. Panic set in... *What if I can't find them and my phone dies*?! I didn't have a torch either. Sunset was in 15 minutes, and I was 3km away from the upper cable station - about an hour's walk in good light! That thought jolted a serious boost of adrenaline into my legs. Luckily, I made up some time running to reach Maclears Beacon, I checked the pin and started down what

I thought was Smuts track, it was unchartered territory. The path quickly descended into Echo Valley and became a twisting labyrinth through boulders that were now in the shadow of the summit above. Still, I couldn't see anyone, and I couldn't run on the wet rocks that dotted the shadowy path because that would be certain disaster – and we don't need to add another hiker to the list.

I turned a corner and stumbled into the emergency scene. A woman sat distraught, hugging her legs, shaken and in tears. The mountain ranger, Aslam, was assisting another woman on her back. Another SANParks ranger watched as Aslam on the radio spoke to rescue teams, updating them on their progress and asking about helicopter support. I'd been added to the rescuers WhatsApp group to keep everyone updated while Aslam gave medical attention to the stricken hiker.

Feeling incredibly awkward, I introduced myself and shared who sent me. I took my phone out to notify the rescue group of my arrival. Shortly after that, it occurred to me that things were a lot more serious. Further adding to the distress was the fact that the helicopter couldn't land due to the steep angle of the slope we were on. Teams of rescuers were starting to head up the cable car to walk across and assist. Every minute felt like it was dissolving as fast as the light.

The other four hikers were distraught and in no state to navigate themselves safely off the mountain, then I heard Aslam asking the other ranger to take them back down Skeleton Gorge. He never responded, perhaps a bit shell-shocked.

Silence, so I interjected...

'I can take them but taking them down Skeleton Gorge would be darker and riskier. Are you able to radio the cable company to stay open for us? We could walk along the top section and be far safer.'

The last cable car down would be 19:30. We were about 400m away from Maclears, which was an hour's walk in daylight. We'd never make it in time in the dark. Aslam agreed and radioed them.

'Everyone ready?' I asked.

A terrible question under the circumstances. The young girl stood up, still crying, and started heading up the path followed by one of the men and then the other woman. The last gentleman lingered to ask a few questions.

'Where will you be taking her?' He asked Aslam.

'The ground crew will walk her back down to Echo Valley and head towards the Overseers huts. An ambulance will be waiting there. They'll most likely take her to the Salt River morgue'

'What about her things?' his voice says shakily.

'You can take them now.'

He carefully removed her watch, mobile phone, and ring, placing it in his own backpack.

I was stunned. I was completely unprepared to hear the word morgue. It never occurred to me she might be dead. I just thought she was in bad shape lying quietly. My heart sank as I watched the man stand back up after collecting her belongings – not knowing if he'd just lost a wife, daughter, colleague, or friend.

He thanked Aslam for his help, I did too – a solemn nod of his head acknowledging us. Time to go. After a few turns, we caught up to the other four. While not exactly as easy as walking on a sidewalk, reaching the top before dark drastically improved our chances of getting back safely without injury, especially under such duress. Trying to be sensitive to what they'd just experienced, I did my best to reassure them that we'd reach the summit in the light and make it back to the cable station. Teary eyes, silence, and a nod back of understanding.

I couldn't imagine what they were going through. I had no idea what to say. Barely at Maclears Beacon, the last drop of light disappeared. Darkness joined the stillness, as the twinkling city lights came into view below the mountain. A stark contrast to the black Atlantic.

With just my phone's light as a guide, I held it above shoulder height while crab walking to provide as many of us light as possible. Thankfully, it wasn't long before we hit the first group of rescuers. They had a spare torch, which we handed to the ladies to share.

'Just give it back to the station set up at the lower cable station.' 'Will do.'

As quickly as they appeared, they were gone again and merged with the darkness. There was an intensity to the silent walk back, which felt worse than speaking about what they'd just experienced. Eventually, I mustered the courage to speak.

'I'm terribly sorry about your loss – my condolences to all of you.'

Those words never feel like they do justice to such gravity, but I meant them sincerely. It opened the door, and we started talking. They were all friends; the two ladies were from France out on holiday visiting. It was such a beautiful day, that they decided to hike up from Kirstenbosch via Skeleton Gorge and then on to the cable station. The plan was to catch a taxi back to their car once they'd completed their hike. They made it up Skeleton Gorge without any incident and started climbing up Smuts track. One of the members in their group, feeling slightly distressed, asked to rest, so they paused to give her a couple of minutes. Shortly after, she stated she was ready to continue. Then not long after setting off again, she asked for another break, only this time, she laid down for her rest. A few moments went by, and then the group asked her if she was ready to continue, but this time............ no reply.

What unfolded was devastating for the group, this is not how trips to the mountain are supposed to go! The thought of the poor family receiving the news sent shivers down my spine.

The top of Table Mountain, while appearing flat from far, is dotted with weathered rocks of all shapes, sizes, and heights. SANParks have built sections of wooden paths to give safe passage across what often becomes a mini swampland during the wet months. This section was a welcomed guide as we made our way back in less-than-ideal conditions. About halfway to Platteklip Gorge, another team passed us and, thankfully, also had a spare torch for us. Two torches and my iPhone were all we had between the six of us to get back. Then we also had the lights of the upper cable station acting as a beacon for us to measure how close we were. The trickiest section to navigate is the crack separating the east and west tables of the mountain at the top of Platteklip Gorge, so we had to be careful there. Luckily the cable company was aware of our situation, and they were ready to support us. This reassured me, and gave us the freedom to take these sections slower than usual. We made it down into the crack safely, and I knew the worst was over. The last climb up the chains signalled we were close. This was normally a ten-minute walk on a much more manicured path for tourists with all types of shoes, prams, and wheelchairs which gave everyone a fair opportunity to explore the Western table. Once we got up here, the trickiest sections were done, and I could safely tell them so.

The sight of staff packing up the last remaining items and closing the umbrellas was a huge relief. I felt a bit better in the knowledge that at least my group was in a safer place. They'd just witnessed their friend leave this earth in front of them on a day they'd planned to experience the beauty of the mountain.

Safely down, I exchanged numbers with the gent in case he needed anything further. They all shared their heartfelt appreciation for the assistance and handed back the headlamps. I continued onwards, and once I found the rescuer's base camp; I handed back the lamps. With 5% battery life on my phone, I sent my last message for the day...... *Safely off the mountain – thanks for tracking.*

I'd just been given a lesson on perspective and a stern reminder of how precious our lives are. I didn't think I needed reminding, but my gratitude for being able to experience Table Mountain through this challenge in pursuit of empowering others took on a whole new meaning.

With the marketing manager for One Heart and his girlfriend joining the next morning, I made my way back home to eat, get some sleep, and put my torch back in the bag.

My solo climb on #108 gave me time to process Monday's experiences, with the eyesores of the graffiti popping up again and again and again. I knew getting angry was just sapping my energy and did nothing but ruin my climb as well as my mood. It wouldn't affect the people who did this, so I had to make a choice, I had to find another way to mentally approach this. Whoever did this surely wasn't in a good place, perhaps they'd suffered abuse. If so, it didn't absolve them for what they'd done, and I definitely didn't condone it, but Ubuntu was about trying to get people back to their true nature. In fact, there were no jails in African culture. People would be put at the centre of the village so that everyone could remind them of all the beauty they had inside, and they'd be helped back to their true essence. A thought popped into my head; every time I walked past any of the painted rocks, I'd say out loud, 'Sending you love buddy'. It would be genuine and come straight from the heart. I knew they needed it.

The strong wind swept my words away and served as a reminder of how much worse Monday could've been but also meant walking past 28 graffiti points as I endured my 21st down climb.

Safely down, I felt happy that I hadn't let each painted mess irritate me. I also contemplated how often I'd said 'sending you love buddy' out loud before this. Perhaps never. Besides changing my outlook and trying to offer love to someone clearly needing it, I'd also just sent myself love 28 times in one outing. I got more than I'd asked for – graffiti had just given me a lesson on self-love.

A week or so later I was contacted by the gent from the group I'd guided back to safety the night of the rescue. He reached out to offer the rescuers and I tickets to do the Fish River Canyon hike up in Namibia. I obviously couldn't accept but passed on the invitation to Michael who'd been in touch with me to help in the first place. It was a beautiful gesture – especially considering these

CHAPTER 8
APRIL - LEARNING THE HARSH REALITY OF EXTREMES

rescuers were all volunteers working in their own time to carry out rescues and recoveries. His heartfelt gratitude was appreciated.

I finally got my opportunity to experience Left Face Mystery B on Saturday the 21st of April. It was climb 111 which also happened to be the Platteklip Charity Challenge Day! The same challenge that had handed me the most severe beating back in 2012. Almost 200 athletes tackled the steep incline which kept the route exceptionally busy all day. Predicted to be overcast and cool, it turned out to be clear and hot with no wind. I was hoping to high-five Achmat, Blake, or Nazeem as they pushed themselves to multiple summits. Alas, I saw none before veering off the path.

Left Face Mystery B takes a detour exactly where my sister took a break and named her rock, which meant I was still able to say hello to 'everybody' up to that point. Lisa (on climb 14) joined to get a new perspective of the mountain. Before the climb though, I sought advice from Hendre (one of the mountain guides I see every week) about the route. She reassured me it was easy to follow.

That afternoon, our friends Pieter and Danielle (also American!) were getting married at *The Roundhouse* - a perfectly positioned venue I drive past every day on my way to the mountain. Pieter was one of the early cheerleaders and bought me a full body massage in January to help keep my body fresh.

Being on a route rarely used made for a very different experience. For one thing, there was no graffiti, but even better than that - there was no trash. It was exciting to see alternative views, particularly looking down onto Platteklip. It was also a far cry steeper, with some intense scrambling which justified my decision to delay the climb. Seeing *The Guardian* close up and from another angle was a bonus. In hindsight, I wish I'd walked the short distance across to take a photo with him. But perhaps some things are only meant to be admired from afar.

Then it was time to climb one of the steepest gullies I'd ever seen on the mountain. Thankfully, there were plenty of the 'hiker's friends' to grab on to.

With winter approaching, I imagined this route would become a raging torrent of water with the way it was structured. After the initial zigzagging lower down, it was time to go straight up. Reaching the top, we were high above halfway rock on Platteklip, watching the different coloured shirts making their way for the challenge! From where we were, it must have been a drop-off of at least 300m before hitting the lower slopes. From below, it looked ridiculous that anyone would even attempt taking this route, which made me enjoy looking down even more – a view I'd save for tomorrow's climb, this time from Platteklip's perspective.

With the yellow footprints painted on the rocks as guides disappearing, we suddenly felt like we were off the 'beaten track'. Overgrown with nothing but sheer cliff faces above us, and completely bemused at how we missed it. Our search attempts to find the path again stole half an hour of our time, which meant getting ready for the wedding would not be a calm and leisurely affair. Finally, we found a way up.

We heard people talking above, so we knew we were so close. Problem was it all looked pretty sketchy, something a free solo climber like Alex Honnold would love. We, on the other hand, had our hearts jumping out of our chests at the mere thought of hanging from a cliff face! At about 4 hours and 21 minutes this was a much longer and tougher climb, I still felt energised by the extraordinary views and the different perspective it gave me of Platteklip. Besides the wobble at the end, I'd thoroughly enjoyed my reward.

We got a cable car down, and who did we bump into? None other than Jamie! What a hoot. He hadn't been back to Platteklip since his achievement in August 2016. This time he was a pacer on a few climbs for an athlete who was attempting to break a record. It was good to see him in our 'natural' environment, both of us geared up, sweaty, and enjoying a laugh about our different day's experiences on the same mountain.

On to the wedding, it was a FABULOUS celebration made extra special as I enjoyed a glass of wine under the backdrop of the mountain. They couldn't have ordered better weather too. I was having an absolute ball and feeling overjoyed that I was about to complete the first third of the year. I definitely took the festivities a bit too far, considering the effort from the morning as well as missing the food as it made its way around. I was too busy catching up with special friends I hadn't seen in a while. Thankfully, my Uber was a short 7-minute ride to my welcoming bed, where I passed out with loads of alarms set for the next morning.

Joshua's brother climbed with me on Friday but sadly headed back home soon after. As a small show of appreciation for all Joshua's help, I'd send him a '100' Ubuntu shirt.

April wasn't over yet, though – there were still extra special memories just around the corner.

After just five solo climbs in three weeks, I enjoyed having five days alone again, starting with a self-induced shocker of an afternoon climb on Sunday 22nd. It's just what I needed.

My solo climb on Thursday became my third wet and rainy climb of the year, something I'd hoped might become more frequent post Easter.

Friday was Freedom Day, commemorating 24 years of freedom since South Africa held its first free and fair elections for all – everyone got an opportunity to vote. Our democracy became official when Nelson Mandela was sworn in as our first President, fulfilling a 42-year-old prophecy he made back in 1952 when he stated, "I will be the country's first black president based on majority rule." Mandela gave me more synchronicity for the year: this would've been his 100th birthday. Every time someone donated cash on the cable car, the mountain, or wherever they generously opened their wallets, his smiling face would shine up at me. His example of dedication and commitment over a period of 67 years set a standard of what we could aspire to.

I was joined by a wonderful couple from Holland on a misty and cold day. They were excited to be part of the climb, and the weather didn't deter them one bit.

Aslam arrived with a banner and a massive flag for us to hold as pictures were taken as part of their mission to each of the major trails along Tafelberg Road. The couple were a bit challenged though, the husband started getting dizzy spells at the first waterfall, which was now in full flow thanks to the previous day's rain. We began heading down to support him, but he reassured us he'd be fine and ventured the short distance to the road alone, promising to catch the cable car and meet us at the top. Mervi, his wife, soldiered on with us in the fine cold mist, choosing the rock for climb 117.

As cold as we were, it would've been a lot worse if the wind had picked up. When we reached the top, our luck ran out as a brisk wind made the water sticking to us feel like ice, luckily, it wasn't blowing hard enough to stop the cable car. We smartly made our way to the 'viewing' deck, where I snapped the 24th photo of the year with a weather-restricted view. So far, that was 1 in every 5 days, and winter was only just scratching the surface.

Soaked, we met Mervi's husband and enjoyed a much-needed coffee and hot chocolate indoors above the cable car. Aslam also made his way up and enjoyed the shelter with us. It was hard to believe that it was already 11 days since I last saw him at the sad incident that saw a hiker pass away. He and his team are always busy assisting people who've run into some sort of trouble on the mountain. Heavily understaffed, trying to cover this gigantic space is like one man trying to stop flood water at the river mouth from reaching the ocean.

But just because tasks are difficult, it doesn't mean we give up.

Aslam, like many others, are the real heroes in life we should be celebrating and rewarding so that their impact can be even greater.

Having started just before 11 am that day, we were all starved, but these two beautiful humans treated me to lunch at the Roundhouse and handed me their donation in cash. Suddenly the day was much less cold and miserable as my heart was warmed by their generous support. It was the perfect way to celebrate Freedom Day.

CHAPTER 8
APRIL - LEARNING THE HARSH REALITY OF EXTREMES

The gifts kept rolling in as my cousin Grant, who was in town on business, stayed extra days to join so he could add his rock to the family pile. This climb gave us a clearer day, but it was bitterly cold, and the swirling winds that lashed the mountain prevented the cable cars from running. It was just the two of us, many years had passed since we last saw each other, so this was the best kind of catch-up in the outdoors, with ample opportunity to talk about our lives and add another rock to the growing pile. Every member's support and love acted like a breeze at my back and helped me up the mountain.

April would also see the fruits of people working tirelessly in the shadows to support me. In this instance it was Allan from LA Barista Coffee. He was also a monthly donor and had contacts at Cape Union Mart, one of the largest outdoor retailers in South Africa. Thanks to ninety-odd consecutive climbs behind my name, he knew they'd take what I was doing seriously, so he asked me for a brief outline of what I was doing.

'Bud, I can't promise anything – but give me a proposal of what you're doing and why. Maybe we can get you sponsored by them.'

I must be honest, my mind went beyond the sponsorship. I mean, that was a fantastic idea, but I began thinking and hoping that they would jump on board and use their network of 140 stores countrywide to get people involved. I'd learned to remain calm when approached about sponsorships because of some of my previous engagements with other companies who'd sent me faulty products, or generally just never lived up to their end of the agreement. These were all lessons to not get over-excited until 'the money was in the bank'.

Cape Union Mart came through with flying colours! They usually sponsored trail runners and extreme athletes with their brand K-Way. Blake from Love Our Trails was one of those sponsored athletes. After getting completely drenched and only having the raincoat my folks bought me, I was getting concerned about my ability to navigate the stormy climbs which were fast heading my way.

I was deeply grateful for their sponsorship split over May and June, as it solved my three basic concerns: a waterproof bag, waterproof pants, and waterproof boots – my Adidas boots were starting to look pretty thin on the soles too.

All this was beautifully rounded off as April ended, and I finally got to watch the full moon rise on top of the mountain. It was third time lucky, and it rewarded my patience as a third of the year closed off. I began to think of our general lack of patience and how it contributed to the divide we often experienced in society. Understanding it from this perspective really resonated with me. I know I've got patience, but that doesn't mean I won't be tested again and again.

This understanding gave me a deeper appreciation for teachers too. To sit year in and year out teaching the same principles with students grasping it at different speeds was a beautiful commitment and surely deserved to be one of the highest-paid jobs around.

To teach, and never be weary. Is love. ~Unknown

With sunset at 18:07 we had ample time to relax at the top before the moon rose at 18:46. The spectacular sunset entered its final act and ushered in the main attraction for the evening. The others were nowhere to be found, and the lack of signal rendered our phones useless. Usually, I would've spent the time missioning around trying to find them, but I wasn't prepared to miss the very reason I came – so Imogen and I sat down, cracked open a bottle of wine between us and enjoyed the stillness while the city lights twinkled far below. I hope everyone at some stage in their lives gets to enjoy a sunset from the top of Table Mountain. What an exquisite experience it is to be a kilometre above the sea with the city neatly fitting onto the lower contours of the mountain. Then the moon emerged from the horizon, gliding effortlessly into the black pool. The Cape's finest has never tasted so good. This was a year of celebrations.

Celebrations for every summit.

Celebrations for every month completed.

CHAPTER 8
APRIL – LEARNING THE HARSH REALITY OF EXTREMES

Celebrations for each donation.

Celebrations for each new donor for DKMS Africa.

Celebrations for each book that would help children learn to read.

Celebrations for a home to become someone's new castle.

For the first time this year, the moon rose in total darkness. It justified my previous decisions to watch it from halfway down. I can't imagine climbing down in such darkness – torch or no torch!

My brain couldn't fathom what I'd achieved to date – but my legs could, the fatigue was becoming more noticeable with each climb. I wondered how the next third would progress, it could possibly be the toughest 123 days all year. Only time would tell.

I'd also soon learn that the next few months would become some of the hardest of my life.

April Stats:

120 / 365

People Joined: 50 / 218

12 days 14 hours 1 minute 28 seconds / 820km / 23 equivalent Everest Summits / 58 solo climbs (51,7%) / 23 Up & Down

(19,2%) TOTAL DONATIONS: R175 683.71

Kym & Karl: "Wow look at these donations!!! Keep going!"

Chris: "Keep it up. Keep posting your beautiful pics. Will hopefully do one with you."

Melanie: "Super well done on 100 climbs Andrew, wishing you everything of the best for today and loads of Mana (strength) for the next 100." NZ

Not all storms come to disrupt your life, some come to clear the path
~~ Unknown

CHAPTER 9
MAY – THE POWER OF PERSPECTIVE

The sun's migration continued. I watched keenly as it rose and set further north each day creating a lower arc across the sky. This meant cooler days with the option of midday climbs; a welcomed mental relief as I juggled winter's approaching storms. The mountain was changing. The weather was changing. I was changing. To avoid climbing in the dark, I could no longer start before the morning traffic. This made life easier for those joining me. Previously, I had to wake up at the crack of sparrows to navigate the insane city traffic.

After a week of early climbs in temperate weather, Sunday's climb was at 15:30 with Page. She was introduced to us by Tamzyn who'd been visiting us from America. There was plenty of time to reach the summit and catch the final car down, or so I thought. I learned a valuable lesson about paying closer attention to detail, which was a gift that, in the future, would prevent me from overlooking things in worse conditions. With hardly anyone else climbing, we enjoyed a slower summit. The overcast conditions created the perfect lighting for Page to immortalise her memories of Climb 126.

CHAPTER 9
MAY - THE POWER OF PERSPECTIVE

My calmness was shattered when I heard a dreaded sound close to Ubuntu rock.

The siren....

Then the PANIC kicked in!

The siren only goes off when they warn people the wind is picking up and they'll be shutting down, or as a reminder that the last car down for the day would be in 30 minutes.

It was 17:30. I had made a rookie error. I thought the last car moved from 19:30 to 19:00 from April to May, but I was wrong, it moved to 18:00. Now we were between a rock and a hard place! Miss that car, and we'd have to climb back down in the dark. Not something a novice would enjoy, even though I had torches for us. I subtly picked up the pace, embarrassed about my gaff and reluctant to cause Page unnecessary stress. *Maybe we could make it.*

Finally on the top, we walked briskly – we were cutting it fine. An empty mountain wasn't a good sign either. The upper cable car photo was the quickest so far. Then, as we got closer, my eyes were blessed with the most glorious sight ever: a queue snaking out of the upper station. A queue! I never expected to be this happy to see one in my life. Usually, this painful sight signalled at least an hour-long wait, maybe two. Today looked like 30 minutes. We might have made it in time, but my misjudgment denied her the opportunity to leisurely enjoy the vistas.

The queue was a get-out-of-jail card, and I suggested I wait in the line, showing her the loop to walk around to get the best of the western and southern views. The queue gave me time to reflect on how lucky we were to have made it.

I couldn't afford mistakes like this in the future, especially with our first major storm arriving the following day. I messaged her when I was 10 minutes from the front (roughly two cable car trips or 130 people). It's one of only three cable cars in the world with a rotating floor. Engelberg, Switzerland, and Palm

Springs, USA, have the other two. I chuckled every time visitors rushed to the windows for the 'best' views, only for the floor to start rotating as we set off. It was ingenious because it allowed everyone to enjoy an incredible 360 view in one trip. Flying high above the India Venster route, you often saw climbers slowly making their way up or down.

Page's luck turned into Mark's misfortune. The storms were forecast to make landfall in the afternoon, so we both opted for a dry, but blustery cold morning climb.

Climb 127 had an added layer of uniqueness for me. Mark was part of a group celebrating a friend's 30th in Gansbaai back in 2017. That was my first weekend as a 'free man' from corporate life. Alone up the mountain, he took me through his side of the experience, from hearing about my idea, to witnessing my discipline to training each morning on our weekend away at Eagles Nest in the mountains of MacGregor until today, becoming climber 229. It's not often I get to hear a perspective like this, especially his honest feedback on his initial feelings. He wasn't convinced this would pan out – but watching it unfold, he finally saw the complete puzzle instead of just one piece. The conversation reminded me of how I decided to take on this challenge even if no one supported me because I knew a full year would allow me to build trust and demonstrate the impact of each investment.

The conversation with Mark was more powerful than he realised because I was still battling self-doubt issues, demons, and insecurities about my ability to build support and raise as much money as possible. Although high school was a different challenge to this, the same insecurities around being accepted had manifested. Hearing him candidly share his mind's journey about my idea put a crack in my negative belief system. And it was also enough to encourage some action for the next week.

Mark's willingness to endure a down climb was rewarded. I introduced him to the pyramid, where he helped me move week 18's rocks across.

CHAPTER 9
MAY – THE POWER OF PERSPECTIVE

They carry added weight with some valuable lessons learned:
1. There was no room for error.
2. Trust the process in others as much as within.

That trust was injected with purpose by the first use of funds with DKMS Africa. The plan was always to distribute them throughout the year as soon as they accumulated to a significant amount for the various charities. I arrived at opportunity #1.

Hitting R100k in April, I coordinated with Virginia, who promptly swung into action, putting a donor drive together at N1 City Mall. Incredibly too, 'The Hit 30' show on Goodhope FM was broadcasting live to amplify awareness.

With such a diverse ethnic population, South Africa has added pressure to find willing donors in each segment for potential matches with patients. Registered nurses were on site to draw blood and immediately put new donors into the system. In an anonymized form, the laboratory analysed tissue types and added people's details to DKMS Africa, partnered with DKMS's stem cell registry. The process was a costly exercise and not something every donor could afford, and it's where fundraising came in to remove the barrier to becoming a donor. Their details would then be part of blood stem cell donor searches for people worldwide who needed a genetic match to get a second chance at life. Research showed that the genomic variances between people of African descent were greater than those observed between European populations. This genetic diversity in African populations posed practical challenges for the transplantation medical community to find HLA-matched unrelated donors for patients in need of life-saving stem cell transplants.

Meeting a survivor at my previous corporate company's year-end function completely blew my mind as a donor and fundraiser. She had been clear for five years, and her donor had come from Germany. Interestingly, only 25% of positive matches usually happened within families, and as in her case, the other 75% came from strangers. Genetically, the likelihood of finding a suitable unrelated matched donor was considerably greater within the same ethnic background.

It was humbling and inspiring to feel her gratitude for having a second chance. I considered myself fortunate as first-hand experiences demonstrated the impact what giving had on another's life. Without it, I wasn't sure I'd have the stamina to keep climbing.

After Climb 132, I was greeted by a sea of radiant DKMS Africa staff smiles. I was introduced to Mariska, a leukaemia survivor, who also lent her support to attract more donors. Her story was invaluable because it allowed prospective donors to see the impact they could have. 100% of donations received cover the costs of adding new donors, which were *R3 000 per test. Donors were asked to contribute what they could to this expense, but the fundraising efforts primarily covered the full cost or shortfall. At the end of the day, 15 new people signed up. I hoped they'd be a match and give someone already desperately waiting for a second chance. *R3,000 was the amount to add per person to the registry in 2018.

Week 20 was a rollercoaster of emotions. Firstly, Francoise, my kinesiologist, made a beautiful contribution and emailed her entire client contact list, inviting them to get involved. An action that took a few minutes but made a massive impact and added another brick of gratitude to my challenge.

Habitat for Humanity had their climb the next day, which became an emotional one as news of their ex-colleague's death reached them before we started. Sadly, Sue had lost her ten-year battle with cancer. Felicity had planned to catch the cable car up to meet us, but distraught with the news, she felt compelled to climb in her honour. She'd never done the climb, but her determination, coupled with our guidance, got her safely to the top in about 4 hours.

Tears were shed, anecdotes shared, and respect was paid to a woman who left this world a little better than how she'd found it. Climbing together in a shared purpose for a common goal created a richer experience for us to develop our relationship. I witnessed their incredible inner strength and heard how Felicity worked her way out of the townships and empowered others with opportunities to do the same.

On the climb, I was profoundly struck by the depth of our conversations, and by the fact that some of the staff were moving on ahead. Remaining behind helped lead me to an epiphany about patience. How many times have you wished for more patience? Or heard someone call out for it? My understanding of patience was impacted in my 20s when I heard someone say, 'If you ask for patience, God will send you opportunities to practise it.' Patience is an action. It's not something we wait for, it's something we build. Like asking for a house and continually getting bricks.

It felt like I wanted patience to reduce my stress for a better quality of life. Yet it wasn't the lack of stress that helped, it was the depth of these conversations with Felicity and Lea that did. **Therein lay the epiphany: Impatience would've robbed me of an opportunity to learn.**

I could easily have pushed on with the others, but something tells me I wouldn't have had the epiphany or even written about it now. Instead of fixating on the summit, this experience layered on top of all my others, teaching me a valuable lesson. I was learning to embrace the process and practise patience inwards. Patience was the gatekeeper to **amplified meaningful experiences by which to grow.**

More time on the mountain meant more time to explore the landscape. I started seeing faces in the cliffs; first, an open-mouthed skull stuck out. Later, a Mayan mask appeared above him, and then the Wicked Witch of the West (ironically on the west wall!) with her mouth agape cackling away. She even had a wart on her nose! 136 climbs it took, and now I had three faces keeping me company on my solo climbs. Patience, I was learning rapidly, was one of the greatest teachers of all.

Sarah, a journalist, and avid hiker herself, joined Habitat thanks to an introduction through my cousin Charles, an editor for a major publication in Johannesburg. She'd been taking pictures and keenly talking to the various staff members. It was wonderful for her to meet the people the funds were being collected for.

In a video on the summit, Lea shared her love of mountains and even greeted the mountain, "Hello you beauty," as she drove up. I learned something new too, as she shared Habitat's ethos on teaching people to take ownership of their lives. Habitat does this through skills development and knowledge, assisting people to become confident in their abilities to improve themselves, their future, and their families. Habitat resonates with people's hearts. Their patience is demonstrated every day, every year, as they tirelessly invest time into each person they support. I'm profoundly grateful to partner with them and excited to see how many lives we can change together.

Their money will take longer to accumulate sufficiently to build a home – but it's worth the wait.

A skiing accident back in 2004 taught me a valuable lesson about being careful with my words. I wanted to say, 'I plan on skiing all day, as much as possible, until I'm tired. So tired they'll have to push me around Geneva airport in a wheelchair.' What came out was, 'I'm going to ski so hard; they're going to have to wheel me through Geneva airport in a wheelchair.' That wish was fulfilled when I almost broke my leg and incurred a hematoma. I never ever ever ever EVER say things like, 'What more could go wrong?' I'm not about to poke fate in the ribs like that!

I genuinely wished to see a rockfall on the mountain — but from a safe distance. See what a difference that extra wording makes?

My friend Stefan met two tourists from Belgium, Alec and Sarah, while on holiday up the Garden route. Hearing their desire to climb the mountain, he naturally connected us. I was blessed that my friends acted as ambassadors and sent people my way to become part of the Ubuntu Family.

CHAPTER 9
MAY – THE POWER OF PERSPECTIVE

On calm days like these, I took new summiteers to a favourite spot on the west side of the plateau. It was a tiny rocky outcrop the size of a medium dining room table that required a step over an intimidating crack. Dropping away on three sides, it was to be avoided on windy days. Peering over its edge gave us a magnificent view of Platteklip – all the way from the contour path snaking its way up to the final section through Stairway to Heaven. It is a dramatic view to behold if you don't fear heights.

Peering over the edge today, though, brought a fearsome sight: white rocks littered amongst a boulder field. The splintered rocks lying around the impact point looked like tiny fragments, but some of those original boulders were bigger than a fridge – a shudder went down my spine thinking about what could've happened if they hadn't stopped in that boulder field. I saw evidence of how a smaller rock fall decimated the path just a few turns below.

When did this happen??? I wondered. At least this week.

Alone on Friday, I desperately tried to see what it looked like from the path while passing the boulder field. The path bent away, making it almost impossible to see without bundu bashing through the thick fynbos. I decided against veering off the path and chose rather to get the pictures up top. It must've been at least a three-second free fall, maybe four. I'd often wondered what I'd do if confronted with a rockfall, knowing that on Table Mountain, they'd already killed and injured people.

My dinner plans for that night were postponed. Chantelle had mumps, the disease that, at age five, took away the rest of what little hearing I had in my left ear. I kept that information to myself when I responded to Chantelle. Mumps is highly contagious, so she was housebound for at least a week. I'd had six solo climbs since Mark joined and was contemplating how exhausting self-doubt was. These daily climbs up Platteklip Gorge forced me to confront them with real exhaustion. I wished I had another paragraph to say how I easily overcame it, but I was battling to let go of the debilitating negative beliefs that kept creeping up.

Even after 138 successful climbs, I was still thinking, 'okay maybe I'll be taken seriously when........', and always thinking of 'what if's.' I was tired of constantly battling and following the thoughts that popped into my head, and I decided to perform a symbolic ceremony to release my negative thoughts. I asked my trusted friend Linda for advice. She suggested burning a black candle, representing all the past and negative attachments, followed by burning a white candle, representing an end to those patterns and welcoming a new future.

I firmly believe we can train our minds and take control of our lives. Looking back now, I realise how that ceremony should've been one of self-love. I should've asked myself a more important question: *Why am I not as patient with myself as I am with others?* Because I was trying to force an outcome again, and I was allowing my brain to attach meaning to the number of people we want to help. After the donor drive and the Habitats climb the past week, the reality was I desperately wanted to raise the money I dreamed of. I had another vivid dream, this time clearly showing me the total: R6.8 million. My bruised ego calculated how far away I was: only 2.9% raised. Ouch....

Nevertheless, hindsight is a beautiful thing. I still believed I was doing something 'wrong'. My old companion of self-doubt was what was holding me back. My kinesiologist, Francoise, had been instrumental in helping me release trauma from my cells passed down through our lineage. Consciously, we can work towards a desired outcome, but subconsciously, we'll fight it and destroy the very thing we want. It's no use writing down something a million times or saying it if you don't believe and feel it deep down. Simply put by Lao Tzu, your destiny is shaped by your character, which is shaped by your habits, which in turn are shaped by your actions, shaped by your words – which all come from a thought. I was fascinated by our complex nature, and the more I learned about what affected our daily lives, the more I realised how little I know.

I decided to act on my intuition on the mountain and started the ceremony later that evening. It was time to step into my power within. I had a 37-page document Linda gave me when she painted my soul portrait in 2016, the introduction

CHAPTER 9
MAY - THE POWER OF PERSPECTIVE

from which our friendship blossomed. Soul portraits are one of Linda's many gifts to the world, tapping into your energy through your name and birth date to create a painting around your essence, gifts, and lessons to embrace. My painting hangs in the middle of my lounge – two sets of eyes staring directly at me: The Eagle at the top of my totem and the bear. I chose these two aspects of my painting to re-read as part of my ceremony.

As I started reading about my Eagle, my eye caught the heading "Raven's Feather." – I read this, too, as I often saw crows gliding on the thermals high above me while climbing. While not entirely the same animal – it stirred me enough to read its significance.

Shamans know the power of an unexpected piercing sound in shifting consciousness. Ravens have this power, giving out varied sounds, and can assist us in shifting our consciousness into various dimensional realms. Ravens represent transformational energy, revealing to us how to rid ourselves of our inner fears. Ravens will show you how to go within yourself, into the dark areas, and then illuminate them, making you 'sparkle' and bringing out your true self. Inner conflicts should then be resolved, however long buried they are, this is the deepest healing. Raven awakens the energy of magic, linking it to our will and intention.

My phone vibrated to life; and I was dumbfounded by the message from a friend in Blouberg across Table Bay.

Table Mountain's on fire again!

I looked at the candles in disbelief. *What are the odds???*

'Reports' of arsonists started circulating as it intensified and rapidly spread across the front face of the mountain. The crazy timing of the fourth fire for the year was not lost on me.

My 5 am start the next day was to join a high school friend, Gerhard, for school rugby out in Stellenbosch. Kyle, his son, was at Paul Roos, one of the oldest schools in the country, and they were playing Paarl Boys High in a rivalry that stretched back more than a hundred years, which was reminiscent of our rivalry at King Edward VII School (KES) in Johannesburg against Jeppe.

With sunrise still two hours away, it may as well have been midnight, eerily creating the perfect canvas for the fire still raging on the front face. Lines of orange flames seemed to hang as though attached to an invisible kite. It had been burning for almost eight hours. Would I be able to climb Platteklip Gorge? Currently, three people were on standby to join me. I needed to message them about the potential route change and decide which one to do.

The morning was a great distraction, enjoying schoolboy rugby while Gerhard and I reminisced about our time at KES. The first team game was mid-morning, and Paul Roos pummelled their opponents 44-8 in a shock upset. Thankfully, I was the passenger on the drive back. My phone buzzed with activity, checking in with Safety Mountain tracking about the fire, while updating my potential climbers on the possibility of climbing India Venster as my first choice. If the fires blocked that route too, then we'd revisit the pipe track and up via Kasteelspoort.

Chantelle and Gerhard had been a great support, donating and checking in with me, so with her awake and Safety Mountain tracking's message that the fire was under control, it meant I didn't have to rush off and had an opportunity to chat with her. Platteklip was 'open for business,' and it was perfect timing. She made me promise not to laugh before I walked in about her puffy cheeks. At least her spirits were up a bit. I couldn't stay too long, being past 2 pm already, so I changed into my gear and left. A high layer of dark cloud blotted out the sun, and the thin wisps of smoke still rose out of the gorge directly in front of me as I drove back from their home. One by one, the people joining dropped off. It became my 67th solo climb out of 139.

The charred mountainside high above was already visible as I walked along the road from the lower cable station. It was burned all the way to the top. I

CHAPTER 9
MAY - THE POWER OF PERSPECTIVE

had no idea what to expect. I knew the fynbos needed fire, but I couldn't help feeling a sense of sadness at the destruction. It was at least 40 years since it last burned on Platteklip, so it desperately needed this fire for its ongoing cycle of regeneration. I mulled over last night's candle ceremony. I had focused on imagining the flames only burning to ash whatever didn't serve me. This would allow new empowering growth to rise from the ash. Just as the fynbos seed remained and used the ash as nourishment to grow.

It was the fourth fire in five months, and as fire trucks whizzed past me, I wondered what the path's new makeover would look like. My gratitude ritual included Platteklip being open to climb, my weary legs made sure to include it! Passing my sister's rock, I was just a couple zig zags from the base of Ascension Corner, and already the air was thick with char. I was completely unprepared for what I saw next - puffs of dust surrounding deep scratches and cracks on the path. Another rockfall. *It must've been caused by the fire, no doubt.*

A chill ran down my spine while climbing Ascension Corner, that first puff of dust became one of about eight on the steep vertical section. Had this been during the day, anyone on the path would've been in bad shape with nowhere to hide. I didn't discount that the fire could cause more rockfalls - so no music today. My ear was on high alert for boulders careening down the mountainside. One thing about climbing every day is you know a route intricately well, and halfway up this steep section, one step had been cracked wide open. The immense power of the boulder hurtling down in the cover of darkness clearly showed no mercy. Can you imagine the noise this must have made?

The next corner revealed another crime scene, trees on either side of the path looked as though they'd been brutally assaulted. How many boulders came careening down the hillside? A few steps on hundreds of tiny shards of rock littered an exposed boulder. Clearly, one of the rocks smashed into it. One piece was big though, about the size of a handheld vacuum. It looked like an ancient rock tool carved with the top rounded and the bottom pointed. One side showed the weathered walls of the boulder contrasting against the newly cracked open white rock inside. Inspecting it closely, I could see each speck that, in time, would become grains of sand. It was wild to think this mountain was made of trillions upon trillions of tiny pieces like this, compressed together thanks to millions of years of pressure.

Mangled fences, used to keep hikers on the path and not take shortcuts, joined the scarred terrain. More splintered trees. More dust. I couldn't help but analyse the debris like a detective hot on a serial killer's trail. Two things were still a mystery – where did this start, and where on earth did it stop?! The rockfall spanned a wide path down the mountain. The evidence provided a welcome distraction from my screaming legs. Truthfully, I was mesmerised. Halfway rock had its own horrors, a sizeable crack coated in about ten dinner plates worth of dust. I thought this was where an original large boulder split and created smaller ones, giving birth to new assassins terrorising the mountain below. I selected a hand-sized chard as rock 139, thin and flattish – one side was weathered while the other was clean. Less than thirty paces up the path from the halfway rock, it appeared some culprits didn't get away, two boulders and another jagged piece lay handcuffed on the path. In my head, where they lay was exactly where I'd dive for cover, hoping the slope above would be enough for the motoring boulders to fly over me. Clearly, I'd have been wrong. Would I even know what the noise was or where it was coming from?

I'd climbed close to 100 vertical metres since the first puffs of dust, and I still wasn't even at the fire source. There were six more switchbacks before I could see the ash I'd been smelling. The mountainside had an avalanche of ash that had cascaded down from the top of Guardian Corner, almost a perfect line framed the bottom. The sky above suddenly filled with the ominous sounds of crows. Too many to count but it could easily have been 60. Alone, I experienced this incredible sight and sound of crows diving and circling. The thick smell of ash dominated my senses. Yet again, the fire happened on a day with minimal wind.

Steadily, I made my way up between the cliffs and arrived at where the fire started. The ash still smouldered next to the path. The mountainside where the 'avalanche' stopped lower down was treacherous and next to impossible to reach during the day, never mind at night, with nothing but a headlamp. Something didn't seem right about an arsonist starting the fire there. The gorge was like a tale of two cities – the destitute left side: completely burnt, black, and 'destroyed.' The opulent right-hand side: green, lush, and teaming with bush, grass, and life. The contrast was hauntingly beautiful, the left side naked and bare, revealing every rock and gully previously hidden for decades. The higher I got, the more revealing the devastation was. Smaller rocks became hot coals, and with no underbrush stopping them, fell below starting the next wave of fires.

I took a moment to sit on Ubuntu Rock, watching the crows and reflecting on how quickly things changed. I was eager to re-read about the significance of the crow feather on my portrait because this 'coincidence' was surreal. It would have meant something to me even if there was one crow. Considering I'd never seen more than six or seven flying together previously, this many certainly had my attention. Eventually, I placed stone 139 and continued to the top.

Running into one of the fire marshals allowed me to ask if the perpetrator had been caught, seeing as there was only one way up or down Platteklip. Surely, they'd caught him.

"It wasn't an arsonist. It was started by a rockfall."

It was hard to believe, but the mountain had been doing this for millennia. Fun fact – The cliffs of Table Mountain are receding at a rate of ten metres every million years. Questions from later groups asked whether wind or rain played a part in this fire. Neither. Nothing abnormal happened leading up to that day, except that I'd spotted another rockfall and had taken pictures of it the day before! Gravity simply won a small battle against the mountain.

The mountain is a living, breathing organism. Rocks heat up and expand during the day while cooling down and contracting at night. A microscopic version of breathing – but breathing, nonetheless. Mix in erosion and the plant root systems' constant exploring of cracks to seek out nutrients and strengthen the plants against the insane winds experienced in summer, and you have a perfect recipe for rock falls. Then throw in a three-year drought, and the tiniest spark is like a kid let loose in a candy store. Life doesn't stop because we modernise the slopes below the mountains. Again, the proximity to the city belies the wild nature of this quiet giant.

The biggest storms of winter haven't even arrived yet. I wondered what would happen now that large sections of steep mountainside lay exposed and with nothing holding the top together. There could be many more rock falls or even mudslides on the way. I began to think my earphone-wearing days on solo climbs were over. I couldn't take the risk. I may not be able to get out of the way of falling debris, but I sure as hell would have a better chance if I heard something happen before it appeared in front of me.

I was forced to reconcile my need to constantly multitask or cram in as many activities into a time slot as possible without truly experiencing one of them wholeheartedly. Like climbing up Table Mountain. The point should be to experience nature for all its value with all my senses. Listening to the sounds, experiencing our surroundings and enjoying life in action, feeling connected to everything happening around us. Listening to music for the rest of the year would've robbed me of that experience. Who knows what else I'd already missed? At first, I felt music helped pump me up to get me moving up the mountain; but all I was doing was missing out on hearing all the different birds chirping. I felt like the fire smacked me across the face and woke me up to what I'd been missing out on.

My next four climbs were all gloomy and overcast, so another lesson from nature was quite unexpected. I'd already been given tiny gifts, like watching flowers bloom, only to vanish three days later. I enjoyed witnessing these subtle changes that only a daily practice could bring. This was highlighted on climb 143. Sjnólaug, a woman I met while travelling in Iceland, was in town with her friend and had been watching my adventure. While in Austria with Carl and Maddy, her sister

CHAPTER 9
MAY - THE POWER OF PERSPECTIVE

Kordula, went to school for a brief stint in America with Sjnólaug's sister, Iris. It was a treat interacting with locals in Iceland, so I'd snap up any chance for an introduction. This was how I met Sjnólaug. I loved learning directly from locals about their culture and history. Incredibly, Sjnólaug had spent three months in South Africa already and loved it so much that she drove her family crazy about her desire to come back. And here she was 18 months later.

Unfortunately, the misty and cold weather persisted. An incoming storm hit us with a vicious wind at the top. No rain at least meant a safer climb back down, my 27th already. We laughed at the top as I showed them my photo from Saturday on the viewing deck. They got their phones out and took a photo of my photo, a perfect way to sum up their experience.

The biggest, unexpected treat was that nature and fynbos had sneakily planned a surprise party, and the mountainside became alive with freshly bloomed Nitida Proteas. The beauty was an infusion of yellow and luminous green with some earthy streaks of rock and soil. It had fine, almost tentacle-like, petals radiating around its nectar-filled centre. It looked as if touching the centre would cause it to close like a Venus fly trap. The bees hadn't wasted any time working furiously between all the thin petals. It was a grave reminder of the mountain's missing bugs.

It was wonderful to see the bees working their magic, but bizarre how my mind played games, and it made me wonder if I'd missed them the previous days. Today was just a snapshot in time for the people walking past and witnessing the stage the flowers were at. One might even be so inclined to think they were blooming on time while the buds were in fact slower than usual. Fast forward a month, and those early bloomers would turn black as they died.

Walking past at any particular moment was very different to day one of blooming, one could easily point out, 'these died quickly, these are perfect, and these were too slow', but that's just a snapshot. Nature's bigger picture doesn't care about first, second, or last. It's all in perfect harmony doing exactly what it needs to do, when it's needed for those that need it. Like watching a symphony. This is such a perfect metaphor for us humans. Just because some learn or grow faster than others, it doesn't make them better or worse. It depends on what snapshot you're looking at. The real picture can only be observed when everything's viewed in its entirety, then we see the magic. Everything blooms when it's supposed to, and it all works together. Imagine if all these flowers bloomed in one go with an oversupply of nectar for the bees and sunflower birds, and then had nothing afterwards?

Secondly, it didn't matter that all the flowers had access to the same nutrients, climate, water, and sunlight – they still grew at different rates. They all had equal access to those ingredients. Imagine what the mountainside would look like if the flowers were plagued by the same inconsistencies we have: less sunlight (opportunity), Water (toilets), climate (education & jobs), and nutrients (homes). Everyone's on their own journey. There's no right or wrong way – we can just do our best with the above ingredients to shape our future. Maybe society would move further along if we focused on the ingredients instead of the results? Or maybe I was falling into the trap again – and each of us (the flowers) was being given exactly what we needed, when we needed to bloom.

Our first severe storm hit us the very next day. Torrential downpours all day meant no escape, and I'd be able to test out my new kit from K-Way. Waterproof pants, a new pair of waterproof shoes, and gloves. I decided on a 14:30 start to avoid the worst part of the storm and allow myself to see waterfalls. It's amazing what a difference having dry legs and non-squelching shoes can make – I already had my eye on the next prize: a waterproof backpack to keep extra warm goodies like gloves, beanies, and extra jackets dry. I was feeling blessed; thanks to Allan for following through on his idea and the owners of Cape Union Mart for supporting me personally.

I could certainly use some of LA Barista's coffee at the top. The icy wind felt like thousands of pinpricks on my exposed cheeks. Climbing up in extreme cold was negated by the exertion needed to climb. Of course, that rapidly changed

CHAPTER 9
MAY – THE POWER OF PERSPECTIVE

once I stopped at the top, my core temperature dropped dramatically. This was a potential risk, especially if I needed to climb back down, which on days like these was more likely. Exposed on the summit, the wind sliced through me, keeping my core temperature low. Usually, as soon as rain started falling, I'd put on everything I was carrying underneath my rain jacket to keep it dry. No point in carrying wet clothes! Today, I wore everything and just kept my torch and some water in my bag. My layers included a long sleeve compression top under a T-shirt, a warm jacket, a rain jacket, a cap, and two sets of gloves (tight ones and ski gloves in case it got extra cold). I was learning to improve my heat retention by adding layers two corners before I reached the top instead of on top in the wind. I learned that the hard way after taking my rain jacket off exposed to the wind, no amount of rushing to get a jacket underneath helped me get warm again. The damage had been done. I froze along the top and the entire climb back down.

It was my second time completely alone up and down on the mountain. Three hours of solitude. It allowed me to think about when the indigenous Khoisan lived here, and I might've been one of the boys alone up here completing my right of passage – minus the manicured path and clothes.

My shoes and pants changed the experience of wet and cold conditions and taught me yet another valuable lesson:

There's no such thing as bad weather – just bad preparation.

Climbing down in wet conditions was possibly the most dangerous of all for me. With all my weight transferred to the leg that searched for the step below, one slip could end in disastrous consequences. I'd seen the most experienced climbers slip, so I was acutely aware there was no room for error or time to zone out. I realised how important my barefoot climbs had been. Their unintended consequence of heightened awareness was invaluable for days like this. I had visions of me tripping and falling in certain places too, which made me pay more attention to the mountain and forced me to take extra time stepping down sideways, a far safer way to fall than backwards.

On my way back down, I was excited to explore a new route. On the contour path, I'd usually turn left, but now I was turning right towards Devil's Peak. Since my idea to climb every day, I knew one of my benefits would be days like today – an opportunity to experience the waterfalls on the mountain up close. I knew they were in full force because even from afar, I could see the white water cascading down like a seasoned sculptor carving deeper to create its masterpiece. One such waterfall was called Silverstream. I'd heard stories about it, which motivated me to take this route today.

The eastern table acted as its shepherd, herding the rain drops down its slopes into the gorge below, forcing millions of litres of water down the mountain. A great man, Dave Irish from Mr Suits, had sponsored me with a GoPro, and this was the perfect opportunity to test it out, especially as the water gushed all around me. The loud roar was music to my ears, knowing our thirsty dams were getting their fill!

Unsure of how far Silverstream was from the intersection, at the start of my climb, I decided to explore after summit 144 and then turned right into uncharted territory. With no earphones blaring music, I was amazed at the constant sound of water cascading down from one layer to the next. It was even more prominent between the cliffs as it fell hundreds of metres, echoing and creating an aura of peace. I promised myself that I'd enjoy these moments to the absolute maximum. While most label these days as 'horrible' – I focused on them being a new experience I wouldn't have had indoors sitting on my couch.

Considering our hectic drought, I was irked by the fact that the local government had still not implemented plans to collect this water. The mountain made it no secret as to how it gets to the ocean and even provided one handy collection point further down the mountain.

The rumble of the water tickled my ear. I was completely unprepared for the scale, though, as the waterfall emerged around the corner out of the mist... It was magnificent! It reminded me of the amazing waterfalls I'd been privileged

CHAPTER 9
MAY – THE POWER OF PERSPECTIVE

to see in Iceland and Yosemite. This ranked right up there with them. I was filled with awe, wonder, respect, and a healthy dose of fear. The cascading water sprayed mist, soaking me. I was mesmerised. I could've sat there for hours if it wasn't for the approaching sunset. Carefully studying the raging torrent, I navigated the contour path without getting my feet soaked. To my left, the view transformed as the late sun streamed through a gap in the clouds, lighting up the mountain and raindrops, creating diamonds. I kept heading east along the contour path to see the other three rivers in full force.

The first river cut through the March fire zone, and since my last trip to this side of the mountain was in December, it was a welcomed change of scenery. Turning around, I had the perfect angle, looking up at Platteklip. It had only been a couple of months since the March fire, and yet the fire-ravaged landscape was bursting with life again, not quite completely green, but a far healthier colour than a few weeks ago. Rain, rainbows, and sunlight followed me, the perfect end to a memorable and wet climb. My heart was warm, knowing this kind of flow was happening, pushing out the dreaded 'Day Zero.'

After an extra hour enjoying the vastly different scenery, I headed back along Tafelberg Road to my car. Some boulders had dislodged and rolled down the mountain and came to rest on the road. A massive one had crossed the road and rested against the wire fence, while others were strewn across the road. I moved them into the gutter and out of the way of any cars using the road.

Could this year get any better?!

I didn't have to wait long for that question to be answered, even though I was battling the demons of 'not doing enough' having 'just' 14 donors in May. The most destructive thought was always, *'Maybe when I hit x number of climbs... then they'll donate?'*

There was no 'when'; I just needed to keep doing what I was doing, exercise patience, and a little more self-love!

I had two special guests for Climb 145.

Compared to yesterday's storm, the day's gorgeous sunshine made me feel like I was in a time warp, and yesterday's climb was months ago. I remember zipping through the city streets on my way to pick Elliot up at the train station, feeling empowered by the sunshine and guests joining me. Elliot was one of three security guards in our building; their rotating shifts were brutal - two days on, two nights on, two days off. Repeat. I'd been in my building seven years and, having worked security desks in London, knew what it was like to be looked down on and ignored as people walked past. That experience taught me about the impact of a simple smile and greeting. Elliot rang my buzzer in March, thrilled to see my photo in the newspaper but stunned to read what I was doing.

'Is this you???' He asked, bewildered.

Bear in mind he'd never been up Table Mountain. We needed to change this.

'When are you joining me?' I asked.

'When I have a day off, I'll join you.' He replied earnestly.

There are complexities that living in a township brings; it's not as simple as saying, 'I'm starting at 8 am'. That means he'd have to get up at 3 am to stand in line for a taxi for an hour to the train station into town and then another taxi, possibly two more, to get to the cable station. When I say taxi, it's not what you see in Europe or America, where individuals ride. These mini-buses hold up to 15-20 people at a time. Elliot was so grateful and excited he dismissed the stress of the early start and said he'd be in town whenever I needed him there.

The day had arrived, and I collected him in town outside the train station around 8:30 am and then drove us to the lower cable station to meet Lifa, special guest number two. Lifa was in Cape Town receiving treatment at the Sports Science Institute. He'd had a tragic accident during a rugby game in June 2017 that left him with a broken neck. He had to learn how to walk again — a much bigger mountain to climb. Lifa heard about me through *The Chris Burger*

CHAPTER 9
MAY - THE POWER OF PERSPECTIVE

Petro Jackson Players' Fund, a company helping sportsmen like him and their families on the journey of adapting to a "new normal." They work hard to uplift and encourage injured athletes to focus on their abilities as they reintegrate into their communities.

I had met several employees at an event with the *Sustainable Development Network*, and knowing my story, they shared it with him after he expressed his desire to climb Table Mountain. He connected with me on Facebook and shared his story and desire to climb Table Mountain with me. A Durban native, he'd been in Cape Town for three months to tackle a gruelling physiotherapy schedule.

I entertained his wish only because he successfully climbed up and down Lions Head — with the aid of crutches and his friends — back on April 12th. Ubuntu is about community and I'm yet to deny someone with 'you can't join.' This was no different. In fact, I was honoured when people chose to participate, no matter their fitness.

Reaching Tafelberg Road, Elliot's excitement bubbled over, his generous and warm face lit up with that all too familiar smile I'd come to love.

"I've never even been this high before."

A gentle reminder of how something as simple as this, still hadn't been experienced by many. Not knowing what to expect, I suggested a 7 am start to Lifa to provide enough time to reach the top safely. With his final physical therapy session that morning, he'd only be able to make it around 10:30 a.m. I had no idea what to expect or how this would play out, so I agreed, having learned to relinquish expectations for each climb.

The minute he stepped out of the Uber, a tremendous smile radiated off his face. For me, a smile that would come to define the essence of the human spirit.

In May, the last cable car down was 6:00 pm; it was the only thing we needed to beat. As usual, we met at the lower cable station, the 2km walk along the road, and the 'warm up' to the climb. Seeing Lifa walking with his crutches made me question whether we were doing the right thing today by walking on the road.

"We don't have to walk across – I can drive us to the start if you like?" I said skeptically.

"How far is it?" He asked.

"It's 2km."

"No – I'm good – I wanna do it the way you usually do it."

"You sure? It's no problem to drive us."

"I'm sure."

Spending time every day in nature sharpened my intuition – and listening to it showed me how it was never wrong. Just the past week, on my ninth barefoot climb, I sat down to rest my feet on one of the exposed portions of a rock that had fallen and cracked open during the fire. About fifteen minutes from the top, I felt an urge to put on my shoes. As I tied my second shoelace, it started raining. I remember laughing at the insane perfection of the timing. I decided to always trust my gut, and taking on this climb with Lifa was no different.

I've walked on crutches, I know the pain you experience in your hands, forearms, back, and shoulders.

"Are you in any pain??" I asked.

"No, I'm good," He responded as he smiled.

I expressed my admiration at his tenacity as sweat dripped from his forehead. The flat walk allowed us to learn about him and his experience. Wildly, our two life-changing events were barely 24 hours apart. My retrenchment was on June 30th, and his injury had occurred the previous day.

I thought about everything I'd gone through to get to this point, including the 144 successive climbs, switching to everything he'd been through to get here

CHAPTER 9
MAY - THE POWER OF PERSPECTIVE

– just 329 days later. His herculean effort was poles apart from mine. He'd spent months in hospital, was told he'd never walk again, felt every spectrum of emotion, decided no one would tell him whether he would walk again or not; found support, learned to sit, stand, and now walk with crutches – and finally had chosen to climb with me.

One road bend away from arriving at the start of the climb, I felt uneasy and questioned whether to leave out the section in my gratitude prayer about having 'strong legs that work.' I decided to leave it in. I shared my gratitude prayer as Elliot and Lifa listened intently, smiling and nodding their heads approvingly. I felt a lump in my throat as I was about to express my gratitude for my legs, and instead of the uneasiness I thought I'd experience, Lifa pursed his lips and nodded in agreement at me.

We had no standard climb, so we took some time to briefly plan our attack; I'd start at the front, walking backward to help pull Lifa up while Elliot positioned himself behind as a safety net should he lose balance and fall backward. That nugget of wisdom came from being on crutches in London in 2004, walking up stairs I lost my balance and started the scary fall backward. Thankfully, a saviour was sitting at the bottom of the stairs and was watching me. He leapt up and caught me in time, and I've never been more grateful I wasn't alone. We wouldn't make that mistake with Lifa and had him covered from step one.

Finally, we set off. The glorious sunshine made us sweat more than usual. Our slow and steady climbing meant it was the 8th time this year I'd heard the noon gun blasting while on the mountain. Since 1806, the firing of the cannon has been a historic time signal in Cape Town. It consists of a pair of black powder Dutch naval guns, fired alternatingly with one serving as a backup. The guns are situated on Signal Hill, close to the city centre. That day, the boom sent powerful shock waves through the city, but I was so focused on Lifa, I didn't even hear it.

What are easy steps to climb on Platteklip for most, were a challenge for Lifa. The larger steps required all three of us to work as a team to haul him up. Because of some nerve damage, Lifa had an ankle support on one leg to keep his foot from dangling when he lifted it. Lifa's smile continued to belie pain barriers I could never comprehend, and he always acknowledged the wishes of support from people walking past us coming back down or starting.

Team Lifa was making steady progress! The first section was tough, but by no means was it the toughest of the climb. We reached the first waterfall, still flowing strongly, although nothing compared to the day before.

It was just past 13:00. We hoisted Lifa up the toughest section of the mountain, and after such extreme effort, it was the perfect place to catch our breaths. Seeing 13:00 on my watch though, jolted me.

As I did the numbers, I got that sinking feeling. We had five hours left to get to the upper cable car and we'd taken an hour to reach the first waterfall. A guesstimate told me we'd take another six hours simply to reach the top of Platteklip. I based this calculation on the fact that we were now 1/7th of the way up. We were not going to make it. So, sitting enjoying the view of Cape Town bathed in gorgeous sunshine, I re-calculated repeatedly, hoping I was wrong. I had to make the single hardest decision of the year, and I broke the news to Lifa and Elliot.

"I have some bad news. At this rate we're not going to make it. Judging by the time it took us to get here and the distance ahead – we'll miss the cable car by two hours."

I took the safety and health of everyone climbing with me seriously. There was no point in going any further, knowing it would jeopardise Lifa's safety on the treacherous climb back down. When you are tired, fatigue hits the brain. And when the brain has a lapse in concentration, accidents happen. For twenty minutes, Lifa sat devastated, trying to come to terms with the news, pleading that he'd go faster and take fewer breaks. But we both knew that wouldn't work.

CHAPTER 9
MAY - THE POWER OF PERSPECTIVE

The truth is, we needed to start earlier to make it. If we had, Lifa would've made it.

Being in his presence, seeing his effort, felt like watching someone climb Everest without oxygen. I let him know it wasn't because of capabilities, it was because of time. I hated giving him news that seemed to dampen his spirits, especially since he may have placed enormous importance on getting to the top of Table Mountain. Lifa's effort showed me where his future was headed.

Reason prevailed, and we began to climb back down. Tired and hot, more effort was required on my part as I kept him from toppling down and each step reinforced I'd made the right decision. As the three of us edged down in silence, I had two choices: let Lifa stew in his disappointment – or challenge it.

I chose the latter.

Knowing we had at least an hour until we reached the road again, I believed we could help him process his feelings. I asked him what he'd share about his experience, knowing he was mentally stuck on not reaching the top. He needed to know the difference between not making it up due to planning versus physical abilities. So, we spoke it out and reframed his disappointment. We turned it into an accomplishment to be proud of.

Elliot, too, had been a true champion, his face a constant picture of calm with a beaming smile. And his patience was exemplary – especially for someone who's never climbed Table Mountain. His time would come though, on another landmark day.

"Andrew... remember you asked if my shoulders were sore on the road walking here?" Asked Lifa

"I certainly do."

"Well, I lied, they were already hurting when you asked me."

That meant he finished the 2km walk and he climbed for an hour, fully focussed on reaching the top with all that pain. Now, I was an even bigger fan and grateful for the time together. His story is important and was by far the most popular with future groups. His message of what's possible when we challenge our circumstances head on, is just the beginning of his impact on the world to come.

Our climb was wrapped up, and as we made our way along the road, I realised how unnecessary it was to keep walking, so I suggested we call an Uber to whisk him away.

"You've earned that drink sir." I told Lifa.

"*I think it's going to be more than one!*" He responded as he smiled and disappeared with his lift home.

Elliot and I felt a surge of admiration as Lifa drove away.

"Elliot – I can't thank you enough for your patience and help."

"*No worries Andrew – I'm glad I could be here to help.*"

"Ready to give it another go?" I asked.

"*Actually, it's getting late now, I need to get back home please.*"

Knowing his disappointment, I replied... "Sorry we didn't get you to the top today."

"*I'm here Andrew – I'll have another opportunity on another day off.*" He said, beaming his trademark smile.

With that, we walked back to the car, drove to the station and I waved him goodbye before driving straight back to the mountain.

Back on the road and ready to start it all over again gave me a sense of Déjà vu. Round two kicked off at 15:00, and Lifa's efforts were forever imprinted in my soul and escalated my level of appreciation for my able legs that were strong enough to do this daily. He'd be shared with the groups to come, all 115 of them, over the 220 days ahead.

CHAPTER 9
MAY - THE POWER OF PERSPECTIVE

Walking up face first again, I marvelled at what he'd accomplished barely an hour earlier on exhausted shoulders. This was a sobering reminder to be grateful for all I had. And even as my mind came up with excuses, I returned to the fact that Lifa had just demolished a monumental obstacle. I passed the rock he sat on as we convinced him we needed to head back down and realised its significance — so I named it Lifa's Rock to honour his accomplishment.

Reaching the top, I was rewarded with one of my best pictures from the viewing deck. Not a cloud in the sky. The sun's journey north meant it was low enough to be included in the photo. Its golden trail lit the ocean perfectly and aligned with the front edge of the cable station. I was filled with immense gratitude and began to think about the next day's climb with Business Matters. Thankfully, it was only due to start at 14:00, a beautiful opportunity to crash and sleep like a log tonight.

Lifa had some profound words about his experience:

"In 2018 I had the privilege of getting into contact with Andrew Patterson after hearing he had been hiking up Table Mountain every day for 365 days to raise funds for different charity organisations. Needless to say - I was blown away by his initiative and determination to help others, and this inspired me to join him on his next hike up the mountain. Now is a great time to mention, at that point, it had been 11 months since the day I'd injured my spinal cord playing rugby in Durban. My doctors told me I may never walk again, but, after intense Physio sessions and sheer grit, I began to walk with the aid of crutches.

A few weeks prior to my meeting with Andrew I had hiked up Lions Head with a group of friends and supporters I had met in Cape Town. I was tired, but eager to push the envelope - I knew joining Andrew on one of his hikes would help me fulfil my desire to go further.

As the saying goes - The first few steps up the mountain are the hardest. I knew I would have some difficulty, but I really underestimated the path. We hiked and crawled and shuffled up the mountain. The point came when Andrew realised, we probably wouldn't get to the top before the cable car closes, and hiking down would be far too dangerous in the dark. Although I was disappointed at the prospect of not reaching my goal to push my own physical boundaries, I felt a deep sense of respect for Andrew for his efforts to give so much of himself for the benefit of others. This encouraged me to broaden my goals to include helping others transition into living with disabilities, and of course I was determined to return to conquer the entire Table Mountain feat.

A year later, in November 2019 I returned to Cape Town stronger, fitter, and even more relentless. I had upgraded from walking with the aid of crutches to hiking poles — which was coincidentally better suited to help get me up Table Mountain. The Gorge route was just as difficult as I could remember, but, this time, I'd left myself no option but to reach the top. Again - I walked, crawled, and shuffled my way up the mountain. With each level of difficulty - I remembered my first hike with Andrew and it gave me the encouragement I needed to power forward. My ascent to the peak brought with it nostalgic thoughts of my personal journey - going from an energetic rugby player; being injured, vulnerable and scared; battling into my transition as a person living with quadriplegia; to now growing in strength, passion, and confidence.

I reached the top with a deep sense of gratitude at the realisation that we all have our mountains to climb. We may not be able to climb them as quickly as we'd like, but we always have it in us to do so if we just allow ourselves to try again.

Lifa.

I told you he'd make it to the top! I was over the moon when my sister forwarded this post to me. I respect people taking on tough challenges that would push them outside their comfort zones. I was inspired by people who returned to conquer what was left undone. Lifa is a real hero that we can all learn from. Just his final paragraph alone speaks volumes to his character. I hope it inspires you to take your first step toward a goal you've been putting off.

No days off were starting to grab my attention and reminded me of my Platteklip Charity Challenge event six years earlier — Five summits over 7 hours and 33 minutes, a total assault on my legs. But Lifa's perseverance yesterday gave me the gift of perspective. Even though my legs felt battered, I was deeply inspired and grateful because I knew he would give anything to feel this pain in his legs again and take this climb on. Any rumblings of self-pity and internal complaints were quickly vaporised. He'd single-handedly injected his perspective into my focused attention, reminding me of what was important and pushing me to get through the next 220 days.

The following day brought another first...

I was always grateful for the group climbs, and the support garnered from all the work I put in both on and off the mountain. And although it wasn't a year of 9-5, it was starting to feel like I was always on and grinding. Recording data for statistics, networking, taking photos, social media, interviews, media, and meetings with partners for team building, organising and appropriately allocating funds for each organisation required as much perseverance as climbing the mountain.

It was difficult to put a specific donation value to the impact of each conversation touchpoint. Still, I knew more money came from networking and sharing my story in front of people than all the media and online coverage combined. Going into this challenge, I knew that as simple as the idea to donate R1 per climb was, people only got involved when it resonated. People were more likely to contribute if their hearts were touched or if they experienced relatable challenges.

Exhibit A: the children from Amoyo.

Finally, Climb 146 with Business Matters rolled around! It was my first group joining from a networking event where I shared my journey over their Friday breakfast session. Roy coordinated the group's climb and donated on their behalf. They were the first group to do so. It was a brilliant experience, and the first time I shared Lifa's grit and determination with a group.

'This is Lifa's rock. A reminder to me of the human spirit in action.'

All 14 were in awe and complete appreciation of his effort.

The group had a wide range of fitness levels, but we kept moving steadily up the mountain. Our next break was on the contour path, and my clock-watching the previous day had made me extra vigilant for today's climb – especially for a late afternoon climb. It wasn't just about getting up safely, but ensuring everyone made it to the upper cable station by 18:00. The time on my phone said 15:20, not terrible, but late enough to be concerned. But after covering just four more switchbacks in 24 minutes, that sinking feeling from yesterday returned. At this rate, we weren't going to make it.

For the second time in two days, I headed to the back and made an executive decision. Explaining the difficulty of the situation, I suggested the struggling pair walk back down to the contour path and keep on it to enjoy the splendid views instead of using the road to the lower cable station. The path under the cable cars would be their final climb down. I could sense the disappointment, but in truth, there were still 219 climbs left to try again with me. I re-joined the group and explained what had happened. And if anyone was concerned about the time remaining, they could turn back too. Everyone was good, and by keeping a decent pace we'd be able to reach the top with half an hour to spare.

Another journalist joined us, tracking behind me, and after paying close attention to my feet, commented how they seemed to glide up, as though they'd become one with the mountain. An interesting observation considering just that week, I'd realised what a difference sound had on my physiology. I noticed my steps seemed louder, so I placed them more intentionally and quietly. Almost immediately, the climb felt 'easier' as though my feet were somehow lighter. The quietness profoundly affected my psyche and tricked my body into feeling lighter, thus enabling me to glide up.

CHAPTER 9
MAY – THE POWER OF PERSPECTIVE

Applying the same thing day after day, step after step, in a heightened state of awareness and gratitude, allowed me to learn these deeper truths and improved my performance on the spot. And instead of complaining about my daily experience, I was looking for the valuable tools hidden in challenges. I knew they'd help me up my next mountain. Like writing this book, I could slouch over and feel tired, or I could sit up straight and tell my body I was still energised, even after eight hours of writing.

Just four climbs later though, the end of May arrived like a prelim exam for winter. Climb 150 on May 30th was shrouded in misty weather, so instead of taking on a different route for the milestone, it was back to Platteklip. Cape Union Mart did a great job of promoting it to get people to join, but only two showed up. Something I'd become accustomed to when weather like this hit.

While hiking, one of the ladies posed a question I was sure many people would feel.

'It's been 24 years since Apartheid ended – can't we just move on?'

This simple sentence led us into an intense discussion. She shared how her husband started with nothing but had built a successful company. It was easy to hear an anecdote like this and assume his process would produce the same result for everyone. I understood that. My idyllic younger self saw things in black and white. Too young to understand nuance, circumstances, history, and other factors. I kept learning about the two big gaps in my knowledge: I don't know what I don't know; and I do know what I don't know. I can demonstrate the latter by saying I don't know what injustices from apartheid kept people back. Even though 24 years sounds like a long time, that could mean different things depending on which side of injustice you're on.

I think privilege is associated with 'came easy to you' – I see it as a fortunate set of circumstances that empowered me to be where I am. Just as meeting an idol of mine would draw the phrase 'it's a privilege to meet you.' I highly recommend reading Malcolm Gladwell's book 'Outliers.' He does a wonderful job of explaining how influential circumstances have helped shape men like Bill

Gates. It doesn't take anything away from the fact that he still applied himself and did the work – it simply shows that without access to opportunity, the same diligent behaviour and work might not have produced the same result.

To be honest, I butchered my answer to her. It triggered me in a way I wish it hadn't. However, it showed me I hadn't developed the deeper understanding I have now. The truth is that the way I dismissed her question was exactly the way she dismissed people still living in shacks. Reducing someone's circumstances to being the result of actions like laziness is, in fact, laziness on our part. It tells us not to be supportive because the onus is on the 'lazy' person to empower themselves. At university, I failed Accountancy, and my lecturer phoned my mother and told her it was because I was lazy. My mom laughed at her, 'You clearly don't know my son, it's not because he's lazy.'

She was right. I'm the type of person who needs someone to show me how to solve complex issues. Once I understand how the principle works – I'm up and running. I enrolled in introductory basic accountancy courses for six months, learning what most do at school. I went back the following year and passed.

Poverty and inequality are too complex to break down here. My aim isn't to solve the issue... it's just to do my best to rally us towards empowering others while instilling the understanding that success isn't guaranteed just because you have the opportunity. Just look at the many examples of children from the same family where one becomes successful and the other struggles. These issues demand more respect from our questions, thinking, and time. It's so complex that it hasn't been sorted out in the 24 years since apartheid ended, and continuing to ask that question (or dismissing it in my case) keeps us from engaging around the problem and hashing out solutions.

Almost three hours later, we squeaked into the cable car in the nick of time – and thanks to the 'miserable' weather, there were no queues. As we descended out of the clouds, I hoped my lifetime would bring a time when our collective minds would descend out of the fog of separateness into the clarity of supporting one another.

CHAPTER 9
MAY - THE POWER OF PERSPECTIVE

I was exhausted when I got home. Mentally drained, physically beat, emotionally holding on, and spiritually committed. Sarah, the journalist who joined Habitats climb, had confirmed she would join me the next morning. I had decided that only experienced hikers with the correct gear could join me when storms came through.

'There's another storm moving through. Going to be cold and wet – do you have rain gear?' I asked.

'I certainly do, and I love the rain.'

'Guess I'll see you at 8 am at Platteklip – the cable car won't be running.'

For the first time this year, I overslept. I hated the panicked feeling I got when it happened; particularly when it affected someone else. I woke up five minutes before I was due to arrive. I apologised profusely over the phone, and she very kindly waved it off, stating:

'I'll start up slowly and wait for you, I've got Salvador and Precious with me.'

Precious is from Malawi, and Salvador is a gorgeous black Alsatian that may as well be a wolf.

Thankfully, it was only a twenty-minute drive and Sarah happened to be running late too. In my head they were already halfway as I started. The weather was miserable, low clouds hugged the cliffs, but the fresh puddles from the earlier burst of rain highlighted my gratitude to start dry as I got out of the car and messaged Safety Mountain tracking. I'd become good at slipping into training mode, 'resigning' myself to my 30th climb back down.

I'd finally reached a full month's worth of climbs back down.

Not wanting to keep Sarah waiting and unprepared to run into them just after the contour path, I pushed harder than normal. I whipped off my jacket as the sweat poured from my face. I was trying not to drench my jacket internally

199

because I knew it would be at least 10 degrees (about 50 degrees Fahrenheit) colder at the top.

Sarah and Precious were talking to two men in jeans carrying a plastic bag when I reached them. I later heard from Sarah the bag had beer in it, and they reeked of booze. I knew they were tourists, and thought they'd simply misjudged the day to climb, realised their mistake, and were now on their way down safely.

Wrong! They picked up their bag to follow us.

'You're not going back down?' I asked?

'No, we'll follow you,' one of them replied.

'You know it's going to be far colder up top – what other jackets do you have?'

'None – but we'll be fine.'

I shook my head in disbelief and started up. Salvador was in doggy heaven and bounded up ahead of us. In less than ten minutes, the temperature dropped significantly enough to make me stop and put my warm jacket on – Sarah and Precious did the same. Just before Ascension Corner, there's an exceptionally massive rock that, if it were a meteor, would've decimated a continent. Okay, maybe it wasn't that big, just a solid granite delivery van.

As we reached the mammoth stone, the drizzle arrived, accompanying the wind, so I immediately stopped again to put my rain jacket over my warm one. Mr tourist sat down under the safety of the big rock, nicely sheltered from the rain but with the most forlorn look on his face. He was no longer having fun.

'It's only going to get colder and wetter the further we go. This is the last time I'm stopping. I'm doing this every day for the whole year and I'm not putting it in jeopardy for you by stopping every time you get tired, especially when I've told you to go back down. You're not dressed for this, you're not prepared. Your best option is to go back down. I'm not waiting again.'

It was ludicrous that it took hearing 'I'm doing this every day for a year' supported by Sarah for the 'credibility' to take me seriously. Hypothermia isn't a joke. It can hit you in under ten minutes, especially when you're already wet with a cold wind blowing on you.

It blows my mind that people explore mountains with no clue as to what they're heading into and without any preparation. Again – the mountain's proximity to the city is a blessing – and a curse.

He dropped his head. I reiterated while putting my backpack on and zipping up.

'I'm not waiting for you. I strongly suggest you head back down.'

Eventually, he nodded meekly in agreement and said,

'Okay, we'll head back down.'

Salvador treated it like a summer's day on the beach, zooming all over the mountain, probably doing the equivalent of three summits, while us mere mortals pushed against the cold biting wind and rain. I still didn't have a waterproof bag, but I was grateful for my shoes and pants, which held up and took all the hits. Up top, Salvador continued to zoom around like a cartoon dog, hardly touching the ground. *Where the hell was his energy coming from??*

My hands were so cold that my iPhone's screen didn't recognise my finger. I had to get my 4th consecutive topside photo of grey mist with Sarah's phone. We were soaked to the bone! Thankfully, the following day's forecast was clear, so I could use my old shoes and leave the wet ones in the sun to dry.

Climb 151 was a test for what was to come. Mental health would take centre stage. It was hard to stop my brain rushing into future mode, thinking, 'Oh my god what if the next 100 days are like this?' Climbing back down while the rain pelted us, I turned my head to protect my cheeks and kept repeating... 'one day at a time, step by step by step.'

May finished with climber 276, 277, and a dog! I created new friends, new experiences to breed new perspectives and gained new insights that would help me prepare for some of my toughest challenges yet. The challenges of weather and life were about to dramatically ramp up, my roller coaster banking sharply down into loops towards the halfway mark.

Use the first half of the year as training for the second half of the year!

Halfway? That was still 32 climbs away.

MAY STATS: 151 / 365

People Joined: 59 / 277

16 days 4 hours 43 minute 22 seconds / 1029,65 km / 29,38 equivalent Everest Summits /

71 solo climbs (51,7%) / 30 Up & Down (19,2%) TOTAL DONATIONS: R206 436.86

Nicolene: "Thank you for living the ubuntu spirit & may the support keep on rolling in to help you push beyond your goal(s) !!!"

Francoise: "Spread the love"

Kirsty: "It's not how long or how you get there, but did you enjoy the journey?"

> *Everything will be okay in the end. If it's not okay, it's not the end*
> *~~ John Lennon*

CHAPTER 10
JUNE – THE IMPORTANCE OF MENTAL WELL-BEING

Mental fatigue was starting to become an issue and began to impact the concentration I had available for each step. I was physically exhausted; the weather was grinding me down and my mental health was becoming a little bit shaky. Apart from the accident, the rescue, and the graffiti, I hadn't been tested too much on this front. I also hadn't really thought about the end of this journey and my world post 365 Ubuntu Climbs. I was doing everything I could to stay present and focused on today.

June's climb launched with Charlotte, a new friend who had come into my life thanks to an introduction from Bronwyn. In 162 days, she walked a path across South Africa in the shape of a heart, raising money and awareness for charities. It's crazy to think that was 10 days away from my June 11th. With just the two of us on a clear and icy Friday afternoon, we discussed the vulnerability of being alone on long challenges. She spoke candidly about the difficulties of not being 'supported' as much as she would've liked and the difficulty she had with her transition after finishing. I appreciated her honesty with these extremely personal stories, and it got me thinking about my finish line. It didn't remove me from my day-to-day focus – but rather planted a seed that enabled me to think about how I'd look back on the year – hopefully, with no regrets.

The understanding that it would all end eventually, together with my daily gratitude practice, was what kept me grounded. I was already getting questions about what I was going to do when it was all over, which I purposefully deflected. I had a long way to go. It was a balancing act of appreciating what I'd completed and dissolving the stress of what was still to come. I had to be aware of potential problems like depression, and I had to spend time on the mountain contemplating how it could happen to me and how I could avoid it. It would eventually lead to one of my greatest lessons.

Of course, hindsight is a wonderful thing, and while I couldn't appreciate how perfect the timing of my messenger was, I saw the importance, knowing June would become the most challenging month of all. When the student is ready, the master appears! In June, a barrage of storms hammer the Cape while the daily temperatures drop consistently to single figures (Celsius). The climbing window hovers around 10 hours for the month as the winter solstice brings the shortest day of the year – just 9 hours and 53 minutes long.

Five months of mental training was about to be tested. My two and a half hours with Charlotte was the perfect 'warm up', and prepared my mind to stay razor sharp.

Love our Trails, in conjunction with K-Way, sponsored a Platteklip clean-up, and brought materials to clean the graffiti that remained. The empty parking lot on wet days was a reminder that my character would be tested, but it would be worth it. It was a gloomy, cold wet day, but 16 of us, together with SANParks rangers pushed on. Once again, Karel, my coach, showed his true colours and joined as part of the clean-up crew.

It's hard not to harp on about this, but the litter on Platteklip was disgusting. I can't believe human beings can be so callous in such beautiful surroundings. I put this down to a greater societal issue: A lack of respect. If you don't respect yourself, you won't have respect for your home and those who share it with you. As painful as it was to see the mountain in such a poor state every day, I had a choice; I could let it anger me – or I could do something about it.

I chose the latter and every climb, I picked up whatever I could that would fit into a plastic shopping bag. The usual suspects were tissues, cigarette butts, plastic bottles and plastic caps. That was just on the path, and filled the bag to 99% even before I reached halfway. This day was different though, we moved off the path to pick up everything, which amounted to a dozen or so full-sized rubbish bags worth of trash. It breaks my heart thinking about all the sad people tossing rubbish as if it means nothing. I hope they find some light in their darkness and reconnect with both the amazing human beings they truly are, and the gift that is our home.

Blake had an expensive graffiti remover all the way from the States to help with the cleanup. Armed with wire brushes, we vigorously worked to remove the graffiti. *Sending you love buddy.*

There were gale-force winds higher up, so the long hours on the mountain were rewarded with a climb back down. It took us about three hours to pick up rubbish, clean graffiti methodically, and reach the same rock where Mr Tourist turned back around just two days ago. The bags were full, and the drizzle started to intensify. Blake joined me as I continued up for summit #153, carrying all the supplies and continuing our 'off the beaten track' cleanup.

Blake started *Love Our Trails* when he decided to organise his first clean-up on Platteklip after being disheartened by all the trash. His initiative has now grown to make an even bigger impact as he builds relationships with SANParks and the government to provide safe, clean trails around the country. I was eternally grateful it was just the two of us as he spoke about the environmental conference he enjoyed on his recent trip to Japan. He had also just come back from another conference in Johannesburg with luminaries such as Thuli Madonsela – a former Public Protector. The most interesting nugget was how everyone spoke openly about their privilege. It wasn't mandated – it just happened organically. This was important to me because of how the word 'privilege' caused most people to become defensive. Blake tried to put his own privilege into perspective by arranging to stay on top of Table Mountain in one of the huts in January for a week. He did this to simulate township living: no electricity or running water, and added travel time with increased difficulty to get to work in Century City. He had to trail run down the mountain to get to a car park, where the bike he used to get to work was chained up. He also couldn't use his cell phone for that week. This experiment gave him a deeper understanding of how other people lived, and it helped him look at his privilege in a new way. It wasn't a gimmick, he used that knowledge to improve the lives of others, and I was proud to have him as climber #279.

We had two bags filled with rubbish as we began our descent. People's reactions to seeing the bags were always inspiring, especially if I was on my own and my arms were filled with all types of plastic bottles. I hoped that this got the perpetrators to stop doing it and that it encouraged more people to do their part. Whenever I feel disheartened by all the troubles in the world, this example gives me hope. While it takes many people to trash the mountain – just one person can make a difference cleaning it up. People offered me bags for the bottles under my arms, but I preferred them to see just how much crap was dropped. The bottles also acted as mini bins to shove smaller wrappers, cigarette buts, and dry tissues in. It also created some heart-warming moments as children would tap me on the leg, handing me a piece of rubber or plastic that I'd missed. Another seed planted. The cutest by far, was a little boy who loudly asked his dad what I was doing.

Then I hit the jackpot after some ponce left a Pringles can on the trail – the wide mouth of the tin was the perfect solution to the small neck of a plastic bottle problem. Especially for those damned tissues! Sadly, the only days I didn't see any trash was on an early morning climb after being the last person up the night before.

I have angry days where I feel the shock factor needs to be dialled up. I dream of emptying trash over the first few stairs, forcing people to acknowledge it and walk in it. *Is this what you want the path to become? Please keep all your trash and throw it away in bins provided at the top.* Imagine the difference it would make if everyone on Earth just decided to use a trash can for every piece of trash? Imagine how clean the world would be.

The fire cleared the vegetation and made it easier to spot trash, it was an eerie walk through the burned sections, seeing plastic bottles contorted and fried. It was like a rabbit hole, I'd see trash and head over to pick it up, then I'd find another three pieces along the way, and when I reached those, more would appear ahead of me.

Blake is an inspirational doer, it's wonderful to learn from one of South Africa's true leaders who shares this philosophy: stop blaming or waiting for the government to sort problems out and get stuck in.

That doesn't mean we don't hold them accountable, it means we just have to stop using their misgivings as an excuse to give up.

With engaging conversation and hard work removing graffiti, the six hours flew by, and it was already mid-afternoon when we hit the road again. My heart was happy, my soul aligned, and my mind expanded. Even though I was feeling good about my mental health, discussions about it were far from over.

Radio interviews took the lead for awareness of 365 Ubuntu Climbs. I'd become accustomed to DJs or radio personalities paying lip service to what I was doing by inviting others to participate. My response... *'I look forward to hosting you on a climb.'* Only two had followed through though. Eunice from *Tafelberg Radio* and Sara-Jayne Makwala King, an author with an incredible story (I highly recommend reading *Killing Karoline*) and a talk show host on *CapeTalk Radio*. SJ joined climb 158 with Nigel, a friend of mine originally from the UK. Although SJ was born in South Africa, she was adopted in the UK.

Nigel had been a long-time supporter of my cycle rides, and now, these climbs. SJ had just joined the Ubuntu family. Since first interviewing me in May, she regularly checked in for updates and invited me to the studio for deeper discussions into the 'why.' I appreciated her directness. On air, she spoke frankly about being unfit and that it would take a long time. I explained how many climbs I'd done with varying fitness levels. She trusted me and followed through on her promise.

On the mountain, she shared details about her childhood and the trauma she experienced, which raised the topic of anxiety. They both had experience with it, and I was confronted with how little I knew about it.

What are the first things that come to mind when I ask you to name issues related to health and wellness? 'Wellness', in my experience, focuses on the physical. It's interesting that early on in training, I realised the challenge of my mental game would be tougher than the physical aspect.

SJ articulated the difference between depression and anxiety beautifully.

'Anxiety is a result of stress, caused from apprehension or fear about things in the future. Depression is the constant stress about an experience in the past.'

I appreciated learning with her on the mountain. She surprised herself and earned some bragging rights as we reached the summit in under two hours. And although some curse words were flung my way, it was her look of satisfaction and achievement that still lives with me. Little did I know this conversation would prepare me to confront the harsh reality of both anxiety and depression.

Two days later, on Saturday morning, I woke up to several missed calls from Astrid. Something was wrong. I knew it. I sat staring at the phone, mustering up the courage to phone back, and then it rang again.

CHAPTER 10
JUNE – THE IMPORTANCE OF MENTAL WELL-BEING

"Andrew, I have some terrible news."

A dread-filled feeling of helplessness washed over me.

"Josh committed suicide last night."

5 Months Earlier

Josh lost his wife Roxanne to complications with prescription drugs earlier in January. 2018 had given him an insurmountable challenge. His soul mate literally died in his arms. I couldn't begin to imagine the pain. He flew her body back from Australia to be with her family in Cape Town, a place they both loved. This was where he met Astrid. Full of compassion and heart, he understood his return to Australia would be tough, as 'normal' life resumed. Dark times and hours would come. Being eight hours behind meant that while friends in Australia slept, we in South Africa were awake to talk. He'd instantly shared one of my videos Astrid sent him and had been checking in on my project.

He was one of the most vociferous supporters, racking up big interest from down under. As an air steward for Virgin Australia, he was sharing my climbs with passengers. Thanks to modern communication, we were able to chat via video and get to know each other across the big Indian pond. An incredibly kind and dynamic man, the enthusiasm and passion he exuded was inspiring. We spoke at length about Roxanne and relationships, and he always seemed upbeat about the future, connecting dots on business opportunities to build them globally through his network. I questioned him that it didn't seem 'normal' to keep having such inspiring days. Almost daily, I woke up to messages about his inspired ideas, like when he met a café owner and wanted to help expand her business, which included feeding the homeless. Or when he discussed the use of drones to help his uncle in Mozambique combat elephant poachers. He was even in talks with a professional golfer he knew to host a golf day in support of 365 Ubuntu Climbs.

I didn't think his constant upbeat highs were sustainable or 'normal,' but then again, I had no frame of reference of what he was like before Roxanne's death. Who was I to question how someone dealt with their traumatic experience? I wasn't alone though. A lot of us felt that and questioned him about it. He always acknowledged and addressed us the same way – assuring us he was good.

Not being in his presence was hard, but we tried to provide support as best we could. June rolled around, and he was dealt another tragic blow. A colleague of his committed suicide. A man that had been a rock of support and who was present for him during his own grief, was now gone. Josh's daily climb was given more weight, and it pulled him down every waking moment.

Hindsight and 'what more could we have done' will always plague those of us who remain behind, but I believe not seeking professional advice after Roxanne's passing contributed to his eventual suicide. I wish he'd sought professional help. Taking that step helped me deal with the robbery situation I experienced and helped me gain peace of mind.

Earlier that week, he'd received his honorary special edition 365 Ubuntu Climbs shirt commemorating 100 successful climbs in a row – 10th April 2018. It fitted perfectly, and he was excited to wear it on his first hike in Los Angeles. The smile on his face in the mirror as he took the picture made me incredibly happy. His message underneath read:

'Fits perfectly my friend thank you, I'm gonna go find a mountain that does it justice and take a picture!'

After my climb with SJ and Nigel, Josh and I spoke late Thursday night into Friday morning until, eventually I had to say goodbye to go to bed. His excitement boiled over about successfully listing Sealand, a Cape Town brand, into one of Australia's largest department stores. Their website described them as *innovators in upcycling, which is the practice of creating a usable product from waste or unwanted items or adapting existing spent materials in some way that's useful, creative, and adds value. The essence of upcycling is the reduction*

CHAPTER 10
JUNE - THE IMPORTANCE OF MENTAL WELL-BEING

of waste through the prolongation of the use of its properties, thus achieving efficiency gains in resource use. Their website is www.sealandgear.com

The conversation ended with him discussing a Cape Town climbing trip with friends and to visit us. I couldn't wait to finally meet him in person. That was my final message to him before I went to sleep. His response... *'Man it's going to be epic.'*

How quickly things change. I had a distressed message from a mutual friend, Virginia, in Florida. She'd been up all night talking to him because he'd used the phrase 'going to end it' - or something to that effect that scared her. I immediately phoned him. No answer. I hastily sent a message, eventually getting a reply, but his tone was completely different from the energy and excitement of the night before. He told me that he needed to get out of the house. The pain lingering there must have been taking its toll. I only had a couple of hours before meeting Lisa for climb #159, and he isn't answering my calls. Also, his text messages were flat and full of despair. The feeling of helplessness was awful. I called Astrid to share what was happening, and she promised to keep me updated while I was on the mountain.

Both Astrid and Claire had a spare room in Cape Town, and we wanted to provide him with a safe space to heal and find a way to move on despite the pain. He was dejected and broken. For the first time, we saw the pain behind the mask. He assured me he was okay one last time before I left for my climb. All extremely worried, we did our best to surround him in a cocoon of support and love to 'sit' with him and ensure he didn't feel alone.

He'd sent me three screenshots via messenger, which I could only read when I was on my laptop after my climb. That turned out to be too late. I was on the mountain with Lisa. Her 18th summit turned into a gift for my weary legs as she gave them a much-needed leg massage - one of her many talents that she and her business partner, Bianca, turned into a business called Massage in Motion.

I received Josh's screenshots moments before he died. To this day, I don't know what he was trying to express with them. Why hadn't he sent it via WhatsApp? I opened my last message to him checking in…

"Hey buddy, how are you holding up?"

One grey tick. Not delivered. Not read.

At the beginning of the year, my 'confinement' to Cape Town had made me wonder about death. Especially with friends and family who were a two-hour flight away in Johannesburg. Death is a natural part of life, and none of us are exempt from it. I'd never met Josh in person, nor could I thank him in person for sharing my journey with passengers on his flights to and from LA and for trying to promote it to Richard Branson. Josh was back with his soul mate, and with the heavy rain, it felt as though Cape Town was weeping too. I'd fallen asleep nestled on the couch at a friend's house, while the night's fire kept the room toasty warm. The rain was scheduled till around 14:00 the next day, with gaps later in the afternoon. The plan was to start at 15:00. This would become my hardest day to leave home.

In one of the toughest conversations of my life, Josh's mom, Susan, called me. My heart broke for her. Tears flowed listening to the final conversation she had with her son on the phone moments before it happened. All I could do was offer my sincerest condolences and any help she needed, even from far away. It felt so hollow to say all of this because nothing was going to bring him back. The toughest moment came when she thanked me for the way I'd helped him over his last few months. *If only I could've done more.*

The driving wind and rain poured down in buckets outside. It was a welcomed relief for our drought-stricken region, but added to the complexity of just getting out the door. I just wanted to curl up in bed. Thankfully, once again, the timing of a guest was just what I needed. My dear friend Andrew was an avid fan of being in the mountains and doing physical activity, and we'd shared many hikes and climbs together. He committed to joining me rain or shine. He

CHAPTER 10
JUNE - THE IMPORTANCE OF MENTAL WELL-BEING

later shared how close he came to postponing. If he had, I'm not sure I would've left the house.

Lately, he'd been battling fatigue and health issues, which prevented him from going to the gym, nevermind attempting the strenuous climb up Table Mountain. I didn't know this at the time, but such was his commitment to supporting me, that he decided today was the day, and he wouldn't let the storm stop him. Our relationship had become strained as they can when people go through their own experiences and don't communicate it effectively. Thankfully, we corrected our mistake. Writing this, I realise how important it was that he made it, he had been my shepherd and helped get me out of the house to do one of the toughest climbs of my life.

Not thinking clearly, I left my rain pants at home, believing the 'minimal' rain forecast. Well, I was quickly educated that when a small amount of rain was predicted for that hour – it could fall over the whole hour in a fine light mist – or a serious downpour in two minutes. Today was the latter, and Andrew had no rain gear! I was in shorts. It was a miserable start, getting absolutely soaked. Waterproof shoes? Well, the shorts on my legs acted as gutters, so they may as well have been flippers as water ran down my legs into the shoes. We trudged to halfway, and almost at the top of Ascension Corner, Andrew's heart was racing dangerously. His body wasn't out of the woods yet, so we agreed he should head back down.

As I continued alone in despair, colder, wetter, and windier conditions waited for me up top, and it would be the 32nd time I'd have to climb back down, alone with my thoughts. Replaying the last 24 hours over and over. I was numb everywhere, inside and out. All alone at the top. There was no whoop of excitement for another successful summit, only driving wind throwing the stinging rain into my face. In winter, the wind came from the northwest directly off the ocean – making my walk to the cable station and viewing deck for my photo miserable. I had to drop my head to shield my face. I usually enjoyed the days walking around alone at the top, but not today. I plodded on to the viewing deck, and battled the cold to get a picture of 'view' #160. Not even the cable station was visible. Walking back to Platteklip, the wind shepherded me back. There was no one on my way back down.

It's a weird space to be in when your body and mind want to get back to the sanctity and warmth of the fire, but you just don't have the push in you. Cold to the bone, I was grateful to make it back down seven minutes after sunset. Climbs like these were often followed by Josh checking in to see how it had gone. This time, it was just a teary message to Safety Mountain tracking.

'Safely off the mountain – thanks for watching over me.'

Sunday

In true rookie style, I left my boots too close to the fire, the smell of burning fibre wafted into the air as one of the ankle supports burnt. Branded as a solemn reminder for the rest of the year. Even after an all-nighter next to the fire – my shoes were still too wet, forcing me to use my old weathered boots. I wasn't sure how I was going to cope with 10 people scheduled today. Maybe I'd be lucky, and they'd all cancel? I didn't feel like explaining or talking about what I was feeling. I had, however, decided to always be honest in answering the question of how I was doing. Amazingly, I was spared as no one asked the question today.

Yesterday's downpour provided an awesome opportunity to witness the power of Silverstream Waterfall. I changed our route to take advantage of all the water still gushing off the mountain. We started up India Venster, heading directly under the cable cars to the contour path. Everyone loved seeing all the water, which I'm sure was a symptom of being starved of it through the drought. All six rivers were still in full flow, including the gorgeous Union Gorge River, which flowed overhead like a curtain of water obscuring the view as the path cut into the mountain like a mini cave. Too beautiful for words.

CHAPTER 10
JUNE - THE IMPORTANCE OF MENTAL WELL-BEING

Josh and I shared a love of eagles, and magically, for only the second time this year and the closest I'd ever experienced it, a rock kestrel soared above me with its wings easily capturing the breeze to glide above us.

It was amazing how often the very thing I didn't want, ended up being the very thing that would help me. Priscilla and Tracy's energy and delight at finally climbing the mountain energised me. They'd followed through on their promise to climb after hearing me at a networking event in May, and they brought some friends with them. Thanks to DKMS Africa, it was also an opportunity for me to meet Ray, another Leukaemia survivor. His energy and zest for life reminded me who these climbs were for. His gratitude and appreciation for life was heightened to another level. We spent almost four hours on the mountain together, completing week 23. Having started 15 hours after yesterday's climb, my legs were screaming for a relaxing afternoon on the couch. My heart, head, and legs were all aching in unison.

My next two climbs were solo climbs, and with Monday being the 11th – became my 10th barefoot climb of the year. During training, I'd named a massive rock at the top of Ascension Corner 'lean on me' rock – because of how I'd lean forward to rest one hand on it before stepping down. Roughly the size of a car, it was hard to miss. I decided to sit atop quietly processing the events of the past few days to think about my friend Josh. While embracing the silence, I decided to rename 'lean on me' after Josh; and just as I greeted my family and Jessie every day – Josh would get a 'hello' too.

Back off the mountain and I was ready to enjoy a hearty dinner. Miriam contacted me, saying she was ready to finally join me. I'd met her at a birthday party back in April, and as a keen hiker and volunteer rescuer, she had been intrigued by my challenge. Tragically, she'd suffered the unexpected loss of a dear friend the previous month, too. With the wounds still fresh, she was able to provide comfort and share her grief and pain. Her timing, honestly, was just ridiculous. I'd always struggled to comfort others with words in times of pain. I knew nothing I said was going to help. All I could do was sit with someone in their pain and let them know they were not alone. I'd just be there for them and let them know they had a sympathetic ear to share whatever emotions and memories came up. No judgement, no desire to 'fix'. Just an outlet for overwhelming grief. I was grateful for her timing and her openness to talk about her loss as well. Having started at sunrise, we were able to bask in the early morning sun at the top, enjoying some special coffee she'd brewed. Perched on the western table above Platteklip, we had a clear view of the fire's scar, with all the nooks and crannies revealed in the early morning light.

As an avid mountain lover, Miriam organised phenomenal hikes and climbs, exploring some of the trickier routes in the Cape. Her crew, The Mountain Slayers, have developed quite the reputation in Cape Town, and it was a treat to meet and join forces to climb with them. She also happened to be on my Safety Mountain WhatsApp group. She was instrumental in helping me navigate milestone climbs #200 and #350 up different routes to complete the box set for 365 Ubuntu Climbs. But 150 still remained empty as poor weather persisted.

The following day, another storm arrived, a much stronger one. Miriam joined again to see the waterfalls in full flight. Unlike my other days in these conditions, we purposefully chose the worst part of the storm to see what it was like. No surprise, we were the only two people on the mountain.

On a previous day, when I thought the wind was too strong for the cable car, and having already taken my top picture, I decided to do a lap towards the upper cable station and around the café before heading back down Platteklip. I had zero expectations of seeing the cable car working. Concerned, I saw three familiar faces huddled at the door. Don, 67, did Platteklip twice a week and threw in some routes around Lions Head for extra activity. For him, it was the perfect way to keep the body in great condition. The problem was, his knees were in no shape to go back down. They'd misjudged the weather, thinking the cable car would work.

'We've phoned the control room to ask them to please come and pick us up!' he said.

CHAPTER 10
JUNE - THE IMPORTANCE OF MENTAL WELL-BEING

I had no idea this was even an option! I banked that titbit of information.
'Have you been to have coffee yet?' he asked.

'Coffee? Uh – the café's definitely closed,' I responded.

'Don't you have the code to get into the men's bathroom? The cupboard has a kettle, coffee, and tea if you like.'

This was the first time I heard of the emergency room the mountain rescue used for people stranded on the top. When the weather was too dangerous to send emergency services up, people were given the code to take refuge from the cold. It had blankets and hot beverages to sustain you through the night. While we certainly weren't in distress, the insane weather was the perfect opportunity for Miriam and me to enjoy a break from the vicious storm. As I typed the code, I briefly wondered if they'd pranked me. Thankfully, the code worked, and the keys sat nestled inside, just waiting to be used.

Funny story, going back to the three huddling out the wind, desperately waiting for the cable car to 'rescue' them? Well, I stuck around partly for my own benefit to get a ride down, but also in case I was needed to support Don and get him down safely. Two staff members appeared inside, walking towards us. Don was over the moon! The door slid open with the sweetest sound.

'Are you here to take us down?' he pleaded.

'I'm sorry sir, we're just doing a test and due to health and safety reasons, can't take you down just yet.'

'Please!!!?!?! We'll sign anything you need – I can't climb back down with my knees – I just can't.'

I must be honest, I understood why the rules existed, but I was struggling to see how they couldn't help these people when they themselves would be in the cable car?! I'd even climb back down if it would help get them onto the cable car. Rieyaaz, the manager, exclaimed... 'I'm sorry sir, we have strict policies about this.'

Don was desperately trying every angle to get on that cable car, while the others joined him in chorus. Suddenly, the other staff member burst out laughing, he just couldn't hold it anymore. Then, a massive smile replaced Rieyaaz's deadpan expression.

'I was just kidding - we're here to take you back down.'

They did a good job keeping that up for so long and, having played pranks in my life, I appreciated the fact that they took it as far as they did. We all enjoyed a good laugh in the safety of the cable car as we descended out of the clouds.

I was introduced to Mark, creator of Vuka Sports - another man with a fascinating story on overcoming depression, and coming out the other side as a beacon of light for others. I heard about the year he took to work with children and promote sports in impoverished areas. I was blessed to have some solo climbs with him to discuss his background. Exactly one week after I woke up to the worst news all year, I was able to talk about it with someone experienced in dealing with traumatic experiences. I'm always blown away by people's ability to deal with trauma and then speak so openly with strangers.

Interestingly, Mark had just moved down from Johannesburg and had heard me on one of my radio interviews, so he committed to joining me when he arrived. Here's what he had to say about his experience climbing:

'After seeing Andrew's story on the news and knowing that I would be relocating to Cape Town from Johannesburg the year that he started his journey - I had pencilled in to meet this interesting South African & join one of the hikes. I never imagined that we would have similar interests nor become connected as friends.

I was diagnosed with bi-polar disorder in 2015 at age 35. Sport & fitness is one of the pillars key to managing my mental illness on a day to day basis. Our talks on various topics on the journey up & at times down was also helpful. Andrew is an example of a person who not only talks about breaking down stereotypes but does so with action - our continued friendship is proof of that. Living with bi-polar is tough because most people don't take the time to try to understand a topic that can make you feel uncomfortable.

I climb Table Mountain on a regular basis & often smile as I pass by certain points where we stopped for a breather or to take in the scenery. I snap a quick photo & tag Andrew on Instagram. Andrew & the hikes up Table Mountain helped restore my faith in people - & reaffirm that embracing my mental illness is nothing to be ashamed of. In the process I also felt good about myself in contributing to a worthy cause.'

Josh's memorial

Part of my conversation with Josh's mom was around his memorial taking place on Monday the 18th of June, which coincidentally was my Grans 94th birthday. A day of greatly contrasting emotions, celebrating my gran and mourning my friend. I spoke to her before the climb, I could feel the smiles through the phone as she told me about her new reclining chair. Spending most of her day sitting, it was perfect.

Today was my 36th climb up and down. I decided to move last week's stones across on my way back down. I lit a candle and sat on Ubuntu Rock, quietly sitting in the mist, thinking about two special people. I not only picked a new step to represent Gran - but also a stone for the family pile. It felt fitting to pick one for Josh too. I was flooded with memories of how supportive Gran had been, always asking Mom for daily updates on how I was doing. I missed her and couldn't wait to hug her again. I knew that day would happen when I was done. In the meantime, my gratitude overflowed at how privileged I was to still have a grandparent in my life.

Susan decided to ask people to honour Josh's memory by getting involved and donating because of the positive influence that 365 Ubuntu Climbs had on him. Of course, this just made me cry even more. A woman of immense strength, she was instrumental in carrying the torch in Australia, just as Josh had done. With so many of his friends around the world, they planned to stream the memorial service via Facebook so we could all be part of it.

Once again, it was another rainy day in Cape Town as we mourned the loss of our friend. The tributes were incredible, and I was especially grateful to hear that Virgin Australia, who had employed Josh, sponsored Susan's counselling over the tragic death of her son.

Josh, as well as Roxy, would eventually fulfil his wish of climbing with me, as Susan, his brother Matthew and some other friends and family flew to Cape Town in January 2019.

I asked Matt if he'd kept the Ubuntu shirt I'd given for Josh.

'No mate – we cremated him with it. It had to go with him.'

Even as I write this now, it brings tears.

Roxanne's sisters and uncle joined us on the memorial climb while her mom met us at the top. The ceremonial climb in their honour happened on January 26th, which was Australia Day and their ashes were scattered together at the top overlooking her hometown, Hout Bay. I was incredibly moved to be included in such a private family honouring. Susan asked me to read a letter Josh had scribbled just before his death, speaking about how to live with positivity and all the beauty that existed in the world.

They'd be forever bound to the beauty of the mountain, hopefully holding hands, and laughing atop one of the seven natural wonders of the world.

Being a keen observer of nature, I was able to see the small changes that were taking place each day – like following the sun's journey across the sky. Doing so introduced me to spectacles like the shadow of Lions Head neatly sitting on Devil's Peak. A mountain within a mountain, just for a few days before the angles change and it vanishes into thin air.

As the luckiest traveller in the world, I 'happened' to visit Stonehenge on the winter solstice in 2016 with my dear friend Carl. This experience of seeing the sun perfectly aligning with a man-made monument got my mind rolling, and I wondered if the sun rose between the gap at the top of Platteklip on June 21st?

CHAPTER 10
JUNE - THE IMPORTANCE OF MENTAL WELL-BEING

I guess there was only one way to find out.

Alas, of all the days to miss my alarm again – it happened on June 21st. This day also happened to be the first glorious day in a week, the perfect opportunity to put my theory to the test. Only starting at 8 am though meant the sun had been up for 9 minutes already, and I'd blown my chance. And tomorrow? Overcast and rainy conditions would set in for the next four days, delaying my theory. Thankfully, my patience was well-oiled. Mainly because the internet had taught me that the sun rose from the same position for most of the month. Still, I would've preferred my 'Table Mountainhenge' pics on the solstice. I settled for June 26th on climb #177.

Desperate to try to see it on the 22nd – I started in the dark even though it was forecast to be cloudy. This reminded me of my very first climb. While it was fruitless in terms of watching the sunrise, the significance of the date was worth trying. It was incredible reaching the top of Platteklip at the same time the original idea to launch this project had popped into my head 365 days ago. I was eternally grateful that I listened to my gut and took the retrenchment to follow this idea. While unsure of where it would end up, I genuinely believed in the power of this project and believed it was preparing me for my journey and my purpose to connect people, inspire action, and live my best purpose-driven life. That wish seemed to be fulfilled as Iona became climber #300 and joined me on Saturday, which inspired me to ask...

'What was your favourite takeaway from our climb today?'

'Ubuntu Rock and the accumulation of love it has that turns the walk into a prayer of love, hope and connection.' she responded.

After a full weekend of getting soaked, Monday was always going to be a late afternoon climb so I could get some extra rest. My late climb turned out to be a godsend for three travellers, two from New York and one Brit living in Bordeaux. A bitterly cold day, the clear skies belied the icy conditions as the wind hounded the mountain.

I knew it would be an up and down, my 8th for the month already. I knew I had limited time to make it back just before dark, so seeing a German tourist casually snapping pictures at the top, I politely suggested he should start making his way down. I understood why he was taking his time, it was a phenomenal view with high clouds wisping across the sky, a sure sign our sunset would be splashed with colour.

I wasn't sure if it was because of me seeing the tourist earlier or just my intuition, but something made me do a wide sweep towards the upper station and past the café along the southernmost path back to Platteklip. I would've loved to get a sunset picture with these clouds, but I wasn't prepared to chance a dark descent. Just then I ran into the three unsuspecting climbers, and something made me blurt out...

'Just to let you know the cable cars are closed!'

'What?! Are you kidding??' they responded.

'I wish I was, you need to climb back down and soon, before the sun sets.'

The panic was splashed across all three of their faces.

'We've just spent five hours climbing up from Kirstenbosch, we really wanted to catch the cable car.' they said distressingly.

I wasn't exactly thrilled at having to climb down for the 38th time – but here we are. Something made me ask them how they were planning to head down, and thankfully I did, because it turns out they only knew the way they'd come up.

Not even Jamie, on his fastest trail run, could cover that distance before the sun set. The only option was to go down Platteklip with me. A beautiful day on the mountain almost ended badly for them. We barely made it down in the light – making our timing that much more fortuitous as the final section from Lifa's rock down was almost in darkness. As I expected though, we were treated to one of the best sunsets with a range of pinks, oranges, yellows, and lilacs. It was wonderful to experience it, especially after consecutive miserable days.

CHAPTER 10
JUNE - THE IMPORTANCE OF MENTAL WELL-BEING

It had been a treat hearing about their projects in SA and how Jeff's first child was on its way. They were staying in Observatory, and as luck would have it, that night, I was staying with Beth in Vredehoek. Instead of Ubering all the way, I offered to take them to Vredehoek, which left about a third of the way to go. They were all extremely grateful and gleefully handed over some notes to donate to the cause. It made my heart beam with gratitude.

'Thank you!' I said.

That went into my 'treasure box' housing all the cash donations to split between the charities at the end in a ceremonial handover. We bid our farewells, and I headed over to Beth and Richard's place. There'd been a spate of break-ins recently, and Beth had actually come face to face with someone who was trying to break in through their gate. She was understandably nervous on her own while Richard was away on business, so I was happy to stay. She treated us to some pizzas while we caught up with vino aplenty. Thankfully, we kept it pretty clean because the next day, I'd be testing my 'Platteklip Henge' theory.

Gratefully, I never overslept the next morning, and I quietly left the house into another pitch-black start to reach the summit in time. While walking along the road under a blanket of stars, I gazed up and said out loud...

'How do you explain this to people?'

As I navigated the path I'd become accustomed to, I couldn't help but think about everything that had happened since my first climb in the dark, just like this one. I had a mini wobble, worrying whether I'd given myself enough time to see the sun rising at 7:52! Nothing like some added motivation to encourage my weary legs. It had been a grind today, with less than 12 hours since my last summit. I reached the top with ample time to get pictures and a time-lapse video.

It wasn't perfectly centred – but it certainly rose between the cliffs! And even more spectacular; it was perfectly aligned with the summer solstice sunset, too, on December 21st. How incredible is THAT?!?!?!

As if I needed any bonuses, some low clouds rolled in, creating a beautiful white carpet glowing in the sunrise and covering Lions Head in a game of hide and seek. Low clouds always made me feel like I was higher than I actually was, and it added to the heavenly feel.

I was incredibly grateful to witness all this extraordinary beauty. It soaked into every cell of my body. I watched the sun become brighter and light up the stairs on the stairway to heaven for about 15 minutes before I headed over to the cable car. Climb #177 complete, and just 188 left.

I loved the fact that all the staff were as appreciative of the view as I was. They gleefully shared their experiences from the past, and even teased me about how beautiful it was on the 21st. The way they greeted me every day was a joy! Hopefully, the company appreciates what great ambassadors they are.

I was four days away from being spoiled again. Jessie was due to fly back and visit in support of the halfway mark. Halfway! It didn't compute.

June was the coldest and wettest month by far, no matter how hard I tried to find gaps in the storm. It left me with 8 wet climbs, 8 up-and-down climbs, and just 11 days with company. Interestingly, week 26 was my first entire week alone and would become the longest stretch of solo climbs all year. Perhaps I had too much time to think about how fatigue had contributed to my struggles mentally. Like the way I'd been waking up on the wrong side of the bed. I hoped it was just a phase. I hoped Jessie's spark would be the perfect antidote to help me start the second half of the year with the strongest possible mindset.

If I thought the past 28 days were rough, the next few days were about to say: *Hold my beer...*

The truth? I wasn't sure if I'd be able to fix the crack that was forming in my psyche.

It always seems impossible. Until it's done
*~~ **Nelson Mandela***

CHAPTER 11

JUNE TO JULY - CELEBRATING 100 YEARS OF MADIBA MAGIC

I broke my golden rule. I allowed the stream of concerned messages to divert my attention to the next four days and away from what's served me thus far: the present moment. Storms were coming. The messages had the best intentions and were for my safety, but they created a crack. Superstorms would roll in on Friday and keep coming until Monday afternoon. Making matters worse, Friday's climb didn't start on the best foot.

The higher up Kloof road I drove, the more I was surrounded by mist and rain. Windguru already 'told' me the cable car wouldn't be working for the third time this week. I drove past the lower station with desperate eyes. It was closed tighter than an anaconda on its prey. To make matters worse, I had a meeting booked at 10:30, and I was worried that it would cause me to rush in this weather. I decided to call and reschedule. Fortunately, they agreed to make it later. It wasn't worth risking, and it helped ease my mind.

Typing my message to Safety Mountain Tracking, the sound of the rain kept getting heavier. I probably hadn't helped my cause by constantly preaching...

'Just like golf, it's easy to start dry and get rained on when you're already on the course; but no one wants to start in the rain.'

Well, that ain't happening. I gingerly put my rain jacket on in the car.

Instead of crouching in the rain for my gratitude ritual, I decided to say it out loud as I climbed. It was a weird kind of day; it wasn't freezing, but it was cold enough to warrant warm clothes. It wasn't pouring, but just wet enough to warrant a rain jacket. Trust me, as someone who sweats profusely, I tried climbing without the rain jacket. It was clear that both the jacket and I would be drenched in no time. The problem was, now I was wearing two jackets. This at the start of the climb, was like stepping into a sauna before going to a steam room. I couldn't tell if the water dripping off my nose was rain or sweat. Probably both. Hot and bothered, I unzipped both jackets using my hands as curtain holders to hold them open at my hips. It was unbearable. I couldn't go on like this. With the first gap in the rain, I whipped them both off.

Adding insult to injury, my new long rain pants kept falling down. I must've pulled them up 40 times before I even reached the contour path. Every five steps, I had to pull them up. With my jackets off, I was tempted to get these annoying pants off as well.

My worst sweating episodes were always after break times at school, when my body desperately tried to cool down. The sweat would stain my shirt and drip off me long after the bell went. Now I was overheating, and it was running down my forehead into my eyes. Then my pants fell down. AGAIN! What the actual fuck?! Had the waistband gone already? Did I buy the wrong size?!?! And I still

CHAPTER 11
JUNE TO JULY - CELEBRATING 100 YEARS OF MADIBA MAGIC

had four days of this weather?!? My sense of humour was failing. This was the first of three blood-curdling cries. It was raining again, and I scurried to put the jackets back on. More sweat. More rain. More adjusting.

Was this REALLY going to happen all the way up?!?! AND BACK DOWN TOO?!?!

The second cry of anguish happened when I realised I wasn't even halfway. I imagined all the mountain creatures huddled in their homes, eating popcorn, watching this unfold. The local show, 'Humans Gone Wild' would be the talk of the mountain showing on 'Nestflix'. This was my sixth straight day alone. I jokingly wondered what hallucinations would come with it. Well, towards the top, near Ubuntu Rock, I swear I heard voices and even the rustling of packets. Nothing. *Maybe around the next corner I'd bump into someone*? It Never happened, there was no one else crazy enough to be here with me.

I couldn't see anything further than ten metres. The mist was so thick. I let out a deep, rage-filled cry that echoed between the cliffs as I climbed one of the longest steep sections. I was desperately trying to think of how I could keep my pants up on the way down. Maybe a different motion would help? *Maybe going up was different to down?!*

I was clutching at straws at this point. I was so agitated, annoyed, angry, and frustrated. Consumed with all the worries and fears of dealing with this all weekend. I was descending into a dark place, cursing along the top of the mountain, praying for what would be the greatest miracle of a lifetime - the cable car. This was only the second time I was completely alone on the mountain from start to finish.

Begrudgingly, I trudged along the top to get my picture of the grey cloud. As I Dropped my head, the peak of my cap shielded my face from the rain that was smacking into me. The hood of my rain jacket created a small window. Already this year, I'd been blessed with many small miracles, but I'd quickly trade all of them for one right now. I was pleading in my head, making deals left, right, and centre. I felt like I'd been on the mountain for four hours. I didn't even want to contemplate turning around to climb back down. With the desperation of a man who had nothing to lose, I dawdled towards the station. Finally, it revealed itself in the thick mist.

What is that? Is that the..... side door open?

THERE WAS STAFF WORKING IN THE SHOP!!!!!!!!!

I'd never been so happy to see people doing stock take. Three days from the halfway point, I was given a breather. AND my meeting has been moved to Tuesday. It was a moment that changed everything. A weight was lifted. I was shepherded down the corridor to ask the driver whether I could get a lift. The windows were completely steamed up, I couldn't see anything. Suddenly, the cable car doors opened, and I must've looked like a puppy staring out of a cage begging to be adopted.

Bululani!!!!

Nothing I say can justify how amazing it was to see him. His smile warmed my heart more than my double jackets ever could. He was my 'Uber' driver down the mountain.

Today sir, you're my earth-bound angel, I said.

He just laughed. He's remarkable, and always shared my mission with the other riders over the intercom as we descended. An act that often resulted in cash donations from tourists. It was just us this time, and he asked for an update on how things were going and how much money had been raised. He laughed at my re-enactment of my torturous climb and sudden change in fortune.

He's started his own tourism company with another of my favourites - Siyabonga. They're two brothers whose smiles always give me a boost, and will no doubt succeed in delivering memorable experiences for many tourists. True gentleman.

CHAPTER 11
JUNE TO JULY - CELEBRATING 100 YEARS OF MADIBA MAGIC

Safely down, I gave him the biggest hug, and he humbly shrugged it off, *'For you - anytime my friend.'*

As I walked along the road to fetch my car, my video for today went from bordering on homicidal to buoyant and overjoyed. It was exactly what I needed to snap back into gratitude and celebrate another summit. I was perfectly split down the middle - 90 climbs alone and 90 days with 305 people. It was also my 37th vertical equivalent summit of Mt Everest, and that was seriously insane!

Saturday

What a day! It was my mom's birthday, and it gave me an opportunity to think about how fortunate I was to have the parents I have. How many chance moments had to happen for everything to arrive at this point at the end of June with officially half the number of months completed? But it wasn't halfway for me. I was being finicky as 181 days wasn't half of 365. Monday's climb would be the 'middle day' for me, with both 182 before and 182 remaining.

Jessie was due to arrive later - a moment of importance I doubt I'd ever fully grasp, especially after yesterday's meltdown. Her timing for this visit was perfect. It was hard to believe it had been 63 climbs since I last saw her. The relief of collecting her was offset by the fact that my car was overheating and was in the garage getting sorted. Don came to my rescue (again!), and I used his car to fetch her. Just like that, the 16,475 km separating us dissolved, and we were together again. It was amazing to have her close and to enjoy dinner with her.

The mother of all storms was due to land the following day and would hit just after midnight. There were about four waves of downpours scheduled, with the last one coming at about 13:00. It was guaranteed to be my most arduous day.

Sunday

I opened my eyes to the sight of rain mercilessly pouring down. I was grateful for the warm sanctity of my bed.

While I was crazy, some people were nuts. A group voluntarily climbed during the apex of the storm at around 8 am. Their video, already doing the rounds, showed a raging waterfall of water ripping down the mountain. 'Stairway to Heaven' was a torrent of white foam cascading down the stairs. It made for an impressive video and justified my decision. Thankfully, no one got injured and no poor rescuers had to schlep up and carry them back down.

Even with the right gear, there was no way Jessie would be joining me today. Not after seeing that. She got an opportunity to relax after a 32-hour journey. I was hankering down for the coldest, wettest climb and even switched my thin waterproof pants for my thicker skiing pants I bought in London. I had the inspired thought to take a second waterproof jacket, a Springbok jacket from a team building years back that wasn't entirely waterproof, but was enough.

I took no chances: I had a thermal top, t-shirt, warm jacket, and two rain jackets in my bag. Two sets of gloves, three buffs, a cap, and a beanie, just in case. My decision not to shave my face in early May brought unintended consequences – a functional beard. The only exposed piece of skin was around my eyes and forehead. It's amazing what impact the correct clothing makes on an experience like this. The climb became a front-row seat to the awesome power and beauty of nature. I saw it as a gift, and thought how some of my craziest adrenaline-fuelled experiences had prepared me mentally for this.

Driving in Iceland in winter ranked high on the list. Not only did I drive on the 'wrong' side of the road, but I was alone in a country where the language was so different from English that there may as well have been no signs. The wind was howling around my little rental car and driving in that situation, in arctic winter, on tiny roads covered in snow felt absurd. But I made it out unharmed, and was extremely grateful for that, especially after seeing doors being ripped off cars; roads closed due to high winds, and cars rolled on their roofs in the middle of nowhere.

That was all in my rental car's cocoon, complete with heated seats. This was just me against the elements. I couldn't help thinking about Masande and her family, and how much joy their walls and dry house must give them.

My Uber dropped me at the station at 13:35 and gave me enough time to be as cautious as needed. Walking along the road, I caught glimpses of the rivers cascading down as the mist faded in and out of view. I'd head up Platteklip first before coming back down along the contour path to see the waterfalls up close. After the morning's video, I was excited to see them at their peak.

I reached the base of Platteklip and the little reservoir was the highest I'd ever seen. I was concerned about crossing the stream at Dad's rock but decided to chance it. Mistake! The water was flowing OVER the big boulder, and it took strategic planning to cross safely and dryly. The first waterfall? Insane. White water roared down highlighting every inch of the fall. Its entire path was visible through the trees, which usually blocked the view. The path was alive with water. Everywhere. Reaching the contour path, I gazed upwards for the first time. The gorge was a cauldron of wind, whipping clouds around the kloof just waiting for me to enter.

I was reminded of why my ritual at the bottom was so important in connecting me with the mountain and inspiring gratitude for the lessons awaiting me. This was my spiritual path, and showing respect to the mountain kept me grounded. Most people warned or wished me luck on days like this, but truthfully – the mountain deserves equal respect on all days. All my mindfulness practices were being put to the absolute test.

Ironically, the very thing I always needed to do was being forced on me by these extreme conditions. Focus on each step and take nothing for granted! The middle section of the climbing delivered ferocious winds so I stayed far from the edges and as low as possible. I was taken back to my windiest climb to date – Day 26. The foreboding message on my WhatsApp tracking group confirmed Windguru's purple and dark red wind predictions. I wasn't even one quarter up, and already, this was a climb to remember.

The path was a river and the cloud's edge above seemed to recede at the same pace I was climbing. Strangely – the wind dissipated two-thirds of the way up, and the sound of my jacket thrashing gave way to the calm sounds of water tumbling over the cliffs. I saw one guy at the top who was unsure of how to get down, so I pointed him in the direction of Platteklip and didn't see him again. The dryness and calm of the top lulled me into a false sense of security. The raging torrent from the video was now a baby stream on 'Stairway to Heaven' and reminded me about Friday's forecasted 'easier' climb. Another mistake! Rule #33 on the mountain: I should never make statements about the weather until I was literally off the mountain. Nature, of course, had a surprise in store.

The top was shrouded in grey and even though I couldn't see a thing, I could visualise the views in every direction after all my climbs. Knowing the view is hiding there somewhere almost gives the grey clouds their own aura of beauty.

Climbing down, I was always taken aback by the beautiful view when clouds suddenly parted. I was astounded by the tapestry of grey and green hues of Devil's Peak and its contrast against town and Milnerton. I was wearing my gloves and one rain jacket and had safely negotiated the trickiest parts coming down, with just Ascension Corner the worst of the lot left in front of me. This was when my previous 'observation' came back to bite me in the arse. With no clouds blocking my view, I saw what looked like a swarm of bees, trillions of them, fly around the Kloof turning abruptly and heading straight for me. But, they weren't bees. It was rain. As quickly as I spotted it, I was being pelted with what felt like ice. I desperately turned my back, scrambling for my second rain jacket. The wind tried to rip it out of my hands, but thankfully I pulled the zip up just as the full swarm descended with all of its might. Now I looked like a proper Michelin man! With less than halfway left, I successfully navigated Ascension

Corner. I celebrated a little victory but in no way would I become complacent. I was engrossed in every step.

Reaching the contour path, I continued over the first stream devouring the path. Rocks that were usually prominent barely kept their heads above the water and acted as my guide. A few minutes later I walked past a couple, and the gent tried to warn me about the erratic waterfall coming up. Not even his warning could prepare me for what was around the corner. I proudly declared how I had two rain jackets. He just smiled and carried on.

The wind's ferocity was blowing the waterfall back up the mountain. Slowing down a smidge, it appeared to be a never-ending cresting wave, desperately trying to crash down below. I stood transfixed, witnessing the water flowing again, only for the wind to pick it back up and blow it backwards... sideways... forwards! If I weren't wet enough yet, the waterfall would probably have seen that as a challenge.

Usually, the water poured in front of you creating a curtain of water, allowing a dry passage behind it. There was no such chance today as the wind hurled it around like a Great White shark thrashing its prey from side to side. I tried to time my walk behind the water but it clearly had eyes in the back of its head and caught me!

The next spectacular waterfall I needed to navigate was completely different with layers and more stepping stones to tip-toe across. I stepped on a stone I thought was fixed, but it twisted under my weight and dropped me ankle-deep into the water! Both feet!

Have you seen that scene with Jim Carrey in Bruce Almighty? Well, he's walking into a building and puts one shoe into a puddle. I had the same reaction, with two kilometres left and both feet submerged, I wasn't impressed – especially since tomorrow's climb would be the final day of this wet weekend. The prospect of starting with soaking shoes? Not fun at all.

I finished typing my message to Safety Mountain at 17:17 – after 3 hours and 36 minutes of one of the most intense yet spectacular climbs of the year. It was a long, mentally draining climb, but I was excited that Jessie was waiting for me. I was starved and couldn't wait to order my favourite Chinese food, wrapped in her supportive and loving energy.

Week 26 ended with character-building moments and I felt like the universe rewarded me as Andre Du Toit, The Big Positive Guy, invited me onto his newly launched show on Smile FM. I was grateful for the opportunities that kept coming my way that would help me share my project and build more support.

Monday

Another intense day meant Jessie would sit it out, but her chance to join again would come on climb #184. The afternoon looked like there was a gap at 14:00. My new system for evaluating the weather was Windguru for wind forecasts and YR for rain. YR had been more accurate and said the rain would stop at 14:00, which was hard to believe as I watched wave after wave falling all morning. Right on cue, the rain magically gave way to sunlight and the first sight of blue skies in four days.

Mercifully, Don was home today, so I could use his car and kept a towel in the back. It was my 9th straight solo climb and 40th back down. I took a few minutes to sit at Halfway Rock on the way up. In my video I was lost for words and fumbled horribly trying to express my emotions. I struggled to articulate what I'd accomplished with the climbs; what we'd accomplished together with the donations; how I'd been blessed by all 304 people who'd joined; and the support I'd been shown. It was overwhelming, and the recording didn't do it justice, so I tried again. Long pauses perhaps would better capture the gravity of what I was doing. It was tough to express my gratitude and pride in what I had accomplished. Many times I heard people say, 'I don't think you understand what you've gotten yourself into.' For the first time the gravity of what this really was sank in as I allowed myself to think about the end for the first time.

I took a picture down the mountain symbolising what was behind me. I took another one looking up the gorge, symbolising what was to come. Both had patches of blue sky, acting as little rays of hope. Alone on the mountain, Jamie's words echoed in my ears... *Treat the first half as training for the second half.*

All the experiences of the past 183 climbs flooded my memory. Now I had to do it all over again, but with a body that hasn't rested since 2017. I'd made it this far. THAT'S what mattered most. And now it was time to complete today's climb. As I started, I was motivated by the thought that every step was taking me closer to my goal and further away from the beginning.

After moving week 26's rocks across to the pyramid, I didn't linger, the waterfalls were not flowing, but big icy drops of water were constant enough to make it unpleasant. How incredible that the site I picked for the pyramid was under a waterfall! Every rainy day invigorating them with fresh energy and bathing them together. I enjoyed seeing my eclectic collection of stones uniquely combining to create a pyramid of love and Ubuntu.

At the top, the wind felt like it was straight from Antarctica, so I buried my head in my chest to protect my face. Thankfully my buffs provided some relief for my ears and nose. I was grateful for all the layers that kept me toasty. I could feel there was snow on the mountains, and I was excited to see it in the coming days of clear weather.

A dassie cuddle pile greeted me as I took photo #183 – soaking up as much sun as possible before the night dropped below freezing. All eight of their faces reflected the same disbelieving look that someone chose to be in this weather. Dassie, which is a Rock Hyrax, is Afrikaans for badger, and their closest living relative is – wait for it – the African Elephant. That trivia still blows my mind and is often met with healthy skepticism when I tell tourists.

My alone time climbing down in clearer weather was perfect for deep introspection on what the year had already brought. One thing was blatantly apparent: the most amazing and unexpected opportunities appeared when I took a leap and followed that which set my heart on fire.

Lisa joined us for a halfway celebratory dinner. After being battered the past four days, I was grateful that the glorious sunshine would persist for the rest of the week and we'd have a perfect day to celebrate 'Independence Day' with Jessie on the 4th of July.

My next milestone number was the 200th climb, the day after Nelson Mandela's birthday, which I had no doubt would be special. But looming large on Monday the 23rd, the cableway was due to shut down for its yearly maintenance, this was July's next big challenge. It was one of the biggest tests I'd faced all year. Two weeks of climbing back down every day? That's double what my last week of training was.

July's start was a huge contrast to the stormy weather that had just passed. It was crazy to be wearing shorts and a T-shirt again. The best news was how the dams were performing, their levels rising slowly but steadily. The gorgeous line of snow-capped mountains in the distance would also play their part in filling the dams. I'd never seen this much snow in the Western Cape, with the Hottentots mountains to the South, the Boland mountains behind Paarl and then the Cederberg range in the north appearing as one long white line of jewels against the African Blue sky which was truly spectacular on these clear days.

Jessie would smash another six consecutive climbs taking her tally up to 13 for the year. I asked her what she thought she'd finish on. Both in sync, we said about 30. She helped me pick out my waterproof bag with my new voucher from Cape Union Mart, and my cousin Linda bought me another pair of boots. Now I could switch between the two. I got another smaller lightweight torch and two space blankets. I wasn't taking any chances with another two, maybe even three months of storms like the past weekend potentially still ahead. Space blankets provide insulation from the cold, and double up to signal helicopters by reflecting sunlight on clear days too.

July the 4th turned out to be one of my favourite days with Jessie, when Carrey and her son Josh joined. We met a tourist from Holland on the road where the climb starts and invited him to join us. William was a fascinating young man. He chose a long-haul destination flight every year to immerse himself in culture, language, food, and history; for an entire month, South Africa was his second destination after visiting Nepal last year.

He had a tattoo on his forearm of a Nepalese saying which translated to: ***everyone you meet is superior to you in some way***. I loved this! It resonated with me as I thought about the 310 climbers that had joined me and all had something of value to share. It was a beautiful reminder that applied everywhere, not just on the majestic mountain. I'll never forget it. What an amazing gift to decide to give yourself at 24.

Followed by another solo climb with Jessie, I was blown away by her fitness and ability to glide up the steep incline. I was extremely fortunate to be on the receiving end of her love and support which uplifted me and gave me fuel for the legs. She treated us to some full body massages – the bulk of which I asked to be done on my legs and upper back.

Elliot had been super excited to join us on Friday, especially now that Jessie was here, but alas for the second time, it wasn't meant to be. His wife had woken up in severe pain, so he messaged to say he'd be staying behind to make sure she was okay and to get her to the doctor if need be. Thankfully, it wasn't anything too serious, and we'd just have to try again. Third time lucky I guess.

He certainly didn't miss anything on the climb. If anything he saved himself. Dave and Mark joined us, Mark being part of an elite group of people who'd joined on more than one occasion. Our light-hearted conversation came to a screeching halt. I had no idea what this person could've eaten, but on Ascension Corner under one of the trees used for shelter from the sun, someone's bowls had exploded. And I do mean – exploded. There was shit splatter on the path like nothing I'd ever seen. Alas, the first rain to help 'clean' this up would only arrive in a week too. As yet, I haven't had such trouble on the mountain, and long may that continue!

It provided a moment of lightheartedness a few days later when I took the largest group so far for the year. 16 of us tackled climb #189 to complete week 27 on an unseasonably warm winter's day. It felt like Spring, the proof being the rapidly disappearing snow on the distant mountains.

Dom was an ex-colleague I worked with on projects for Pick n Pay. Her son Jake had been following my progress. We met up back in March to discuss how to prepare, and how to get others involved. He listened intently as I explained how I trained and gave suggestions on what to do. Who knew a winter's day could be warmer than spring? He bought some friends, and another colleague, Christelle, surprised me too and joined. It was crazy to hear that a year later after being laid off, they still hadn't filled my old position. It didn't surprise me though. I sent a quiet message of thanks for letting me go.

Richard joined and brought Paddy along - his Jack Russel. Paddy had an unending supply of energy, and seemed to have done at least five laps with all his bundu bashing while chasing sticks up and down the path. I was super excited to chat with Richard about my upcoming meeting. As one of Cape Town's best tour guides, his relationship with a prestige company had opened the door for me. We'd be chatting on the 11th to discuss how to collaborate and give their clients a different experience to what most mountain guides could provide.

Today marked the day I'd been educated about the speed of human erosion on the mountain. Part of my toolbox to avoid injury was to keenly observe the changes on the mountain. I'd seen some smaller rocks crumble but nothing too concerning yet.

On Friday's climb up Ascension Corner, I spotted a gap forming between two steps, the larger one below the crack, was precariously poised to roll some distance down the hill. I dropped a pin and notified the Safety Mountain Tracking guys in the hopes that it could be avoided. On Saturday, that gap had grown enough to make the entire step wobble.

CHAPTER 11
JUNE TO JULY - CELEBRATING 100 YEARS OF MADIBA MAGIC

How long would it take to dislodge?

My guess, with no intervention, it would come apart by Monday. I was off by 24 hours. Sunday revealed a gaping hole as the stone lay several steps below. I hoped no one had been injured when they dislodged it. This created a domino effect for the steps above because now there was nothing to support them. Unfortunately, this wouldn't be the only spot. As more people spent time on Platteklip, more attention would need to be given to managing the path.

The end of climb #189 brought with it the sad realisation that all that was left was taking Jessie back to the airport. 'Goodbyes' are always hard but this one felt so much harder. Not having a clear date to look forward to her return yet. Maybe it was just my heart preparing me for the 160 climbs before we could see each other again. I was grateful she'd been able to meet repeat climbers.

With Jessie gone I had some solo climbs to contemplate how meeting her a year ago was perfect timing. She never doubted my climbs for a second and while long distance made it complicated, she was certainly teaching me loads about her character. Actions always speak louder than words. For someone who adored visiting new places but was willing to give up her holidays to come back to the same city, which was a 32-hour journey away, AND climb the same mountain: incredible! Her visit was perfectly timed too as my mental state had started to spiral. With her help, I regained control, was out of my nose dive, and was flying again.

The climbs continued, so there was no wallowing. The clear days provided spectacular afternoon climbs. 191's top photo provided one of my favourites – the sun dancing above the upper station, its golden path along the ocean peeking behind the mountain while the cable car hangs effortlessly, bringing another load of people to bask in the sunset up top. It was perfectly balanced against the backdrop of a sunrise climb and the thinnest sliver of the moon floating in the gentle light. This was my 12th barefoot climb for the year with Lisa's 20th climb, which was also barefoot. She finally decided to try it out and enjoyed it as much as I did after initially thinking I was crazy. Dave was on his 7th but happily kept his shoes on.

Lisa has type 2 diabetes, and I'd always appreciated how she never let it rule her life. Unfortunately, this time, she struggled, especially as she hadn't exercised since our last climb. We were prepared for this though, and she ate a bar to help raise her sugar levels enough to get down safely. I was incredibly proud of the fact that I'd never heard her complain about this in all the eight years we'd known each other.

It was interesting to see how the simple addition of my waterproof backpack impacted my mental well-being. Not being forced to wear all my clothes climbing up gave me the freedom to maintain a manageable comfort level, while enjoying the ability to add extra layers when needed. Today, the wind forced me to add the extra jacket just three turns into reaching the cliffs. It really is amazing how quickly the temperature drops. The difference felt far greater than 10 degrees, as the temperature gauge outside the cable station screamed five degrees back at me, and that was excluding the wind chill factor.

The wind rushed up the mountain side as I climbed back down. It was a truly bizarre experience to see the clouds and rain flying uphill! I was grateful to be warm and dry under my jacket, with a huge smile under my buff as I shied away from the stinging rain drops. This was unlike any experience I'd ever had before, and now that I was past halfway, I was more aware that this challenge wouldn't last forever. I was learning to celebrate all the victories along the way, as if each was my final climb and I'd reached my end goal.

For months, I waged an internal struggle as I tried to decide whether to plan an extra 'special' climb dedicated to Madiba on his birthday on July 19th. Something about doing that just felt 'off' to me. I couldn't put my finger on it. It had become an annual custom for people to donate 67 minutes to a cause in honour of the 67 years of public service Mandela gave South Africa.

CHAPTER 11
JUNE TO JULY - CELEBRATING 100 YEARS OF MADIBA MAGIC

I understood the sentiment, but I disagreed with the execution. We shouldn't be honouring a man that gave 67 years with 67 minutes once a year. His birthday should be a day to reflect upon how we as a country are working together as individuals, contributing to a cause that fits in with our value system. It certainly sounded easy for me to say this when I'd dedicated a year. I included myself in this post in 2018 and used his example to drive my thinking to be long-term and multi-layered. I decided the whole year would be a dedication to Mandela, and would make every climb as important as the next one. Something I passionately believe and maintain to this day. Day 365 would never exist without Day 79. I chose not to plan anything and let it unfold the way it was supposed to.

Well, it couldn't have worked out better. As I arrived home after finishing week 29, Elliot casually mentioned that his next day off was the following Wednesday. Fingers crossed, third time lucky! It took a couple of days to register, that was Mandela's birthday!

Climb #199 arrived and I wished the stars had aligned perfectly for there to be something special for his 100th birthday. Well, someone was listening because it worked out to be the 100th day that somebody joined me! That wasn't all though, Raquel, a woman from Switzerland, joined the party and became the 360th climber. You couldn't script this, considering my gran was Swiss and would've been 100 if alive today. Incredibly, Raquel found me while Googling 'Outdoor Activities in Cape Town', and a 365 Ubuntu Climbs article popped up. Thanks to the beauty of social media, she got in touch and today just happened to be her best day to join.

It was a casual climb up as I took them to enjoy Silverstream, which was still flowing after last week's rains. We spent some time talking about apartheid and privilege and what I'd learned from it. It still felt awkward speaking about it in front of black people, but Elliot is a soft soul with great insight and no hatred or resentment. Perhaps if he were resentful, then he wouldn't have joined. Raquel showed great depth as she asked questions with the hope of learning. I'd experienced the full spectrum of people, from talkers, to soft-spoken people, to those that say nothing only to become chatty up top.

241

Elliot's climb was higher than he'd ever been before, his face radiated pure happiness and bliss. They were both thrilled to see the pyramid and smiled as I showed them today's stone, which represented them too. It was a beautiful multi-coloured stone for the 'Rainbow Nation' Madiba and all his freedom fighters fought so hard to achieve.

Happy birthday Madiba!

It was the 3rd time I heard the noonday gun while climbing, but for some reason, it felt like it reverberated more today. It was the perfect salute to Nelson Mandela's life of belief and action.

We finally reached the top, and Elliot was already enamoured by the restricted views on the way up. His mind was blown, admiring the full view. He turned into the latest supermodel as he posed for tons of pictures. Nobody back home believed he'd make it today. Sounds familiar! He did extremely well, and I love how he expressed his emotions, like a kid in a candy store. It was beautiful watching them enjoy every step up to the top and then the spectacular view too. We celebrated with coffee and cake, basking in the sun, and took in all the splendour that Table Mountain offers. I was blessed that both appreciated the significance of the day, and I was grateful that I hadn't 'organised' it. I simply 'let it be.'

I like to think Madiba would be proud of what I was doing. The insight I was gaining, and how I was learning to be of service. I believe he was looking down and saying, 'That seed I planted in 1993, has grown into a great sapling.' While I may not be responsible for the suffering of others, I could certainly do my best to be part of the solution. If not now, then when?

Let's make Madiba proud and honour his legacy.

The early spring weather continued with a smattering of rain. It was another huge load off my mind as Day Zero continued to be pushed out, even with our warmer weather. August and September could still be cold and sneak some wet weather past our defences.

CHAPTER 11
JUNE TO JULY - CELEBRATING 100 YEARS OF MADIBA MAGIC

The Cableway two-week shutdown was due to start the following day.

Saturday's climb provided a much-needed distraction as the two Clare's from 'the Wellness Company' finally joined. They'd previously requested June the 9th for World Wellness Day, but due to the storm, they sensibly postponed it. I was used to people 'disappearing,' so it was refreshing to see some people live up to their desire to climb and reschedule for a later date. They were rewarded with a rare occurrence. Just seconds after being asked how many animals I'd seen, we spotted a Tahr to our left.

He was a massive male with a thick coat and armed with sharpened horns. A Rhodesian ridgeback suddenly dashed up the hill behind us, bounding as though it had spotted a dassie. It disappeared onto a ridge above us but had attracted the attention of the male, his head turned inquisitively to decipher what was going on. He calmly started making his way up the mountain after the dog. I had an awful flash of him bucking the dog off the cliff with his horns.

I think the two women were worried too, heading into the bush desperately calling their dog down. Happily, the dog emerged unharmed, and we all shared a collective sigh of relief. That was the last of the 'action' for the day, and my grateful legs enjoyed their second last cable ride down for a while.

My next climb was on July 22nd, and the weather was clear, so I stripped off my shoes for barefoot climb #13. Allan (LA Barista – 5th climb) and Lisa (20th climb) joined me. I was happy that Lisa took on the barefoot climb challenge too. In all the times people have tried it – I've never had someone put their shoes back on. It was comical hearing them being asked the same questions they'd asked me, as other climbers looked on incredulously.

Mother nature had a real sense of humour. Before reaching the top, she decided today was the perfect time to blow a gale and close the cableway a day early.

Of course! Why on earth would it happen any other way?

I was strengthening my mindset. The more I chose challenges and stepped out of my comfort zone, the better prepared I became to take the unexpected difficulties head on. Exhibit A: the cableway closure. I chose to see it as another mini-challenge within a challenge.

Even the mountain guides had been dreading this time, and jokingly hoped they would get no bookings. It was great to have regulars to share some laughs with about our impending doom. My gratitude for all their support was growing, especially as I heard them say, 'This is the guy I was telling you about.' The support was tremendous.

I was alone for the first three days of the cable car closure, and it allowed me to ease in gently. I told myself that this was what the previous 205 climbs were preparing me for. As requests came in, I understood if first time climbers chose rather to wait for the cable car to run again. After all, there'd still be 147 more opportunities.

I motivated myself a little bit more every morning as I slipped my pounamu over my neck. It was a reminder of all the strength being stored inside. Day by day, one step at a time infusing excitement into what lay ahead. I focused on the lessons I had prepared. Even through the toughest weather conditions, I was unscathed. I was grateful to enter this fortnight with no major joint pain or injuries. This allowed me to put my focus on the important tasks that lay ahead.

Thursday, which was also a down climb, became my longest day on the mountain, even longer than the clean-up day back in June. It was mentally exhausting, even though it was slower. It was so easy for my mind to wander and all it took was a slight lapse in concentration on any one of the 2,579 steps and my year would be at risk.

Jo and two of her friends, Liz and Maryellen from DC and New York, joined climb #140. She spoke about her experience stirring excitement and inspiring the others to join. It was a beautiful cool day with high clouds and minimal people on the mountain. They were very engaging and asked great questions. They even got to experience the cheeky Dassies who relentlessly tried to steal our food during our picnic.

Seeing my shirt and cap, my guests wanted to get some before they left. Today was out of the question, but I'd be able to get some printed and delivered to them the afternoon they were due to leave. I was grateful it worked out, especially after their generous donation. Thank you Jo!

I was almost at the end of week one of up-and-down climbs, and I could feel the extra 40 minutes a day in my legs. I felt like I was on my third lap up Platteklip for the day. It was already my 11th climb back down in July which took my tally up to 49. It's incredible how consistent daily action stacks up on top of each other. I now had 149 kilometres of vertical climbing; the equivalent of 40 Mount Everest Summits. Only 37% of the way up to the International Space Station.

After watching Sara-Jayne being interviewed about her book in June, she introduced me to the organisers. They run a project called '1001 South African Stories'. As they say, *'The aim of the project is to contribute to a more cohesive and inclusive understanding of South African history. Some stories ask us to glance back, others to explore the present, and some inspire dreams of a brighter future.'*

Shenaaz was keen to hear the story behind 365 Ubuntu Climbs at The Book Lounge. I loved seeing how opportunities arose as a ripple effect after being introduced to new people. I was able to return the favour by introducing them to Blake. We chatted about our projects and what it took to get here.

The following day, Sarah and Kerri joined me. They heard about me through Cape Union Mart. They also purchased a T-shirt with 'July 2018' printed on it as their mementos. Salvador joined again and seemed to have even more energy bounding up the mountain than the last time. I wasn't sure what was going on with me though, I felt like I had used up all my words the night before. I had no desire to talk. Luckily, they chatted amongst themselves while I kept my head down quietly admiring how quickly the steps changed. Our early start helped me get back home by lunch time and gave me the advantage of an event-free afternoon on the couch. I'd also get up late the next morning.

Back on the mountain again and I really wished this was a solo climb. Once again, the opposite turned out to be exactly what I needed. Two people cancelled, and I almost got my wish. Only Robert remained, and I 'inquisitively' pushed to see if he'd still be joining. His answer was yes.

Robert found me through social media and became my 376th climber. He shared his inspiring story of how he was a recovered drug addict who now privately tutors a young boy of 15 and speaks at schools about his journey with drugs. He attributes his successful transition to the rehabilitation centre's methods which included writing down and understanding what he did to get to the place where he was no longer adding value.

They taught him to take ownership of his reasons for drug abuse, as well as his recovery. What struck me the most listening to Robert, was his open manner of discussing his journey, yet harbouring no self-judgement about it. Too often, we deviate from a path of self-love and chastise ourselves, when we should rather be exercising more self-love. Would you chastise yourself for taking a class at university that didn't serve you? NO! You'd probably be grateful for something new. That's how I felt about the three years I studied to become a chartered accountant. I was grateful I changed, and learned to become aware of when something no longer served my higher purpose.

We ran into my friend Kathy who is a mountain guide. She told her clients about my project, and they happily contributed. All it took was for her to share it. My private climbs with her provided some entertainment as she thanked me for the fact that my challenge had given her more to talk about with her clients!

My left ankle began nagging me on this climb, and after the break to talk with her clients it was painful. It forced me to focus on the angle of my foot each time I placed it on the step. The third lap felt harder than I remember. My ankle pain wasn't something new though. I often had minor joint issues. Either one of my knees, hips, or legs would act up and force me to put my focus in the right place. I focused on my ankle, thanked it for everything it was doing, and made sure that I kept my weight even on each side.

Being so conscious about my body often transported me to another world. It reminded me how absorbed I got watching TV shows on the inner workings of the body as a little boy. Seeing the blood flowing in the arteries, and how the heart valves opened and closed, all fascinated me. Now I was diving into the magic of how each joint worked together and how the body operates in perfect unison. How the muscles were attached to the tendons and were fed with oxygen and nutrients to drive this machine up the mountain. How the lungs collected the air and acted as a distribution network in partnership with the heart delivering millions of oxygen packages to places that needed it.

My previous injury was because I wasn't focusing on each step. I consciously remembered which side to use on the next big section – even if that meant breaking stride. That injury was my best teacher, and helped me keep the load equally distributed on the left and right sides. And after 210 days? It seemed to be paying off with no major injuries. Thankfully by the time we switched and started climbing down my ankle pain was almost gone. To minimise the risk, I only used my right side turning sideways down each big gap.

A tourist on his way down clutched his wrist, looking very worried, and asked if he needed a tetanus shot. He'd been bitten by a dassie. It doesn't matter how many signs there are about not feeding the dassies, there's always one who knows better. They may look cute and cuddly, but these are wild animals. He knows that now! Their teeth are incredibly sharp from the wild grasses and foliage they snack on that grows out of the rocky mountain. Their teeth look like fangs. I honestly didn't know the answer to his question. I didn't think he needed an injection but thought it best to visit a doctor anyway.

It was glorious at the top, something the maintenance staff must have loved. They knew exactly how cold and wet it could get so they were having an exceptional day at the office.

On a day that started with me wanting to be alone, Robert had been another unexpected pleasure to host. His story and commitment to empowering kids was just what my legs needed. I was really blessed to meet people who were doing incredible things to change their lives. 3 hours and 3 minutes later we took the final step off the mountain, his stories were a magic carpet ride that made it seem far quicker.

That brought an end to the first week of climbs during the cable car closure.

One more to go.

The last day of July was my 212th climb. The number 212 is significant to me ever since Damien, a former business coach of mine asked me if I was a '212er?' Initially I responded with 'HUH?' but fortunately, he explained it to me.

'Water at 211 degrees fahrenheit is extremely hot, but with just one more degree it starts to boil and turns to steam. That extra one degree is all it took. So what is that one extra degree you're giving your business, personal life, relationships or any other area that you're working on? 1-degree Andrew – that's all it takes.'

Stephan, who is the founder of Distance 4 Difference, exemplified this philosophy, and joined me with a great purpose at heart. Back in March, he started formulating an idea to support his own foundation, as well as 365 Ubuntu Climbs. His organisation focuses on a better future for children in need by addressing family life and education. I love this quote on their website www.d4dsa.co.za *Volunteers don't necessarily have the time; They just have the heart.*

Back in 2016 he started running 5 km every day. He hasn't missed a day yet (including the days he rode in the Cape Town Cycle Tour, which is a 110 km road race!) Now that's commitment! On the 23rd of April, with 900 runs in the bag, he started his campaign. For his 1000th run, he chose to climb with me. His goal was to raise R50k over the course of his 100 runs and then split the money 50/50 with me to support my campaign. This generous effort was made even more incredible after I had to cut D4D from the top four national programs I

CHAPTER 11
JUNE TO JULY - CELEBRATING 100 YEARS OF MADIBA MAGIC

was supporting. I wondered how many others would've felt spiteful about being left out instead of seeing an opportunity to piggyback on what I was doing. Not him, he is a special man!

By 20:05 on Monday he'd 'only' raised R41k and decided to post one last video urging people to participate. It clearly worked because he was sitting on R58k when he arrived the next morning. That meant he'd raised 28% of the money in 0,5% of the time! One more video.... That's all it took. Never. Give. Up! This was a reminder that whether money was invested on day one, or the final minute, it would still be used to create the same impact.

The mist returned for Stephan and his brother-in-law, who stuck it out as the others dropped off at the last minute. I wasn't surprised. Our trek started three minutes before sunrise which was at 7:36 am, and it was bitterly cold. But soon we received our first blessing on the cracked rock at Ascension Corner, as the clouds broke slightly and allowed a line of sunshine to illuminate the mountain. It was hauntingly beautiful.

Jan decided to share some more facts he'd just calculated. Climb #212 could be written as 2 x 12 and Stephan's birthday was on 12/12. He also started his runs back in 2016 on my birthday, which made me realise how beautifully connected life is. Stephan's commitment to doing extra extended beyond D4D. He also participated in Pragma's social program to help students of all backgrounds. Pragma is his full-time employment - while D4D is a project he runs in his own time.

A glaring truth was exposed while we chatted openly about South Africa and our challenges. The vast majority of people held perceptions about others that were not rooted in facts and were not from a place of understanding. My brain was working overtime to think about how we could create more dialogue and get more people to work together to build a prosperous South Africa for all.

Complex questions to end my seven months on the mountain. If only we could celebrate each other in the same way that the various types of vegetation co-existed in a rich tapestry of beauty on the mountainside. I appreciated these opportunities to talk about all the challenges and hear the different opinions from people who were actually doing something and not just whining about it. The one benefit of climbing back down was how much easier it was to talk. It was hard to believe that the number had rapidly risen to 54. Stephan must have been feeling cursed – two climbs, both up and down!

He agreed to have a quick chat on video at the bottom so we perched ourselves on the bottom three steps. Hilariously, I took a photo instead of a video! It felt like we made a perfect 10-minute video too, only to realise my error when I pushed 'pause' and took another photo. Of course, I stumbled on the second one trying to remember the gems we spoke about. It was a lesson learned, next time I'd make sure to double-check before recording.

Stephan shared the journey of how he raised over R6 million in 13 years thanks to people stepping out of their own comfort zones with crazy sporting challenges and the generous support of donors who recognised their abundance and acted kindly. He oozed humility and gratitude and it was a true honour to have his support. He ended his special message by encouraging those who felt overwhelmed, to start their own charity or challenge and to get involved by joining me on my campaign.

I loved that he picked up his own rock, and he chose it because it had a crack in the middle, which reminded him that we all had 'cracks' and faults we were dealing with. He beautifully asked people to put their cracks aside and become part of the giving family. After all, everything we did was nothing without YOUR support! Everything good comes from a team effort.

Building up a decent hunger and finishing moments before 11:00, I heard his magic words:

'Would you like to join us for a Wimpy breakfast?'

CHAPTER 11
JUNE TO JULY – CELEBRATING 100 YEARS OF MADIBA MAGIC

Wimpy is an American-style fast food place that always brings back great childhood memories. I gladly accepted. It was the perfect way to end off another mini milestone, and celebrate Stephan's 1000th consecutive 5km run. It was humbling to be on the end of so much love. I'm deeply grateful for his decision to jump on board.

153 days to go..... And five more days before the cable station would open up again!

I wondered what unexpected treasures were lying in wait for me? **JULY STATS:**

212 / 365

People Joined: 74 / 378

22 days 21 hours 57 minutes 40 seconds / 1 442,41 km / 41,25 equivalent Everest Summits

/ 106 solo climbs (50%) / 54 Up & Down (19,2%) TOTAL DONATIONS: R233 473.12

Kerri: 'Nobody can do everything, but everybody can do something.'

Robert: 'It's not much but I must add something to this awesome endeavour. Thanks for letting me tag along and for your inspiration :)'

Clare: 'Action is the only language. Thank you for your heart, your sharing, your dreaming and most importantly: your action.'

> *What you leave behind is not what is engraved in stone monuments, but what is woven into the lives of others*
> *~~ Pericles 429 B.C Greece*

CHAPTER 12

AUGUST AN EDUCATION ON BUILDING A LEGACY

I knew the year was teaching me about legacy. Last month was Nelson Mandela's birthday and it gave me an opportunity to really examine how he built a legacy with 67 years of dedication. What struck and enlightened me the most, was the amount of extraordinary obstacles he overcame – even after the country was born again. Now I see why he was inspired to quote… 'After climbing a great hill, one only finds that there are many more hills to climb.'

His journey helped me appreciate the challenges I was facing and taught me to view them as part of a lifelong picture I couldn't see yet. It felt like I was hunting pieces that could only be retrieved after difficulty. My legs and body certainly felt that. In July, I averaged a climb back down every second day, and the thought of another five more days up and down was unsettling. To give that perspective it was two more days than my two previous longest streaks of three days, but that was on the back of climbing back down for ten days.

CHAPTER 12
SEPTEMBER - UNCONDITIONAL LOVE

It was a foreboding start to August with my 18th wet climb of the year and my 55th down climb. Mark joined me for the 3rd time knowing full well what the conditions meant. Writing this gave me an amazing perspective on how the pieces of support played out at exactly the right moments. I was always grateful for the reflections in my daily journal, but now I had perspective on how the whole year flowed perfectly with all these beautiful experiences naturally unfolding in a way that kept my cup full.

Thanks to my waterproof bag from Cape Union Mart, I could keep my second jacket dry without wearing and overheating in it. Instead, I could take advantage of the trick I developed earlier in the year, where I'd stop two corners from the end of the climb below the walls of sheer rock face to take shelter. It's the perfect position out of the wind and rain. I also used it as a pitstop to steal some water. Walking along the top I felt like an explorer on ice sheets trekking across Antarctica. I often thought of those men and women spending months in atrocious conditions. Human beings have achieved some incredible feats, acts we thought were impossible, now unlocked by some brave souls.

My days on the mountain gave me time to process the positive impact Mark made by being present at the start of the month. 365 Ubuntu Climbs presented me with the opportunity of a lifetime, especially when it came to meeting new people. All the conversations with my fellow Ubuntu champions were my greatest treasures. I was learning to understand the African proverb... *If you want to go fast, go alone. If you want to go far, go together.* I was about to meet a man that embodied all of this and then some.

We had enough money to deliver our first round of books to two schools, as well as cover the cost to track the impact the books made. Most donors wanted to buy books, but few were keen to pay for the evaluations, which to me, were just as important as the books themselves. It's a measurement more nonprofits are required to consider: Return on Impact.

To discuss the handover, Lisa organised our Friday morning meeting with the staff and principal of Klapmuts Primary school, one of the poorest and most under-resourced schools in the Western Cape. My friend Donald, an ex-teacher, helped me out with his car, and showed up as a top investor for 365 Ubuntu Climbs. He'd been a rock of support at our weekly Sunday lunches, a tremendous sounding board for my ideas and he kept me focused on my objectives. I could run away with ideas and in moments of madness where I kept adding layers of complexity to the challenge by adding more beneficiaries, he'd thankfully reign me back in and keep me grounded.

He's always been a shining example of why taking the time to build proper strategies, whether personal or in business, is so critical to overall success. I am forever grateful and blessed to have him as such a dear friend, and for sharing his extraordinary experience.

Arriving at the school, at first glance, you'd be fooled into thinking you were at the Stellenbosch University campus, just 15km down the road. Mr Ronald Frans was responsible for this. His three decades as a headmaster focused on unrelenting relationship building with a selfless desire that ensured his students maximised their growth opportunities. His passion was the reason a renowned architect's firm, Emerging Architects, donated their time to design and build the wing holding the library, computer and media centre.

The school's motto said, *'Liefde en Leer'* - Love and Learning in Afrikaans. We certainly felt it as his warm smile instantly put us at ease welcoming us into his office. Even at 38 there was something intimidating about going to the principal's office. What an amazing man! Whenever I'm asked who my inspirations are – he's in my top three of all time.

He's a true visionary and leader dedicated to the wellbeing of every child at the school. To put 'poorest' into context, the surrounding town is 15 km from Stellenbosch - and most people don't have the money to get a taxi into town, let alone own a car. The high unemployment rate leads to domestic violence and creates harsh conditions for these children. He understands it, having grown up in a similar area. His vision is to create a beacon of hope filled with love and support for the kids coming to school.

I had a feeling my afternoon climb was going to have wings on it. We were taken on a tour of the school. The smiles on all the children's faces were amazing. The neatness of the school painted a picture of respect. I could feel the love, and I could see it in the actions of the women working all day for R1200 a month to feed the children a meal which would sometimes be their only one for the day. I lost count of the times I heard Mr Frans say 'I'm blessed', constantly praising his staff and donors. I fought back tears at least five times on my visit, which eventually poured out at the top of the mountain. It was no wonder this school got donations as big as the media centre – people trusted that their money was being used for exactly what he said it would – for the children.

It took him twelve years of relentless dedication to get a hall donated and built. Then, when he needed computers for the children, he persisted for another seven years. He agreed to share all of this in an interview with the investors of the project, so they too could get a sense of where their money was going and how desperately it was needed. I was inspired by his tremendous leadership and forward thinking. This is how to build a legacy. I understand why there are no broken windows and why the fence is still the original one built with the school.

The beautiful media centre with meeting rooms, books and computers were open to all parents and adults in the community too. After 14:00 every day and all day Saturday this centre is available to the community. The halls are available free, for anyone who needs to host a funeral. It doesn't end there, anybody going for a job interview needing copies of their Identity document can get one for free at the school. Yep, that's real poverty when the cost of a photocopy is a gift. In an area where poverty is rife, it's a miracle they've never had any break ins, but after hearing everything he had instituted – it makes perfect sense. It's everybody's school.

Most of the children there hadn't even been to Stellenbosch, let alone to Cape Town to see Table Mountain almost 50 km away. A tall building is anything bigger than their two-storey media centre. This school provides not just a dream, but an environment where the teachers lovingly hold their hand and walk side by side to cultivate their future's.

The books that One Heart brought over from Australia, were specifically designed to assist the teachers to teach the children to read. These were the books we'd be handing over. As mentioned previously, our national literacy rate at grade 4 level is 26%... that's like knowing a tidal wave is on its way to your coastal town. The books are in English and Afrikaans (the home language here) and are culturally relevant – the teachers love them, and the kids do too! For the first time in my life, I heard stories about children staying back during break times and after school to keep learning to read. That's proof of the environment Ronald and his staff are creating!

One of the teachers shared a story about a parent who messaged her while frantically looking for her daughter. She calmly replied that her daughter was still at school learning to read.

I felt as though I'd been given the freshest legs to climb the mountain with. Don and I sat in silence just staring at each other in the car. If the true measure of a man is asking those he impacts how they feel about him – Mr Frans would be one of the most successful people I've ever met.

My bubble was shattered as the warning light for my water came on while I was still on the freeway. I was clearly delusional to think it was going to get better. I needed to pull into a garage to let the car rest and cool down enough for me to pour more water into it and hopefully get us back the rest of the way. It was also the perfect excuse to have a Wimpy lunch!

The extra delay meant starting at 15:15, but the inspiration of the morning was still running through my veins – the result was a climb completed in 47 minutes and 47 seconds. I was driven by the constant feeling of gratitude and love, the knowledge that there were more schools that needed our help, and the humility of Mr Frans to put his success down to 'being blessed' rather than strutting around like a peacock. These thoughts powered and allowed me to forget about the screams from my legs and lungs. It was as if somehow overriding the screams would do more to raise money. Ok maybe not, but it certainly solidified my commitment to the causes that meant the world to me.

As I walked along the top to get photo #215, I was overwhelmed by Ronald's expression of thanks and heartfelt gratitude toward me for what I was doing. Here was a man who was exposed to some of the harshest circumstances and deepest levels of gratitude. His acknowledgment was a moving experience. I knew I still had 150 days to go, it could just as well be 1000. The charities were injecting a deeper purpose into these climbs by embedding a perspective of what real suffering and challenge was.

I was starting to appreciate and honour how fortunate I was to have had the idea for this project. I saw how using it to discover what I was made of and to empower others was two sides of the same coin.

I was learning that the greatest wealth came from enriching others.

My selfie was filled with tears. My long strands of hair stuck out from my cap and blew in the breeze as I took a moment to sit next to the station high above the city. Even if nothing else had to happen, every single step had been worth it. A beautiful sense of peace washed over me as I sat alone on the mountain - my teacher. The fire in my soul was being stoked as the summits added up day after day.

The book handover took place on Tuesday the 14th August which was also my friend Wes's birthday. It was fitting, because his fundraising efforts in Germany were equivalent to the impact of the books we dropped off. I was joined by Nicci and Don again who wouldn't have missed it for the world after our last visit.

Naturally, there were no arguments from me to go in his car.

We were welcomed into the hall with singing and dancing – one of my favourite reasons for being African. I love our culture and expressiveness. It was a great honour to share my journey with the students – now 225 climbs in with 140 ahead of me. Inside the hall there were six massive murals: The Pyramids, Table Mountain, the 'Big Five' (Lions / Elephants / Leopards / Water Buffalo / Rhinos), A volcanic Island, Statue of Liberty and the Sydney Opera house. They were beautiful reminders of places I too wanted to visit one day.

Their reaction to Mr Frans who shared what I was doing instantly transported me back to my moment in front of Amoyo. It was like watching a cartoon where all the eyes pop out, jaws hit the floor and tongues roll out. Afrikaans wasn't my strong point (my high school teacher must have been rolling her eyes at me – sorry Ms Groenewald!) so they chuckled at my clumsy sentence and asked if I could continue 'in Engels' (In English). I tried to incorporate as many of the views as well as a visual of the route. The best moment was when Lisa handed over the three gift boxes of books – that was our real purpose for being there.

The blessings continued to rain down on me as Melanie's dad (the one in New Zealand that gifted me my pounamu) was in town visiting his brother. Melanie ordered T Shirts and caps back in March which, after checking how ridiculous the cost to ship them was, decided to wait until an opportunity like this arose; albeit six months later. They spoiled me with dinner and I was not surprised by Melanie's generosity after spending time with her dad. Before parting ways, another envelope was handed over. More cash donations were enclosed. I added it to my growing pile of donations in the shoe box. It made me think of all those drug movies with huge piles of cash. Thankfully, this cash wasn't from harming anyone. I estimated that we were easily up to R15k. I hadn't counted it purposefully so I could just practise being grateful for whatever amount we ended up with. My adult's version of a piggy bank made my heart happier though, especially seeing all the smiling Madiba's together. Handing this over in January would be tremendously rewarding.

CHAPTER 12
SEPTEMBER - UNCONDITIONAL LOVE

This is how I collected the pocket money my grandparents gave me as a child. I'd save it for a toy car or maybe Lego. I'd often stand in front of the lego section and dream of owning it all while my mom did her grocery shopping. Whenever I begged for another toy, my mom would explain that we don't have money for that and suggested I save my pocket money. It was one of my greatest lessons because it made me appreciate what I was saving up for.

My second last climb before the shutdown was slow and measured, not like the emotion filled adrenalin rush of the previous day. The trash bin was completely full at the top, which meant I'd be carrying a huge load of bottles down with me. As I entered the stairway to heaven, I was treated to a bit of comedy. A tourist lunged for one of the sports drink bottles which I accidentally dropped.

'Is this yours??' he asked, perhaps hoping to squeeze the last few drops out of it.

'Uh, I wouldn't drink that. I picked it up.' I responded

I put the empty bottles down and swung the bag off my shoulder to offer him a sip of my water. A regular occurrence assisting completely unprepared climbers. Those previous experiences meant I always carried extra, regardless of whether I was alone or with a group. He was like an excited child seeing his dad come home from work. He grabbed it, thanking me over and over.

He was clearly thirsty because he wouldn't give it back! I was about to correct what he thought was happening, but I had another one for the trip down. It wasn't a train smash. His gratitude burst out of him and he insisted on paying me, and took two crumpled notes out of his pocket. It became the most expensive litre of water as he thrust R30 into my hands. I thanked him, knowing it was going into the cash pot!

Now that I had some 'space' I started picking up peels along the way and filled three of the five bottles. I hate to harp on it, but it's not okay to drop naartjie and banana peels on the path. Maybe people thought what I used to think – *'It's natural and will decompose no problem! Just throw them out of sight?'*

Right? Nope. The acidity changes the composition of the soil, destroying the ecosystem that the proteas thrive in. Because they have very shallow root systems, their environments get destroyed. It's why they aren't as bountiful along this path as they once were. It's such a small piece of education with far reaching implications for future generations, that it should be taught in schools. I used to throw apple cores away with the same thinking.

I no longer toss anything away like this, no matter how 'natural' it seems, because many birds on the mountain play the same role as bees by feeding on the plants and nectar, they help with pollination. Throwing peels away changes their eating patterns, and reduces their involvement in pollination too. It's scary how small actions can be so damaging. This is why education is so important. Education and constantly seeking out knowledge is how we gain a deeper understanding and appreciation of the complex and beautiful world we live in.

I had the pleasure of joining Cerina, one of the Future Females founders, in Kalk Bay with the crew celebrating her birthday at Cape to Cuba. I was celebrating too, knowing that the following day would be my last climb back down and number 59 for the year which was an average of once every four days. Well, at least that's what I thought. But Mother Nature seems to have a sense of humour and threw in an extra day – FOR FREE! I wasn't amused.

Both weather apps showed me that the reopening of the cableway would make my down climbs 16 in a row. It was nature's perfect bookend to complete the shutdown. It was a really miserable day too. My thoughts were deep in reflection though, as it was three years to the day my grandad passed away. He was a powerful influence and male role model in my life. I was fortunate to have him support me along with my dad. He adored his golf, and every second year I'd join the family for Christmas in Johannesburg. This provided us with an opportunity to carry on 'the family classic' golf day. Terence and I, who were the youngsters, took on the experienced 'oldies'. It spanned 14 years, and we started hot, winning the first couple before they pulled us back. I think we ended in a 6/5 split with them pipping us in the final game.

CHAPTER 12
SEPTEMBER – UNCONDITIONAL LOVE

Back on the mountain, I picked a stone for the family pile to place next to gran's. It was shaped like the head of an eagle with a black dot perfectly representing an eye. In a beautiful twist of fate, their rocks each had a perfectly flat side – and fit snugly together. They were married for 67 years. His memory warmed my heart and I knew he'd be proud. I'll never forget the principles he quietly instilled in me. To this day I have to raise my cap when meeting another adult and anytime I see someone crying while laughing, I get flooded with memories of him doing it too. I was incredibly fortunate as a child to know all four grandparents and he was in my life for 35 years. I'm even more fortunate with my gran, at the time of writing this, she still worries about me and checks in to make sure I'm eating.

With July being so warm our dams took a worrying dip instead of filling up, but mercifully, the much needed rain returned. While high between the cliffs, the rain flew up the mountain and slammed into my face. I tried to shy away from the thousand little pin pricks attacking me. I was flabbergasted when I walked past a couple tourists climbing in shorts and with no back packs. I didn't have the energy to engage.

As I made my way down, I passed the first rock that I cleaned graffiti off, and also spotted Don's car alone in the car park. I watched a torrential downpour block my view of the car before enveloping me. I was already soaked so there was no use trying to speed up in these slippery conditions. I incorporated the stat about car accidents into my thinking. 80% of accidents happen within 5km of people's homes. I suppose it's because it's all familiar and we switch to autopilot and lose focus.

It had been my 60th climb down and 111th alone, so I had plenty of time to evaluate the cause of slipping and accidents. I had experienced the urge to up my tempo as I hit the contour path back down, 'to get it over and done with', but after having climbed up and down? One wrong step with fatigued muscles could mean the difference between a twisted ankle or worse. Maybe even losing my balance and tumbling down the mountainside with nothing but hard jagged edges waiting for me.

Thursday's climb brought me more reminders of this. I met a climber that was inspired to attempt climbing Table Mountain every day in September. Sadly with just five days to go, he damaged his ankle so badly that he couldn't even walk to the fridge. It was a sobering reminder of how quickly serious accidents could happen. It's why I couldn't lose concentration for a split second and learned to override the internal urges to pick up the pace!! *"Come on!! We're almost down and the rest of the way is easy."* I laughed at the absurdity of it. I'd just taken three hours, what would a few minutes saved over here really make?

As waves of rain descended upon me, I did a weird version of 'singing in the rain' and jumped in puddles on the tarmac like a maniac! It put me in a great mood as I flopped into the car. I was looking for every possible reason to celebrate. With perfect weather waiting for me the next day, I made sure to kiss the cable car at the bottom. What a sight for sore legs.

Thursday the 9th August was Women's Day in South Africa. Inclement weather prevented me from trying a new route as a reward for 150 consecutive climbs. I was excited to climb Right Face Arrow Face for the 200th. Miriam had been sick and the combination of a public holiday and magical weather made my new dream route a reality. Again, I loved the fact that there wasn't anything specific in mind for Women's Day and organically, a woman would lead the climb. Sarah (the journalist) and Seven of *The Mountain Slayers joined.*

The route took us along the contour path, turned right at one of the majestic waterfalls and came down Union Ravine. It's my favourite route up the Table Mountain, because there's no trash to pick up and it's an under-utilised path. The route is only for experienced climbers though. There used to be signs along the contour path depicting each challenging route branching up, but thankfully those have been taken down. I'm sure many unsuspecting people have been fooled by the easy contour path and decided to push up, not knowing what lay ahead.

CHAPTER 12
SEPTEMBER - UNCONDITIONAL LOVE

Table Mountain's deceptively misleading. Accidents happen on Platteklip and that's a relentless staircase. From across the bay, the façade looks like one steep drop off from the contour path up to the top. While there are cliffs, they're staggered and the distance from the contour path to the rim on top of the cliffs is 500m. Five giant buttresses stick out, almost as supporting legs for the table top. It shows you how uniform the rock strata are.

The day's climb took us behind and around those rock strata. I saw why I couldn't have done this for climb #150 and why it was imperative to wait for a clear day. One of the waterfalls cut through this section all the way down to the Atlantic pool. Even now, the ground was soft and squidgy and we had to navigate loose stones. While scrambling up, it's easy to think you may be off the path, especially as the yellow footprints disappear. But luckily this wasn't our group's first rodeo, everyone had scaled steep vertical sections of rock before, so the conversations stayed calm and relaxed but internally my heart was racing. It was a humbling experience to be on this iconic north mountainside, as a tiny spec invisible to the thousands of people recording their sense of wonder and photographing this marvel.

I love how climbing mountains allows you to catch up with friends, and engage in meaningful conversations with new people. Sarah and I ended up chatting with Mogamat as he shared tales of his frequent mountain adventures. He started recounting his fear of dogs and how, while climbing down two weeks back, a huge black dog scared the bejesus out of him. Sarah and I stared at each other immediately.

'Was the dog's name Salvador by any chance?' I asked.

'YES!! I'll never forget that name!' he responded.

'Then we've already met you! He was with us!' exclaimed Sarah. It sparked an interesting discussion around people bringing dogs to the mountain. My only gripe was when owners didn't flick the shit off the path, but Mogamat shared a

263

different perspective on being afraid of dogs. Salvador is a teddy bear, but he looks vicious. This type of dog triggers a lot of fear for many South Africans, as they were used by the police in the townships to attack people. On his last outing, Sarah had to hold him so people that were too terrified to move could pass by.

Dane was from Montana, and was completing his Masters in Urban Planning. He shared how Cape Town reminded him of home with easy access to beautiful mountains. Dwayne was on his own outdoor journey and was seeing how many times he could summit each of the three peaks in 2018. Today was his 7th time up Table Mountain. Gert had been following my journey on Instagram and was inspired to push his own capabilities and climb every day in September. Graham was one I couldn't quite sync my positions with and only got to hear him on our breaks. On this day one of these fine people took my favourite pic of the year. I laid on a comfy rock with my hands behind my head, while Lions Head, the city and the bay sprawled out and bathed in the glorious sunshine below. It was my happy place and you could see it on my face.

India Venster went from one buttress to the next under the cable car, and we climbed some exposed ledges. I wasn't afraid of heights, but the sheer drop was an intense experience which set off some butterflies. How anyone discovered this route was beyond me. As if ledge climbing wasn't enough, we had to crawl through cracks in the mountain. The first one was just wide enough for me to fit through. Thank goodness I'd slimmed down to 103kg from the 110kg I started on! I wasn't sure January Andrew would have made it through here.

There was no turning back now!

The entrance was like an ancient tomb carved with carefully selected stones. Thankfully, it wasn't too dark inside. I was happy to pop out the other side though, only to find another hole to climb through. This one's 'ceiling' was higher and slightly wider than my shoulders. The boulder facing down the mountain could have been a bus. It was huge and it was the only thing between us and the drop down to certain death. I didn't rest on this thought too much, but the reality was that we were surrounded by teetering boulders. I was mesmerised by the new sights, the overhangs and all the rocks 'living on the edge'.

I was relieved to make it out the second stretch but knew there were some tricky and heavily exposed sections to navigate. There was a gap I wouldn't think twice to jump over normally, but the steep drop messed with my mind. We were in no rush and cautiously moved over the gaps one by one. We had the smallest of the three holes back to back to climb through, where I had to remove my backpack to squeeze through. As I reached the opening, I handed my bag through, then took the other backpacks. Finally, I climbed out as if the mountain was giving birth to me. After four body twisting, butterfly inducing hours, we reached the final half an hour mark that connected us to India Venster. As a special treat, we saw two Klipspringer bucks! It was the first time I'd seen these indigenous 'mountain goats' from the cape.

Sarah wore the 365 Ubuntu Climbs cap and T-shirt she bought, this advertising helped the cause and inspired Mandisi and Winnie to buy some too. I was famished after a long arduous climb, so a couple of us headed over to Coco Ola for a well deserved lunch and beers. One thing I enjoyed about burning so many calories was having free reign to smash as many fries as I wanted. Then our discussion took a turn to a quote I'd posted the day before:

When you make a commitment, you build hope. When you keep it, you build trust.

Again, it was interesting to hear others' perspectives on what I was trying to achieve. Especially now that I had a bank of months behind me. It reinstilled belief that perhaps more donations would come at the back end of the year.

I had collected the day's stone in one of the caverns that had a gap which allowed you to view the cable car through. I was looking forward to placing the third rock from a different route with its 220 brothers and sisters.

The next day I woke up enthused to drop off the previous day's rock. My excitement evaporated as my car's red warning light screamed on my way up to the cable station parking. This was bad.

So much for the beautiful synchronicity I was hoping for. At 18:18 my car hit 180 000 km. I was paranoid about my engine exploding and doing all kinds of damage. Nervously, I pulled off to the side of the road. I decided to take the road less travelled and walked along one of the jeep tracks that the mountain bikers loved going down, but cursed going up. Starting lower down on the slopes added serious chunks to my elevation gain but the new section was a breath of fresh air and another opportunity to find a rock on a new path. Rock #222 joined #221 cradled in my hands The path was invisible from the road above me, but I could see the road snaking its way along. I loved that even this late in the year I could have extraordinary experiences on the mountain. With slow and methodical steps, I finally reached Ubuntu Rock and placed them next to the other three for week 32.

I couldn't help but feel a sense of wonder as I reached the top and stood admiring the upper cable station. It looked as though steam from a volcano rose up then disappeared next to us while we baked in the glorious sunshine. It was an extremely unusual sight. Then I set up to take my picture. I had my left foot on plank number three and my right foot on plank number six, while the camera was in line with my nose. A cloud made its way up the front of the mountain and continued to rise well after passing the rim. The upper station looked like it was in danger of being scolded by the 'steam'. Click – I snapped my photo! #222 for the year.

Although my car was a mess, my tracker was still able to make me smile. Climb #222 took 2 hours and 22 minutes! I thanked my thirsty car as I filled up her dry tank with fresh mountain water. The numbers didn't have any earth shattering significance but it was a beautiful reminder that I was being supported and that things would line up without having to be forced. I was reminded of my next climb which was organised by *Empire Wealth* – a company committed to helping investors build their own property investment empire. They were partnered with SA Property Network. Anton, the founder, heard me speak at both events and invested in my project. He then went on to organise a climb with his clients and invited them to donate. It was a healthy group of 16. It was so cold, it felt like there should have been snow on the ground. There was zero chance I was doing my barefoot climb today, so I banked it for another time. This decision was justified as we reached Ascension Corner, where the wind was the coldest I'd ever experienced.

Rogan was an interesting guy and stayed behind with Jamie and I, as we waited for Danielle who was taking some strain. Rogan shared how he almost exhausted himself at his previous company and how he got no reward for his hard work. Only once he resigned did they offer to double his salary and give him a bigger team. It was too little too late. Funny how most companies operate this way. Why not just look after your existing staff in the first place? He used this opportunity to tour the far east, Vietnam, Cambodia and Thailand for seven months and then came back to a job at Empire. His time in Bali was spent reconnecting with himself, and discovering what he wanted to do with his life. It's a common story for many of us who find ourselves chasing a never-ending finish line, seldom taking the time to invest in these three things: ourselves, others and the environment. These elements were my new benchmark for success, ALL three needed a green tick.

It inspired me to hear examples where people discovered their worth and said goodbye to anything that didn't honour them. It reminded me of the different types of mountains we all had to climb. Scarcity mindset and feelings of inadequacy kept me trapped in bad relationships and jobs for too long. It's a tough pattern to break. Awareness is the first step to getting it right. I refuse to be a victim, that's why I search each heartbreak and poor decision for something to learn. I am enough – means I'm ready to give freely, and I am worthy – means I'm ready to receive freely. It's taken me 40 years to believe this at a soul level.

Anton sounded like a great guy and was invested in helping others achieve financial freedom, this is what attracted Rogan. It was no surprise why they got involved and prepared to get up early on a freezing weekend morning to climb for others.

Devil's Peak sat quietly under the deep blue sky like a volcano and with no clouds in sight. Its summit seemed to 'steam' as clouds continued to flow out of sight behind the eastern table. A majestic sight, and one of the hundreds of reasons this challenge was a gift. I was literally seeing the mountain in every possible way and experiencing views most would never see.

Everyone celebrated with a hot chocolate or coffee before heading down. My new favourite was the café's mochaccino. Having this in my hand meant two glorious things: the cable way was open AND we were able to escape the cold. Some decided to walk down, but I wasn't my freshest, so I was happy to abuse my cable car pass.

August's return to 'normality' with a barrage of cold fronts was fabulous news! The total average fill rate across major dams was only at 58% in July, the spring weather gave us less than half the month's usual rainfall. Mercifully though, our latest deluge put the dams at 62% and left us breathing a sigh of relief. The dams were at 33.8% the same time last year in 2017!

Dynamic Group Travel had expressed interest in offering a climb with me to their clients and one of them and his son jumped at the chance. Climb #233 was the day they joined. Two of my friends, David and Kerri, were celebrating their birthdays too. David hadn't climbed Table Mountain in years and was excited to finally be joining. Both he and Kerri would get a free ride down in the cable car – a lovely perk offered to people on their birthdays by the Cable car company.

The father and son from New York that joined, were celebrating the son's 10th birthday on an African trip. I truly loved the dad's philosophy of giving his children experiences instead of presents for their birthdays. Each child could choose any destination in the world they wanted to visit. He chose Cape Town, South

CHAPTER 12
SEPTEMBER - UNCONDITIONAL LOVE

Africa. The son's questions came flying in and I was happy to answer, hoping to impress Richard with my knowledge. Richard was one of those people who perfectly suited his profession. He was an outstanding tour guide, and I had no doubt he created trips of a lifetime for his clients. They loved my cap and I managed to get some printed with their individual numbers before they left. They also donated and it warmed my heart to no end. This is the message they left:

'Andrew, thank you for letting us join you today to become part of your special journey! #233 was awesome and we were so appreciative of your support on our first climb. Donating $233 x 2! Good luck!'

Was the total amount raised important? Yes – the more money I raised, the more people I'd be able to impact. Was it the only thing of importance? No, and my journey was teaching me that.

I wasn't sure why someone would climb and not contribute. Perhaps they felt their 'small' contribution wasn't enough. This is why I invited people to donate R1 per climb. I think one of the greatest tragedies of our time is not getting involved because we dismiss the importance of a 'small' contribution. I put 'small' because the real measure of a donation is not by the size, but by the percentage of their income.

Just think about those children in the township who donated R2 each when they didn't even have R100, versus a billionaire giving R6,900,000. It's difficult to compare this because the higher donation catches our eye as amazing (and it is!) but it's not the whole picture.

Instead of using percentages, I decided to use 24 hours as a standard measure and converted each donation into time. The billionaire gave 9 minutes of his time. The kids from the township? They gave 28 minutes! I now realise why I broke down in my video when they each gave me R2.

I thoroughly enjoyed getting to know the staff working for the Cable Way. Carl was a very interesting man, always checking in on me and, even though the cable car took five minutes, we had deep conversations. I was always excited to find out what gem he was going to share with me next. I remember Carl from my mom and dad's first climb in September 2017. We were sitting enjoying the spectacular sunset. As he walked past he didn't just smile, he took a moment to stop and chat. His nickname should be Mr Consistent because every time I see him, he greets me with that same beaming smile. I love hearing his perspectives on life. He quit a high powered corporate job to work where he is now. They almost didn't hire him stating he was 'overqualified' for the role. It took some explaining, but they finally realised he was serious and his desire to find work in nature surrounded by beauty was a huge reason for his application. It's hard to beat the office views at this company.

Letting go of the urge to control things in favour of trusting that everything will work out, is a process that keeps rewarding me. It reminds me how powerful releasing expectations is. Carl helps to reinforce this.

That night, I was invited to a birthday dinner with an acquaintance. I arrived first and did what I always do – chose the seat to the far left so I had no one to my left and I could hear people speak in a crowded restaurant. Slowly but surely everyone filtered in with just two seats available, one in front of me and one at the end of the table. Liz sat at the head of the table, she was part of a four women crew that successfully rowed across the Pacific from San Francisco to Cairns. She had given a talk about it at a financial services, called Solid Rock, client evening in 2016. Each year the business had an opportunity to thank their clients and invited a speaker who had made an impact. This year, it was my turn!

Ken contacted me through my blog to set it up. His honesty moved me:

'When I heard you were doing this, I was a tad sceptical, as I've been up a few times in my life.... But if you put it out there that it's a goal, then there's stuff called pride, commitment, plain old 'I'll show you', funders and the expectations of others.

Anyway I have a small business in Cape Town (financial planning) and have client appreciation evenings, where we invite people that have done 'stuff' to chat and

CHAPTER 12
SEPTEMBER - UNCONDITIONAL LOVE

inspire. We've had some interesting speakers but no ones that's quite as mal (crazy)! OK, perhaps just as mal! It starts at 6pm and it's all over by 7:30pm. You would have 20 - 30 minutes to chat/tell your story. If you're available for something like this, our next one is the 5th of September.'

When this email was sent, there were ten more days of the shutdown left. Now it was two weeks later and I was sitting next to last year's speaker. I mean, what are the odds of this? Their documentary is called, 'Losing Sight of the Shore,' check it out if you can. Talking to Liz was a worthwhile experience, she told me all about how they processed falling short of their fundraising goals.

It begged the question, 'How much is enough'? Importantly, I was being prepared mentally for the eventuality of falling 'short' and I was being challenged to think about what that meant, what importance I placed on it and crucially, evaluating and redefining my idealistic interpretation of empowering others. I was being shown both sides of the equation and what could happen if I placed emphasis on the wrong reasons for doing something. Let's not forget, the idea was to climb Table Mountain every day. I chose to use it as a platform to raise money. The test was the primary reason, raising money was secondary.

As my first paid talk, this was something new for me. The sharks started swimming around in my head making me question whether I was worthy or not. I left the dinner bewildered by Liz's presence. It felt like someone with knowledge of the future was orchestrating all these divinely timed meetings, and reassuring me that everything was going to be okay. As I write this it still blows my mind how through all the support, I still managed to default back to irrational fears. Yep - even now I still have them.

I always had interesting thoughts on climbs and while practising for Solid Rock on the mountain, I download this thought:

Whenever we speak to someone, our words can become the wind in their sails and take their minds to places they never knew existed.

I realised that I never thought about a statement like that in relation to my self-talk. Why wasn't I putting as much emphasis on being careful with my own words? Now this journey was much more than just climbing a mountain. In my eight months I'd made peace with the difficulty of reaching the summit. I chose to dig deeper and taught myself that no matter what, I could reach my daily summit. I also learned to transfer this motivation to any metaphorical summit.

I was sure that a hairy bearded mountain man frightened a couple of tourists as he slogged up loudly speaking to himself. Rambling out loud helped me channel my thoughts and my flow.

Our heart understands long before the mind can see. When we live by our heart our mind fights because it can't see what's coming. And so, the mind is locked in a constant loop of apologising to the heart and being grateful for where they end up.

Climb #238 was hands down the roughest climb of the year. The pain was all self-inflicted. Darren surprised me with a ticket to watch some friends DJing at a club in town, with a large group from Summer Camp. How could I refuse? What the heck, I said I'd go support, and I'd leave around midnight. I wouldn't take my wallet, that way I couldn't drink.

The weekend was the start of another four-day storm. It was projected to be wetter, windier, and colder than the June experience. It seemed as if the weather was attuned to my feelings. My car was now inoperable and was being assessed to see how much it was worth. Why couldn't that drunk driver have hit it just a little bit harder?? Darren's generosity extended to collecting me which also gave us the opportunity to catch-up over a pre-party drink.

I hoped that my next climb would be my first opportunity to experience snow on the mountain. At this stage, the only thing missing for me to complete the whole set. After climbing back down I knew Sunday would be the same, but the morning had the best forecast for snow. This is what made me decide to let my hair down a tad. It would give me enough time to get home like Cinderella

CHAPTER 12
SEPTEMBER - UNCONDITIONAL LOVE

and rest before meeting Don at 8:15. This way I could drop him off at the gym and head up to the mountain in time.

Everything seemed to line up and I was genuinely excited about a night out with some great music and friends. That all changed in less than ten minutes of arriving. We decided to head over earlier so I wouldn't have to leave after just arriving. This also meant the club was quiet and emptier. Then James entered. He was down from Johannesburg and was dead set on supporting everyone. He pulled me over to the bar, pointed at me and said to the bartender... 'this man doesn't pay for a single drink tonight - he's on my tab!'

With a massive grin he ordered our first round. I hadn't seen him since Pieter and Danielle's wedding in April. If nothing else happened or I saw no one else - this alone would make my night worth it. It was also the first time I'd heard that he saved Danielle's life on their wedding night! Long after I'd left, she almost choked on a sweet that got lodged in her throat. Unable to breath he eventually picked her up and dislodged it. It's scary how quickly things can happen.

Midnight came and went and I hadn't turned into a pumpkin so I stayed to listen to Dave Irish (from Mr suits that donated my GoPro) play a killer set. I probably would've been fine if I'd left then but Jono came on and spun a two hour web of pleasure. With the alcohol flowing just as easily as the music, 03:00 arrived. If I stayed any longer, I'd probably oversleep again and miss my only chance to experience snow on Table Mountain. I quickly called an Uber. Luckily it was just a nine minute drive, but with the storm hitting us, it was terrifying. I was dropped off at the entrance but got soaked as I dashed up to the front door. I looked like a drowned sewer rat. I bid Sam a good night, and rushed upstairs. I decided that sleeping on the couch would increase my chances of hearing the alarms I set, and although it was less comfortable than my bed, it would be easier to sleep with my right ear up. Thankfully, I heard all of the alarms but not even two cups of coffee could help me. I felt rough!

Don drove us to the gym through more torrential rain. My epic night was worth every moment, but I wasn't looking forward to the climb. Safety Mountain Tracking urged me to be extra careful because there was another storm surging towards the Mother City. Finally at 08:47 am I got to the base of Platteklip and inhaled the icy air. My body wasn't happy at all. My heart rate was at least 20 beats per minute faster than usual, and that was just from getting out of the car.

I was glad that I took videos before the massive storm hit the previous day. Now I was able to compare them to the same spot today. The photo ops doubled as extra stops, something I really needed. As soon as I reached the contour path, rain with intermittent hail started falling. It was a prelude of what was to come. I felt the same way as I did months ago when I panicked about reaching the summit in time to witness the sunrise between the cliffs. Worried I may miss my opportunity to see snow, I was in absolutely no shape to increase my pace. My brain said, 'We need to go faster' and my body replied, 'Maybe if you'd given us more sleep we could!'

One of the most ominous clouds creeped over the ocean towards me. It was a breathtaking sight. The sun rays filtered through and illuminated the ocean in front of the storm while the dark gloominess enveloped everything in its path. The ocean disappeared behind the curtain of rain that was headed directly for me. Minutes went by before the waves of water cascaded from the skies and drenched the city with its grey veil. I covered my bag and zipped up my rain jacket, like a gladiator putting protective gear on in anticipation of an assault.

As I reached the first corner closest to the cliffs I was given a unique hail experience. There was no rain, just millions of tiny ice balls bouncing off me and all around as they collided with the mountain. I'd never experienced anything like this before. With my cap under my hood protecting my head, I battled through the energy sapping climb desperately hoping that I wouldn't miss the snow - if there was any. In no time at all, the mountainside was transformed as the hail clumped together making patches of white. It may not have been snow, but it was beautiful.

CHAPTER 12
SEPTEMBER - UNCONDITIONAL LOVE

The hail made me believe that it was too cold for snow, and the higher I got, the more there was. They were especially beautiful at Ubuntu Rock laying alongside my family stones and all the others from week 35.

With my heart about to kick the emergency exit out of my chest, I was grateful to be able to finish the last section in ten minutes. I was battling to breath at the top, I was taking in huge gasps, and each one felt less oxygenated than the last. I was in a sorry state – all self inflicted. I wasn't sure why I took the longer loop around at the top, but I was rewarded thanks to the water and hail. I saw a rock that had a heart carved into it, and it reminded me that some self-love was needed when I got home.

Sadly, there was no happy ending to this fairytale. I could easily have stayed last night, climbed later in the afternoon, and had a far more pleasant time. There was no snow, but at least I tried. The bitter cold up top forced me to rearrange my DKMS Africa buff. I covered my ears and put the cap over it to hold it in place. Finally my heart rate dropped to normal, I focused on getting back down safely to get dry, under blankets, and to some more episodes of Netflix's, *'I am a killer'*.

Today was the first time in 63 down climbs that I decided to choose a stone from the top of Table Mountain to deliver on the way down. It made me realise how easy it was to fall into a pattern. The entire way down, my hands were so cold they didn't register as mine, even under two sets of gloves. Ivwrong. All 26 days in the rain were combined with 41 down climbs while 16 were consecutive. It had taken its toll. The coldest and wettest month by far offered no reprieve, and it was the only month where I hadn't done a barefoot climb.

I was on 243 completed climbs. My brain struggled to compute that, but my body felt it. Physically, I felt fantastic when I was off the mountain, but exhausted when on it. Mentally, I was coping well and felt positive about making it through the toughest third. Emotionally, I felt rooted in my purpose and prepared for any eventuality. Spiritually, I felt more aligned than ever before. My gratitude and fulfilment was matched only by my excitement for September, Spring and a less taxing third of the year. Well, that's what I was hoping for.

AUGUST STATS:

243 / 365

People Joined: 42 / 420

24 days 05 hours 27 minute 34 seconds / 1 640,37 km / 47,28 equivalent Everest Summits

/ 127 solo climbs (50%) / 64 Up & Down (19,2%) TOTAL DONATIONS:

R288 328.70

Campbell: 'It was an honour and a privilege to climb with you today. I am very grateful for the opportunity. Keep up your amazing work and passion for what is an outstanding endeavour.'

Margaret: 'Very happy to donate to such a worthy cause'

Astrid: 'So in awe of what your vision is and what you have accomplished'

When mountain climbing is made too easy, the spiritual effect the mountain exercises vanishes into the air

~~ D.T Susuki

CHAPTER 13
SEPTEMBER - UNCONDITIONAL LOVE

The first climb of the month was a foreboding sign; what started as a beautiful spring day transformed into another frigid summit. Nothing surprised me anymore. The universe dangled magical carrots in front of me as extra motivation for my exhausted legs. What exactly were the carrots? Buddhist Monks all the way from India were due to arrive and I would have the opportunity to host them on top of the mountain. My friend Nicci sent me an email detailing their trip to South Africa, complete with their timelines in Cape Town, Johannesburg, and Durban. This included an invitation for someone to help 'get them up Table Mountain.' No surprise Nicci thought of me. Three of them would be creating a colourful sand mandala in Simons Town while on their trip to Cape Town. The only spare day they had neatly coincided with my final climb of the month at the end of week 39.

Mountains are an important part of their faith, and selfishly, I hoped it would be me to guide them up. It would be a massive honour and experience to learn more about another religion and culture. My passion for more knowledge in this area started the day after my friend Dexter gave me 'The Little Buddha' to watch. After that, I set things in motion.

It's hard to fathom that 40 climbs had passed by since Ken contacted me for Wednesday's talk two days before climb #250 rolled around! The milestones were coming in thick and fast. I loved the fact that my first paid talk was for a company called *Rock Solid*.

My folks arrived on day #250 for another week of emotional support. It wasn't something they planned, it was just a week they settled on. Now they could celebrate climb #250 just as they did #100.

The first week was a tad soul destroying, it was colder and wetter (sometimes a combination of the two) than I'd hoped for. With a miserable final week of August, I had no illusions that 'spring' would somehow flip a switch.

I had a scare too, with exactly one week until my talk, my throat started tingling like back in January. This time, I picked it up quickly and identified it as an insecurity related to not feeling worthy enough to be paid to speak. I thanked my body for the reminder and worked on fixing it.

I used my solo climbs to focus on believing that I was worthy and expressing gratitude to Ken for selecting me for this year's annual gala hosted in Allan Gray's auditorium at the Waterfront. It was always an honour to share, especially after his initial doubts about my commitment. I appreciated his honesty, too. It was a reminder that I was being watched, but every summit I completed built more trust.

Catching my negative self-talk early meant that I could confront my feelings of unworthiness and prevent it from materialising like in January. It's remarkable how our bodies speak to us.

CHAPTER 13
SEPTEMBER - UNCONDITIONAL LOVE

My supportive network of friends was another bow in my quiver. Dave joined on another cold and wet climb, which also happened to be the day of my talk. It was his 8th climb, and I really appreciated it because there was a strong chance we'd be climbing back down. His knees didn't take too kindly to the down climbs, and would suffer for weeks after. Mercifully, the cable car worked, and his unparalleled support was rewarded. Laughing, I completely misread his previous day's text, so I drove to pick him up.

'I'm downstairs when you're ready buddy.' I texted.

'I'm already outside your place.' he responded.

He knew I had car troubles and was trying to help me out. The result was that we'd both driven to collect each other! It was hilarious! So we just made our way to meet at the mountain. His presence wasn't his only support, he also acted as a sounding board as I spoke about my sore throat and insecurities. Dave is not a yes-man, which I appreciate. He always gives it to me straight. His feedback means the world to me.

Our climb went quickly and we were down in under two hours which was great. It gave me time to review my slides and prepare mentally.

Ken told me that I could invite my partner, but Jessie was a million miles away - luckily, I was blessed with Don and Lisa smiling at me in the audience. They were more than just support, they gave me powerful feedback I could use for future talks. One of the reasons I loved this project so much was because I was able to do some public speaking while the 365 Ubuntu Climbs was on. The year-long project still had 117 climbs remaining, so anybody who wanted to talk to me could do so. Sue and her son Matthew spoke to me afterward and pledged to join a climb and donate. This was more than just lip service - they followed through with actions.

There were three milestone climbs remaining and this meant that there were just two new routes up the front face left to discover: Ledges and Kloof Corner.

Another journalist joined me on climb #250. I thought she joined just to take pictures for her article, but she completed the whole climb. Thanks to the freezing wind, It was the coldest climb of the year. Even with two pairs of gloves, my hands went numb. The temperature gauge at the top of the mountain said three degrees but I wasn't buying it – it was definitely below zero. Because it was a milestone climb, I decided to walk down India Venster; something I'd never done before. I knew it was far more dangerous than going down Platteklip, but I felt up for it. Thanks to the mountain shielding us from the wind, it took 45 minutes for my hands to finally thaw out. The light was gorgeous because of the time of year we were in, and climbing down the more exposed route gave us majestic views of the coast and the city. For the 18th time this year, I heard the noon gun going off. We must've been halfway down already when the cableway started working. I didn't get riled up because there was zero chance I could've waited this long at the South Pole. I was just happy to be moving and experiencing this path down for the first time.

The path had far more loose stones and felt more like a single-track path compared to Platteklip's mythical staircase. My foot slid a couple times on the loose gravel, and while I was grateful for a new perspective, I would never come down this way again. Ever! I was also baffled by people who had told me going down India Venster was 'easier' than Platteklip. Even though my longer legs gave me an advantage on Platteklip, I still couldn't agree with them.

It had been 200 climbs since the last time I was here. A rockfall sent a boulder the size of two washing machines hurtling down the mountain, only to become wedged on the path we needed to clamber over. *That wasn't here on climb #50.* This was another reminder of the frequent rockfalls.

It was fascinating seeing the changes unfold from one day to another. Besides the physical shifts, there were more subtle ones, like the new flowers that bloomed, these were just as rewarding. We also saw the first signs of the China Flowers; five satin white petals splashed with a thin line of red down the middle, lured your eye to its delicate stigmas where the bees collected pollen. I'd been gifted with the opportunity to see new flowers bloom all year, but spring was the most spectacular, with at least 60% blooming then.

My parents arrived a few hours later, and I was overjoyed to see their beaming faces again. My dad's official retirement in March was another advantage enjoyed from the timing of my challenge. It removed the urgency to fly down, something Mom didn't enjoy. They were able to experience a more relaxed road trip over the course of a few days, and I was extremely grateful for their visit. Ever since I'd moved to Cape Town, they had made a special trip down. Their support was a constant driving force and got even better over the year. They watched my climbs live in Endomondo, sent messages, checked in daily on my experiences, and my dad even joined Facebook to see the pictures and videos I posted!

I was excited for another family climb on Sunday, climb #252. Their timing was impeccable because it coincided with One Heart's Family Trail run, which we drove out to support. It would also allow me to introduce them to Lisa. I passed the headmaster from the other primary school that we sponsored. He was carrying the books and his face was a picture of pure joy. He called out to me, and expressed his gratitude. This is what it was all about. It's why collaborating with the right organisations was so important to me. I was grateful my folks could experience this.

We had an early lunch before heading to the mountain to start at 15:00. Just as I'd watched the sun move north for the winter months, bringing shorter days, I watched its trek back down south as summer loomed. Sunrise was at 07:00 and sunset was at 18:30, so we were almost back to 12-hour days. By the end of the month sunset would be at 18:48 and would allow the last cable car to come down at 19:00. Having an extra hour for afternoon climbs like this one would be a relief.

We were never in any danger of missing the last cable car, but it was less stressful and meant we could go at a more comfortable pace. Although the air was cold, the afternoon sun was hot and made the first portion tough. Luckily the shade enveloped us in some areas and gave my dad and Don extra comfort.

Don's concern wasn't fitness. As my gym partner, I knew how strong he was. The swims he did three times a week certainly prepared him for the challenge. He was more nervous about his fear of heights, and yet he still joined and showed his support. My mom wasn't feeling up to doing another one and rather caught the cable car up with the aim of walking down to perch herself on 'Ubuntu rock,' where she'd watch our progress on Endomondo. The mountain drops away from you most at Hail Corner, and this is where Don could only look straight up at the mountain. It was inspiring to be in the presence of someone who was pushing through their fears – demonstrating courage with purpose.

It fascinated me that we were naturally inclined to go at a pace that pushed our capabilities more than usual. Unless someone was going slower than that, I'd never seen anyone successfully slow their pace intentionally. My dad cast his mind back to Caroline and Mom's achievement and was in awe once again. Then he looked at me and shook his head, 'I don't know how you do this every day bud,' – and reiterated it while we enjoyed our sushi dinner. I knew how I did it every day, one of the contributing factors was the support I got. Another factor would be made clear two days later.

Masande and her family were in their new home! Habitat invited me to see the final product, so we bought a cake to celebrate. I felt privileged to have witnessed the evolution from the shack, all the way to the completed house. If I needed people that inspired me to climb Table Mountain every day: Masande was one of my biggest inspirations. Meeting her, and experiencing her passion, gratitude, and love, without ever complaining once, really moved me. One thing we don't celebrate enough in South Africa is the resilience of our people. I'm proud to be South African.

In one of the most heart-warming experiences of my life, Masande shared what a difference it had made to spend winter in her new home. The warmth, the

CHAPTER 13
SEPTEMBER - UNCONDITIONAL LOVE

protection, staying dry, and, best of all, having her own toilet and shower. As she proudly gave us the tour, her eyes lit up, and her smile beamed, I felt like I was in the presence of an angel.

There were 111 days left to finish my challenge, but a lifetime of commitment was needed to help everyone. It was as true 2000 years ago as it is today.

The task of perfecting the world is not yours to finish, but neither are you free from taking part in it. And if not now, when?

Knowing we could give other families this kind of life-changing gift was just what I needed. I didn't know it yet, but September was about to become the toughest month to date. It rained as much as it did in June and August, but also brought a mix of extreme hot and cold.

I kept having near misses with snowfall too. I saw posts from the mountain guides where they shared their little snowmen. My hopes were dwindling fast. A spate of consistent early climbs from the 12th to the 18th included a down climb and three in the rain. This left me completely depleted and drained. The following day would be my 4th consecutive solo climb, so I decided not to set an alarm and let my body decide how long my mini coma should be.

As wave upon wave of rain came down, I expressed gratitude that I'd chosen to do a later climb. But that feeling soon changed! As I switched off my phone's Airplane mode, the first message arrived... *'Did you experience the snow on Table Mountain this morning?'*

You've got to be kidding me! Then Richard, the tour guide, phoned me from the top to ask if I was on the mountain being snowed on. Twice in an hour?! Seriously???? Was I the only one that didn't get the memo? Looking like a zombie, I finally got up and fumbled my way around the apartment. Opening my laptop to respond to requests for climbs and donations, I made the mistake of opening Facebook – a live video of snow greeted me! Not once... not twice... THREE TIMES!! I immediately knew I'd blown it. It was like arriving on the platform as the last train started pulling away. I was gutted. I knew this was the last time it would snow. I was right. The one thing I truly wanted to experience had evaded me.

Well – I guess you can't have everything, hey?

Everyone knew about my keen desire to see the snow, so having people ask me what the experience was like, was more comical than actually missing it. Ah man, what a day to decide to do an afternoon climb.

Time marched on, and soon I had climbed the equivalent of 50 Mt Everests. I hit this milestone on a day when the top was completely covered in clouds. These milestone days without views had helped me build appreciation by reminding me that it wasn't the view at the top that was important; but the journey and the insights that mattered.

It was also my 191st trip down in the cable car. With 108 days to go I was curious to see what the final split was between cable car rides down and down climbs. I was already sitting on 66 climbs back down, which was over two full months out of the eight. One of the cableway staff suggested that I contact their marketing department to try and get them involved. Rieyaaz had been outstanding. With a warm and friendly smile, he'd often push me to the front of the queue, and ask what number climb I was on. Now, he'd gone beyond the extra mile to encourage some company involvement. It made sense to set up a collaboration, especially since they had over a million visitors a year. And even though I'd already spoken to them, perhaps another push from an internal source would help get traction.

Thanks to my friend Ally, I got the opportunity to meet with the Managing Director of Native VML back in July. Every year, the company has a global giving day. Branches around the world would invite their staff to help make a difference in people's lives through education-based initiatives. Usually, the MD chooses who they'd support. This year, she challenged the staff to suggest some beneficiaries. This is where Ally came in. She hated speaking in front of people but put that aside to speak about my climbs and who they were helping.

CHAPTER 13
SEPTEMBER - UNCONDITIONAL LOVE

That created the chance to meet the MD and discuss logistics and how they could donate directly to One Heart.

With the global day set on the 27th of September, I initially thought, 'no problem!' But with snow the previous week, I was less optimistic. Hopefully, the weather would play ball. I was invited to the company bar the Friday before, to speak to those that had chosen 365 Ubuntu Climbs. Originally, I'd suggested 10 slots, but five more eagerly jumped on board! I was proud that out of the three options, mine was the most requested. Getting to know everyone and answering their questions was fantastic too. The climbs would also go down as one of the most memorable.

On Saturday the 22nd, I completed climb #265, which was one of the most mind-bending to date. After that summit, the remaining climbs went from triple to double digits. I reflected back to the 10th of April when the numbers were reversed. I sat high above the gorge, and it felt like a near-death experience as hundreds of past moments flashed before my mind's eye and filled me with a deep connected love. The 433 climbers and all the donations to the project stood out the most. Meeting the beneficiaries of the project had been a life-changing experience. I was being taught the true essence of Ubuntu.

It had been an uphill climb to get here, and if you'd asked what my greatest pain had been, my answer may have surprised you. It wasn't the dangerous winds, the battering storms, the fatigue, or even my internal battle with self-doubt. It was my car! Ever since April, it had been a constant thorn in my side, worse, more like a piece of shrapnel that the doctors couldn't remove. Car Service City Sea Point, which was the garage across from Don, demonstrated the kind of honesty I wished everyone had. He did his utmost to help me, and even checked the returns free of charge. Since I got my car back from the accident repairs in June, the pesky overheating warning light had given me unrelenting stress. I'd use two to three water bottles a day and sometimes kept an emergency bottle just in case. Luckily, my drive to the mountain was short. But the time had come to face a painful reality and get rid of it.

Donald and Stefan did their best to help me out. Stefan was amazing and communicated the intricate issues he found and continuously did his best to keep the repair costs down. His words to me never changed... *'If I were you, I'd sell it.'* I didn't have the heart to sell it, knowing the next poor sap would just be saddled with the same issues. The final straw was hearing the cost of the work might be in the region of R30k, and even then, there were no guarantees. My original plan was to sell before heading to San Francisco in January, but this plan was blown out of the water. Stefan introduced me to Irshaad, whose company specialised in projects like this. They've done a lot of business together, and I trusted Stefan. Best of all, he could explain the mechanical issues that had been dealt with over the past few months. Irshaad had all the information he needed to make an offer and take the car off my hands. I was happy that I wouldn't be giving another driver an endless stream of expensive headaches.

The money provided much-needed relief to my depleting reserves and would contribute to the purchase of a scooter. And even though September's weather was foul, October through December was much better for a scooter. Not only would my fuel costs dramatically decrease, parking at the mountain would no longer be an issue.

I enjoyed another stroke of fortune after speaking to Don about my situation. A friend of his was selling her low-mileage scooter for a very reasonable price, and with him moving to Noordhoek, and needing one for quick runs to the shop and beach, it made sense to buy it. Knowing I'd be leaving Cape Town in January, he lent it to me for the remainder of my stay.

As Mr Frans would say, 'I am blessed'. I saved money by cancelling my insurance, which gave me immense pleasure, and my fuel costs dropped from R700 to R50 a week. With winter over, my mind was focused on negotiating the tourist season ahead.

Table Mountain is the third most visited tourist destination in Africa. This meant that the volume of visitors would soon increase, and I'd have to do more afternoon climbs. The later starts would be extra rest for the legs, but required the tricky process of finding parking before the climb. Tafelberg's narrow and winding road hugs the lower slopes of Table Mountain. Only the section leading up to the Cableway has space for one line of cars to park and two lanes for traffic. There's hardly any parking for tourists, and when you throw in staff, tour buses, and thousands of rentals, it becomes a painful process, especially if you arrive any time after 9 am. After multiple poor visibility days the first clear day sees people arrive like ants swarming out of their nest. There's a tiny parking area on the left after the cableway, and another small space after that where cars can park. After that, parking impacts the bus movement. Throw in some impatient drivers parking on red lines, and you have a recipe for painful traffic jams.

Now, I could zip through the traffic, and I'd always be able to find parking less than 10 steps from the base of Platteklip. Besides the winter weather factor, I wondered why I'd never thought of this before?? Especially since I knew I'd be finishing in December. At the end of the year, South Africans and tourists flock to the peninsula, and I was painfully aware of the large masses that were going to descend on our already strained roads. It's an interesting dilemma – the influx brings money and jobs to the region, but it comes with challenges for locals. It's like a switch, one day you'll be able to find parking, and the next day, the city is bursting at the seams. Don was my godsend for tourist season. Unfortunately, those that were joining me would still have to battle for parking.

My 15th barefoot climb coincided with the '100 climbs to go' milestone. It was surreal to arrive at this point, and my logical brain couldn't believe it. At halfway, I had some genuine moments of 'what the hell did I get myself into', and yet just 82 days later, the numbers were stacking up in my favour. The fatigue came in waves and was always felt more on my solo climbs because of the faster pace.

It was a crisp clear day with some snow still clinging to the mountains further inland. It reminded me of what I'd endured up to now. Let's make sure it's not wasted. On my climb, I decided to print out a countdown to tick off the remaining days and create a QR code for anyone wishing to donate via credit card. For the first time, I was beginning to count down.

I had to lasso my wandering mind in, as it kept thinking about climb #365. I still wasn't 100% sure which platform would show up as the best way to scale a business, but the seed and the intent to continue was there and would keep growing. I was learning so much that could be shared to help others empower themselves.

The next day was a year since I'd first picked Jessie up from the airport and enjoyed a magical week of exploring Cape Town with her. It felt like I'd known her for decades. Her daily support was felt from across the Atlantic pond, and her messages, which were read out by Endomondo, were music to my ears. September's her birthday month, and it was also an early birthday present for me as she booked her final trip of the year back to Cape Town. It wasn't just for a week either! She'd be landing on the 15th of December and leaving on the 12th of January! It was unbelievable knowing that she'd be here for a month and I'd have 12 days in January to show her South Africa beyond Table Mountain. I didn't know it was possible, but I felt even more in love.

The day turned out to be my 200th cable car ride of the year, and two of the staff, Bululani and Siyabonga, had organised a group to join on Monday the 24th, which also happened to be my favourite national holiday of the year – Heritage Day. It was my favourite because in years gone by, retail staff had been allowed to wear their traditional clothes, and the result was always a colourful and beautiful expression of our diverse culture. That beauty shone through their eyes as I interacted with them and heard more about the colours, their meanings, and the tribes they belonged to.

They arranged for 10 climbers to join a special Ubuntu Heritage Day climb, which was sponsored by their company, *Corner2Corner* Tours. They arrived armed with bags to collect rubbish too. Sue, from the talk at *Rock Solid*, also joined. She was heading out of the country to participate in Dragon Boat racing and didn't want to wait until she came back.

CHAPTER 13
SEPTEMBER - UNCONDITIONAL LOVE

It was a diverse group of people with varying fitness levels, and we got hit by a heat wave, which after the freezing days of winter, showed just how exhaustive heat could be. *NOW spring decided to show up!* We should've started at sunrise, but that was always the problem when I wasn't in direct contact with the participants. I had no idea what their fitness levels were and couldn't make the needed weather and time adjustments. It was also a blunt reminder of how blessed I was to be 20 minutes away, and not in the townships where I'd have to catch public transport, which could easily take up to three times as long. The latter was a journey with multiple stops and taxi changes. This enhanced my gratitude for Don's scooter ride!

In the past, I'd get irritated with tardy behaviour. I'd probably have made a joke about 'African time.' Now, I found myself more understanding and sympathetic to someone's lateness. The lengthy journey, the time spent waiting to catch a taxi, and the walk to the taxi rank, were painful daily experiences for many. They were arduous, to say the least. I wasn't even close to waking up, and they were probably already waiting in a line. I was trying to be more thoughtful, and understanding of the behaviour from someone else's perspective.

We collected about four bags of garbage. I was grateful everyone listened to Siyabonga and Bulelani and came prepared with sufficient water, because it turned into a scorcher, with temperatures reaching 28.6 degrees Celsius.

At Rock Solid, I joked about my desire to measure the temperature in the gorge for the full duration of a hot summer's day. The resulting data would help me warn climbers of the dangerous and sudden temperature spikes. Lo and behold, a gentleman from a measuring devices company called Testo came over to me after the talk. His company ended up sponsoring me with a device to measure the air temperature. It also had a laser that measured surface temperature. Now I could see how hot the rocks got and look at the extreme contrast between that and my icy winter hands.

Just as the cycle of nature continues, I was introduced to new groups of people, and often, my project would resonate with an individual who would go on to contribute and participate further. I guess the important part was just to get started.

I was learning to trust that if I took action in life, towards my desires, then I'd be supported. Nothing transformational ever came from sitting on the couch.

Being on the receiving end helped me think of better ways to return the favour, and opened my network to assist others in whichever way I could.

It was fitting that *Corner2Corner* Tours joined for my 200th cable car ride of the year. It lined me up with an even split – 67 climbs back down and 267 summits completed. They'd always been really supportive and would share the details of my journey with others, so I asked them to cross off #99 – now it was real. It was the first time someone else crossed a day off. Their smiles filled with gratitude as they handed over the envelope with a cash donation.

Ngiyabonga. (Thank you in Zulu)

My day finished perfectly with dinner at my cousin's house in Constantia. Aunty San, Uncle John, and Aunty Di, had been more powerhouses of support. Back in February, they committed to paying each charity quarterly as I progressed throughout the year. He hadn't missed a payment, and I invited them to join a climb on their next visit. Our climb was two minutes shy of 4 hours. It was important that people were 100% happy physically before they arrived. I hadn't had any injuries to date, and I planned on having a 100% success rate come climb #365. They agreed on the condition that the weather needed to be perfect.

As luck would have it, the next three days descended back into winter and became my fourth stretch of three consecutive down climbs.

CHAPTER 13
SEPTEMBER - UNCONDITIONAL LOVE

Climb #268 – 200 cable cars and 68 climbs down
Climb #269 – 200 cable cars and 69 climbs down
Climb #270 – 200 cable cars and 70 climbs down

While I loved the symmetry, I was quite happy for the cold snap to end, even if it broke the run of perfectly synched numbers. I was particularly devastated for Native VML, who joined on climb #270. Unfortunately, the weather hadn't played ball for their team-building climb, which was on a day set in stone.

After two days of miserable weather and climbing alone, Ally kept checking in with me, while I monitored Wind Guru and YR leading up to their climb. Alas, the forecast only got worse, but incredibly, no staff backed out. Then, in a cruel twist of fate, Ally messaged me the evening before their climb to share her disappointment in not being able to join. Not because of weather – but because of a client's untimely request. I was gutted for her because she'd been such a driving force for their climb.

With a 9 am start, I checked in early to see how everyone was feeling now that they were awake and the reality of rain had sunk in. Still, she said, everyone would be there. I'd heard that before, even on clear days. Don had been kind enough to help me stay dry before climbing and allowed me to use his car. While driving up, I thought that I wouldn't be surprised in the least if people bailed. The weather was foul. Mark was also going to join again, so I knew I wouldn't be alone. Just in case, though, I packed all my buffs and an extra rain jacket. To my genuine amazement, all 14 members not affected by the client's request arrived. Doing what they said they would do warmed my heart, and restored my faith in people. Not only that, but before we began climbing, I shared what the previous two days had been like, giving everyone who was concerned, the opportunity to back out. It only served to solidify everyone's commitment. Then, I handed out the buffs to those that needed it.

This was also the first time I saw people using the opportunity before them as a real team-building exercise. It was almost as though the adverse conditions heightened people's sensitivities to those around them. Climb #270 was about to become one of the most memorable of the year, with Ben (447), Tanya (448), Lihle (449), Jean (450), Kevin (451), Aminah (452), Jason (453), Alex (454), Candace (455), Langelihle (456), Pablo (457), Darren (458), Elizma (459), Nabeelahi (460), and of course Mark (461), all accepting the challenge before us.

With everyone ready and committed, my gratitude talk doubled as a quick tutorial on how to navigate slippery conditions. I highlighted that making smarter decisions and being mindful on each step would serve their safety well.

It wasn't long before they were able to see the value in the climb. The river was racing down the mountain, and the first waterfall was showing off. More spectacles appeared as we continued. We were treated to a scene I'd never witnessed before: a new river flowed around some boulders and down a wall usually reserved for people to rest off the path. Higher up, Waterfall Corner was really living up to its name. Water streamed over the stairs and through our legs and forced us to take a little more care as to where we placed our feet. At the landing above the steep section, we paused for a breather, and just to our right, water cascaded down to the ground, collecting in a pool before finding its way to the path. We were deep inside the cloud with zero visibility when one of the group came to a beautiful realisation and said...

'I can't wait to come back and see what the view looks like from here. It will be so epic to compare it to this.'

Everyone agreed. We were all in this together, and no one complained once. They demonstrated a level of gratitude for the experience that I wasn't used to, and it made my heart smile. At the top, the wind cut through us. The combination of elements made it the 'worst' day of the year. Not the coldest, wettest, or the windiest, but just the worst combination of the three. Needless to say, our hopes for an operational cable car didn't pan out. I tried my luck to see if my 'get out of jail card' might work and phoned Siyabonga, who was working, but there was no such luck. The gusts were too strong, we'd be climbing down.

CHAPTER 13
SEPTEMBER - UNCONDITIONAL LOVE

Everyone accepted it. I gave a quick demonstration on how to climb down sideways. This method of descending is vital to preventing a bad fall on the trickier sections. Then we began our careful descent.

As mentioned before, I was convinced that more accidents happen when the weather is great because people get lulled into a false sense of security and easily lose concentration. That's all it takes. Whereas on appalling days like today, everyone knows the rocks are slippery, and they're hyper-focused. And no one wants to go back down on one leg or get stuck in the cold weather. I had two unused space blankets for emergencies - hopefully, they'd never be used.

After 4 hours and 51 minutes, our feet finally touched down on the tarmac. No slips, no injuries, and nothing but the biggest smiles of gratitude beaming back at me. They all had a deep sense of pride in what they'd just achieved. I also reminded them about the company's donation and how it would go towards teaching children to read. I was immensely proud of the team, especially those who assisted their nervous-footed colleagues at the back.

I reported back to Ally and let her know how incredible the group was. She was upset that she'd missed out, but knew her time would come on another day in December.

I was only four days into week 39 and already just 10 hours short of spending the most time on the mountain. It looked to surpass the cable car shutdown week, which was a mammoth 23 hours, 58 minutes, and 05 seconds. It had been a rough and long start to the week, but with the weather clearing the next day, I'd be able to enjoy the company of John and Di on Friday before they headed back home to Durban.

They experienced the magic of the mountain, still alive with water at every turn. I knew the first waterfall was still raging, so we headed up the same path that Andrew and I chose in June to try to keep our feet as dry as possible. This route gave us a unique perspective of the waterfall. John and Di were well travelled and had also been to Iceland. I enjoyed introducing them to Silverstream, which kept growing as my favourite area on the mountain. They did incredibly well, and, at 74, became the oldest Ubuntu climbers of the year. They selected their own rocks for the family pile and placed them on Caroline's, which was still the centrepiece. These family days seem to be perfectly timed for lifting my spirits.

Setting and working towards mini targets throughout the year, helped the time fly by. My final day of the month was with the monks, and was just such a target. Finally, the day had arrived. The original plan was to climb to the top, but their sweeping heavy robes and full schedules were limited, so we decided to meet up at the top. I was used to racing against time to make the final car down, but this was my first morning climb with a 'time limit.' Because it was Sunday, I recommended the monks arrive early to catch one of the first cars up for an 08:30 meet. This meant forfeiting the twenty-minute walk along the road to the start at Platteklip. I hated holding people up, and every minute saved was a minute's peace of mind. Mountains are sacred to monks, so the plan was to have a ceremony at the top, where we'd pray and give an offering.

Nicci, who was responsible for creating this magic, was unable to join, but Lisa and Alice were 100% keen to come along. Alice heard about me through some friends. She'd never hiked up before meeting me but was now about to complete her third in 15 days. She would become the 6th person to complete three or more with me. I loved hearing stories of how people were pushing their boundaries, especially when they were fully present for the experience. Her message reflected this, and she donated to climbs, '258, 263 & 273... *thank you thank you thank you.*'

Amanda was part of the trio of ladies joining me for this memorable climb, and it was her 43rd birthday. She had also never climbed before. The monks were set, and on their way from Simons Town, so I was on a mission to time the meetup perfectly. The plan was to start at 6:30, which was 10 minutes after sunrise. Alice, Lisa, and I waited and marvelled at the beautiful clear day. The experience was made richer by my past week's challenges. It also meant the mountain was going to be busy. Then unfortunately, we hit our first snag.

CHAPTER 13
SEPTEMBER - UNCONDITIONAL LOVE

Amanda was 15 minutes late. On any other day, it would have been fine, but I took my commitments seriously, and everyone knew what our schedule was. I just hoped it wouldn't keep the monks waiting. Amanda apologised for being late and then said...

'I haven't exercised in a while, so don't go too fast for me, okay?'

My mind tried to brush it off, but only for a split second. Maybe she was just underestimating her abilities? My blood pressure shot up! This climb would take my tally to 273 and would end off with a sacred ceremony at the top. Soon, I realised that she wasn't underestimating anything. Reaching the contour path after half an hour meant that our pace was far too slow. It was 7:15, and we had 75 minutes to get up more than three-quarters of the way. Lisa and Alice had disappeared ahead of us, and as painful as it was, I knew what I had to do.

Then I told her...

'Amanda, on any other day, I wouldn't do this – but today as I explained I have a deadline to be at the top to meet the Buddhist Monks. Unfortunately, at this pace, we're not going to make it.'

She nodded her head quietly.

'I'm going to have to push on, do you have enough water?' I asked

She pointed to her backpack and said yes. I hated being in this position, luckily, she had another 92 days left to join. She also had more than enough battery life on her phone to keep in contact while she continued up alone.

'See you at the top – enjoy it!' she said.

I pushed on ahead, knowing it would be a mini speed test to ensure we made it. I caught up to Lisa and Alice near Left Face Mystery B and explained the situation. With an hour left to reach the upper cable station, both were up to the task. There'd be no more breaks until we reached Ubuntu Rock and transferred week 39's stones to the pyramid. It was also starting to get pretty hot, and there was almost no wind.

My exuberance upon reaching the top knew no bounds. It had been a brutal week and became my 2nd longest of the year in possibly the harshest conditions on the mountain. We scraped in by the skin of our teeth, and arrived 10 minutes before their marron and saffron robes came into view. It was as though the Dalai Lama himself was here. We introduced ourselves. I found it remarkable how each one of their faces was a picture of peace. Had my heart still been pounding, it certainly would've slowed in their presence.

The Tibetan Ambassador and some South African volunteers were escorting them. One monk spoke English and had a dry sense of humour. I was extremely excited to learn about their culture and practices. It wasn't long before the topic of Kundalini yoga was raised, and how it was only practised by monks who'd achieved a certain level of enlightenment. This also happened to be one of Lisa's favourite ways of exercising.

It was their first time at the top, so I took them in an anti-clockwise loop along the rim. They first saw Camps Bay, the Atlantic below us, and the Twelve Apostles flanking Table Mountain like a protective barrier. Next, I showed them the southern view, and the vast mountain range of Chapman's Peak and Constantiaberg rising high.

They were satisfied, and asked for a nice quiet spot to perform a blessing and ceremony. I knew the perfect place. We headed back to the front table, which had spectacular views of the city. I checked in to see how Amanda was doing and to see if I could stall them long enough for her to join, but she was still too far back. We arrived at one of my favourite places, where the sheer cliff drops off a couple hundred metres. There's a large flat boulder that allows you to lie down comfortably and stick your head over the edge. It's a place I never bring people when the winds howling. I shudder just thinking about the consequences.

Geshe, one of the monks, was interested in what I was doing and asked questions about it. It was incredibly humbling to hear his words of encouragement and what he thought would happen going forward. He paid me one of the best compliments of the year.

We settled into this sacred space as they strung up their prayer flags. The blue, white, red, green, and yellow squares flapped in the gentle breeze. Blue represents the sky; white represents the air; red represents fire; green represents water, and yellow represents the earth. Together, they signify balance.

They began to chant, and the monk next to me rang a bell. We were all given crumbs to throw into the air after three 'waves' as an offering to the spirits. Then they shared their picnic basket with us, which Jessie would've loved! Cashews, naartjies, green tea with honey, and some delicious shortbread was passed around. Again, they seemed to effortlessly radiate peace, and their beaming smiles were an invitation to join them.

They shared the magic of their trip, and spoke about how they spent the past three days creating a beautiful sand mandala. Mandalas are a Tibetan Buddhist tradition involving the creation of a spiritual symbol that represents a cosmic universe of celestial bodies made from coloured sand. They painstakingly constructed the sand mandala design Chenrezig, the Buddha of Compassion, to generate a kind and peaceful energy, which was perfectly aligned to their purpose of promoting peace in South Africa.

The four of them worked side by side to create the two-dimensional representation of a three-dimensional universe. Then, after all the detailed work was completed, they swept it up and headed down to the beach to make an offering. The ocean had been perfectly still, but once the offering was made, a wave gently rolled in and sucked the offering out to sea. Magic.

It was another perfectly timed message: releasing attachment to the outcome. The closer I get to the end, the more the seed grows. In the end, I'll start focusing my attention on the causes of depression. I believe this sent my mind down a path that would lead me to realise one of the greatest truths. It was wonderful to learn about their Nepalese culture. Geshe explained the role that the mountains play in Buddhism and why they wanted to visit Table Mountain.

'All the rivers flow from the mountains, the source of life that enables each village down the valley to live. This is why we honour the mountains first before we eat. We feed them, before we feed ourselves.'

I wish practices, religious or otherwise, that come from a place of love and respect, would become infused with everyday living. I know how beneficial this year has been in building a deeper level of respect for our home. These practices helped bring me back to a place of gratitude, which was far better than feeling disconnected from what I didn't have.

I've always had a deep connection to the mountains. I often thought of them as our 'big protectors' and ancient guardians filled with knowledge and understanding, silently laying dormant. After 273 consecutive days with Table Mountain, my appreciation had grown exponentially. It had been a gift to witness life in action as night became day; as seasons gradually melted into one another; and as storms swept across the land bringing danger and life in the same breath. I watched the landscape transform with colour and sounds, and saw how the fire ravaged it, only to blossom again into a brighter beauty than it was before.

This wasn't a year of sacrifice as many saw it, it was an honour. My family was able to visit their sand mandala creation in Johannesburg as they patiently created another masterpiece. They even met Geshe and had a chance to chat. They were able to experience some of the magic they'd created at the end of September.

Amanda reached the top as our ceremony finished. We'd spent nearly two hours there, and normally on days like this, I'd make sure we were at the cable car before 11 am. Most visitors started heading back down early. The queue was just outside of the door, which was about four cable car rides in length. I left the queue to fill up my water bottle, and returned to Lisa and an American having a conversation.

CHAPTER 13
SEPTEMBER - UNCONDITIONAL LOVE

'Every day?!?!' the American asked.

Lisa beamed as she held the $20 note that Jeff donated. He asked if he could take a picture with us and noted the website details so that he could share my story once he got back home. It was a small moment in the grand scheme of things, but after so many days of challenges and blessings, it was heartwarming and special beyond belief. My immense gratitude overflowed, and I made sure he knew that.

Amanda reached us before the queue moved inside. I was proud of her. What a beautiful gift to give herself. At dinner later that week, I got to hear all about it. Once we got back down safely, we bid farewell to Lisa and Alice. We were all in awe of the experience. They were both just as grateful as I was and wanted to join again. What a special memory to be rewarded with for all their efforts.

Next was my friend Cheryse's 50th celebration at Kirstenbosch. It gave me an opportunity to be barefoot on the cool grass after a long arduous week. My feet seemed to smile as they lapped up their dose of ions from the earth. Lisa and I reflected on our morning and shared it with friends. I still felt the same peace that was in me during the ceremony at the top.

Perhaps it was that peace that allowed my relaxed brain to blurt out an idea for the 16 days of activism against violence against children and women, which was due to start in late November. Justin was standing next to us and loved it so much he pledged his support and committed to getting another 10 men involved. The idea had been stewing in my mind for almost a year. The idea was loaded with tremendous power and aimed to get people actively involved. Now, with contacts at Safety Mountain, Love our Trails, and even at City Hall, I felt like it could become a reality.

The plan was to create a manmade chain of people holding hands all the way up Platteklip Gorge. A wave would then be created that would go from the first person all the way up. A wonderful way for more than 3000 people to enjoy the mountain and donate in the process. A drone would capture what would hopefully be a record and a great advertisement for Cape Town! Initially I thought just men should be involved but this was about everyone showing what they stood for, so women and children would be free to walk the earth protected. It developed into a project within a project and would be more publicity for DKMS Africa, Habitat for Humanity and One Heart. Who knows? Maybe the President of South Africa would be available to join too. The reality was that I had lots of work to do.

After returning to the stillness of my flat, I allowed all the recent experiences to wash over me, and I finally began to contemplate the end. Eight days had already been crossed off my countdown – now 92 remained. The last quarter was my final test of perseverance. I collapsed into bed, invigorated from a day filled with gratitude and purpose. I felt like I'd celebrated the end of week 39 as best I could with the knowledge that everything was as it should be. I did my best to take a leaf out of the Buddhist's understanding – I released my expectations.

What a way to end the month and begin a new one with invigorated optimism and purpose. With each climb now feeling like I'm on my fourth lap climbing Platteklip Gorge – I hope the body holds up.

CHAPTER 13
SEPTEMBER - UNCONDITIONAL LOVE

SEPTEMBER STATS:

273 / 365

People Joined: 48 / 468

29 days 08 hours 12 minute 10 seconds / 1 814,12 km / 53,11 equivalent Everest Summits

/ 142 solo climbs (52%) / 70 Up & Down (25.5%)

TOTAL DONATIONS: R312 911.63

Huni: '250 champ, I told you I would and I am. Love you and your work. P.S. It's getting closer to me joining you on the mountain.'

Yolande: 'Thanks for a very special hike & keep inspiring people to do things for the right reason'

Natalie: 'So excited to be part of this!'

Take care of your body. It's the only place you have to live ~~ **Jim Rohn**

CHAPTER 14
OCTOBER - REAPING REWARDS

The business end of the challenge was physically taking its toll and I began to wonder if there'd be any serious implications long term. I wasn't stressed about it, and had already made the decision to deal with whatever consequences came up. For me, it was worth it, even though I felt like I was on my fourth lap. I was learning the value of quality over quantity and I knew my perseverance would be rewarded.

I also realised that October's dates and its corresponding days lined up perfectly with January's. That felt like a lifetime ago, considering how 'wet behind the ears' I was compared to the more recent and brutal months. The great news about all the storms we'd had, was that the dams were recovering, and we could breathe a sigh of relief. At the end of September 2017, the average across the Berg River, Steenbras Lower, Steenbras Upper, Theewaterskloof, Voelvlei, and Wemmershoek dams was 37.4%. Now in 2018, it was 70%.

I was continuously blown away by the efforts of those who supported this project. I was far away from the days of nervousness, and wondering whether it would be supported, as I watched the results flow into Habitat, One Heart,

CHAPTER 14
OCTOBER - REAPING REWARDS

and DKMS Africa. This was perfectly illustrated by my sister, who led the charge with Terence, Dad, and Mom in Joburg on Saturday. They manned a stall at Kingsmead school's fundraising day wearing their Ubuntu T-shirts and caps. It was outside their comfort zones, and magnified my pride and gratitude for their efforts both on and off the mountain.

With the help of Adele at Bastion Graphics, they even printed poster-sized pictures of all my Instagram posts, which gave people visual context to 365 Ubuntu Climbs and its beneficiaries. They raised R3,650!! Of course, I loved that it had '365' in it. The wonderful effort was made possible by Lyndsay at the school, who went the extra mile to support 365 Ubuntu Climbs and registered a stall. After such a successful morning, they headed over to meet the monks and saw their new Mandala creation. I was pleased that they even got the opportunity to speak to Geshe.

With large masses of people coming to celebrate the cable car's 89th birthday on the summit, the queue was at least two hours long, but the staff, with their incredible kindness, ushered me to the front. After it happened a few times, they told me to come directly to the control room. I was deeply grateful for the VIP treatment, and I knew it would save me as the busy season was about to hit.

My good fortune continued to Sunday's climb, when Sandra, her children, and their friends joined. She followed through on her promise after donating on the 25th of June. She had been following me since my interview with Tim Lundy, and said she would love to join me on a climb once she moved to Cape Town. Well, that day arrived, and it was Sunday, the 7th of October, which was climb #280. Lisa and Dave also joined for a back-to-back weekend of climbing. They had joined the previous day with Eunice, who was on her third climb and was the 7th person to join the triple hitter club. It was also Lisa's 25th and Dave's 13th summit. Bronwyn was another avid supporter and joined for her second climb. She gave me one of the greatest joys back in August, when she sent me a picture of her wearing her Ubuntu shirt at the Rainbow Mountain range in Peru. After Josh's, it was my second international picture with a shirt, and they were both for hikes!

Even though we started at 15:30, it was still 32° which made me yearn for the mountain shadows to creep over us quicker. I was extremely impressed with Luca, Anais, Leroy and Jason's manners. Their confidence was something I would've loved when I was their age. They asked engaging questions that most journalists could learn from! One question that really stood out was if I'd ever do this again. I'd never thought about it, and even though the idea made my blood run cold, I took some time to think about it before answering.

Finally, I responded…

'Honestly, my focus is to finish this one. Would I do it again though? No – I know what's gone into this and having already achieved it, I wouldn't see it as something to do again unless the reasons were exceptionally worthwhile. As someone that tries to constantly improve, I'd rather find another challenge worth committing to.'

In the same breath, I wondered if this would ever be achieved again. My idealistic self would love to pass the torch on and have new people commit to it every year. A year is a big commitment, and as of the 31st of December 2018, it represented 2,56% of my life.

Another month into spring meant the sunsets were getting later by one minute every day. Today it was at 18:53, and we were treated to a cloudless sunset that sparked an appreciation for having the ability to see. The view never gets old. It was the perfect close to week 40 and was about to get even better.

Luca and Anais kept the conversation going in the car as they drove home. The seeds planted were already being watered as each decided to donate their pocket money. The message from Sandra read…

'You inspired young minds to look at the small steps they can take in this beautiful world. From picking up the trash when hiking, to knowing that every little contribution makes a difference.'

It was the most gratifying feedback I could get. As if this wasn't enough, Sandra gave me an incredible gift. Moving from Hong Kong, she opened her own holistic movement centre with her business partner. Her gift to me was a body assessment. I initially misunderstood her, and thought it was a massage! Instead, I was treated to a full evaluation of my body. Although she was really booked up for the coming weeks, she promised to fit me in somewhere, and I was extremely grateful for that!

As a team, The Balance Group shares the belief that there are multiple contributors to our body's alignment and performance. Physiotherapists, Biokineticist, Personal Trainers, Yoga Teachers, and Massage Therapists all work within their speciality, but together, their goal is to improve the health of their clients. I like this holistic way of thinking. It views each discipline as part of an orchestra instead of as solo artists. Incredibly, someone cancelled the day after she climbed, so I got the call.

It was one of the greatest gifts I could've received, especially after 282 climbs. Besides the obvious fatigue, my body seemed to be holding up fine. I had niggles here and there but nothing drastic. I was, however, still mindful of the potential for serious damage.

Here's a little bit about Toni-Lynn at The Balance Group:

'In 2016 Toni-Lynne Monger returned to South Africa after spending 5 years working in the UK, Hong Kong and China. She is a physiotherapist with over 15 years of experience. She's deeply intrigued by movement. Her goals go beyond treating the patient's symptoms to finding the root cause of dysfunction. She believes that finding the person's movement faults and imbalances are the key to success. She works on finding each client's uncontrolled movement and restriction, treating the uncontrolled movement with stability type exercises and the restrictions with manual therapy, muscle release techniques, and functional mobility exercises.'

Being checked out by a professional was a massive benefit, and so was the amazing conversation. Listening to someone with experience in Eastern and Western practices was rewarding and insightful. Most importantly she was searching for the cause instead of focusing on the symptom.

After a quick discussion on how my year was going, she focused on my feet, taking my previous problems with hematomas and dislocations into consideration. I was intrigued as she spoke me through what she was checking and why. I was a little apprehensive, it felt like I was writing a test that I hadn't studied for. I think I was scared of hearing distressing news that would jeopardise my project.

I wish I'd recorded everything she said, because her wisdom was incredible. The time flew by, as she put me through various tests and checked my entire body. Her thoroughness gave me the peace of mind that whatever news I got, would come with detailed plans on how to fix or prevent further damage. I was nervous after each answer, not being able to tell if it was going well or not. Finally, all the checks were complete, but I was too terrified to breathe. She placed her hands on her hips, tilted her head, and set me up for the prognosis.

'I'm not sure why Sandra referred you – your body is in fantastic shape.' she said.

The news was like the first breath of oxygen after being starved of it for too long! I was elated! ESPECIALLY after the injury in 2012 that ended my running days. One thing surprised me: she didn't chastise me for not stretching. Her reason astounded me.

'Why would I do that?' she asked.

She went on… *'There's no evidence to support stretching improves performance or reduces the risk of injury.'*

She also explained how we both had the type of joints that, regardless of what we did, we'd never be able to do the splits or certain yoga poses.

I stretched when I first started training for my climbs and stopped to see if it would make any difference. There was no difference to me, and even if there was – it was too small to notice. Admittedly, I started soaking my legs in the frigid Atlantic Ocean once a week for the first three months of the year. This didn't generate any significant results either. And I hadn't stretched once in the past 282 days.

CHAPTER 14
OCTOBER - REAPING REWARDS

It was great talking to a professional, rather than just hearing the opinion of someone who didn't have the same scientific wisdom on the subject, and she really piqued my interest. For more than 20 years, I'd been living an active lifestyle that included multiple sports, and I'd learned so much over the period. My knowledge ramped up significantly when I lived with Jono in London. We followed the world's top drug-free bodybuilders, mimicked their weekly regime, and read as many articles as we could on nutrition, recovery, and training. They taught us two key principles that other bodybuilders scoffed at. Firstly, their daily training sessions were never longer than 45 minutes. Because they had the benefit of working with top doctors and scientists, they learned the value of maximum overload training, which also gave their muscles enough time to repair. Secondly, they took rest seriously. This is another key component that's undervalued by most people I speak to. While my results in the gym are anecdotal, the training methods I used to get there are scientific.

My biggest question was if my feet were showing any uneven load distribution. This was finally answered, and it was a big no. Whew... this was crucial, it showed that I'd learned from the injury to my right hip and that my daily focus on giving equal attention to both legs was working. I had a revelation after she shared another anecdote about 68-year-old men who regularly competed in IronMan competitions. After every race, they'd come to see her massage partner – and not her. One day, when the massage therapist was ill, they were forced to choose Toni-Lynn. This was the gap she was hoping for.

'Why don't you ever come to me instead of the massage therapist? Have you had a bad experience?' she asked them.

Their answer shocked her. They'd been competing since the age of 20. They didn't over-train. It was more of a lifestyle than a fitness program. Their bodies were accustomed to the gruelling demands of a 4km swim, a 180km bike ride, and a 42km marathon. Compare that to someone who had started in their 30s and 40s and was doing something extreme with no fitness base to work from. This stress created opportunities for the body to break down. This nugget gave me a revelation and lifted the floodgates to the memories of the lifestyle I'd lived over the last 20 years.

I trained legs at the gym for a long time, cycled for eight years prior to 365 Ubuntu Climbs too, I did trail running for three years, played touch rugby league for eight years, walked whenever I travelled, and loved hiking. Doing all of this before my mountain training created varying layers of consistent action in my life, and served as the perfect launch pad for this challenge. Couple that with choosing never to 'mask' niggles and pains with injections - and you've got a well-oiled machine. Pain is our body's way of saying, 'Hey! there's a problem!' The cause of the pain is the issue, not the pain itself. Either my technique is wrong, or my thoughts and approach to dealing with emotions are manifesting as a warning. Everything in the body is interconnected. Toni may decide to treat the hip for a neck problem or the neck for an elbow problem. She considered the physical, biological, and behavioural influences of the body in assessing the issue.

Too many people, including professional athletes, take the quick 'fix', which masks the pain in the moment, but causes severe long-lasting problems like knee surgery later on in life. There are no shortcuts. I learned that in 2015 while training for the Cape Town Cycle race when I felt a sudden pain in my left knee. With a voltaren injection out of the question, I gave it a two-week rest and had the physio check it out again. First, I started on a stationary bike with no resistance. As soon as I increased the resistance, I could feel the pain. Although I was fundraising for DKMS Africa again, I came painstakingly close to pulling out of the race, but, after a 70km pain-free road ride two weeks prior, I felt that I was good to go. It was all in vain in the end, though, because the race was cancelled for the first time in its 40-year history. 'The Black South Easter' forced organisers to do the unthinkable.

While sharing this with Toni, I realised something quite profound: copying the Platteklip Charity Challenge's route was a stroke of genius. The 2km walk on the road was the perfect warm-up to get my body, joints, and muscles ready for the

CHAPTER 14
OCTOBER - REAPING REWARDS

assault of climbing, while the walk along to the top was the perfect warm-down. Watch the Tour de France cyclists after a race, do they stretch? Nope, they hop back on a stationary bike for an active recovery to help stimulate blood flow to the legs, which allows them to get rid of waste like lactose build-up and heat.

Who knew that something as simple as the choice of route would have such a profound impact on my body's well-being? My repetitive route allowed me to spot issues and make subtle changes before they became serious injuries. I wish I could take credit for being a strategic thinker and consciously choosing all these things beforehand, but I can't... It was by following my gut and not letting my ego get in the way, combined with my gratitude for a healthy body, feet, and legs, that I'd managed to arrive safely with a clean bill of health. Most importantly, I believed that staying on this path would get me to the finish safely. Saying that I felt relieved, was the biggest understatement since Noah said, 'Looks like rain!'

Oh yes! Before I forget, I have to tell you about Monday's summit! I didn't want to break the flow of magic created by Sandra. One of my fridge magnets is the inspiration for my daily photo at the top: a gorgeous sunset with the upper station, Lion's head, and cable car silhouetted against low cloud flowing like a river; the top of Lion's Head looked like an island in a sea of pink mist. Before climbing, I picked it off the fridge and pondered over whether I'd ever get to see that view in real life. I bought it in 2004 on a trip to Cape Town, 14 years after my first visit to the beautiful Mother City, which had also been my 25th birthday. Who knew that 14 years later, I'd take my own photo just like it?

That's right – by the time I drove up, parked, and climbed for 2 hours and 16 minutes, I was greeted by a nearly identical scene. I couldn't ask for a more rewarding start to week 41. The previous day's weather was almost identical minus the clouds and made it even more memorable.

Earlier I'd seen 'Mountain Lisa' again. She was one of the 'locals' I'd come to know after seeing her on regular mountain climbs. She always climbed as far as possible for 30 minutes before turning around. One of her great achievements was completing Lions Head up and down in 40 minutes, and Platteklip up in 40 minutes.

'Good to see you again – I was just thinking that I haven't seen you for a while,' I told her.

'Yes I've been sick for 2 weeks. I finally got fed up and decided to come today no matter what.' she replied.

Two weeks. That certainly made the 'fridge magnet sunset' all the more sweeter.

There was a noticeable change in the volume of traffic. It was the last month that Don could share his car on rainy days before relocating to Noordhoek. Thanks to my lesson from the rockfall on Platteklip, my ear was treated to the most incredible experience that I wouldn't have believed if not heard.

With no music to distract me, my gratitude ritual was beautifully accompanied by frogs enjoying the mini reservoir. I'd seen and heard them here before, so I didn't pay too much attention. The insane thing was that their croaks never stopped. All the way up to the first waterfall at the contour path – their concert continued. I expected it to stop there. Nope. Their songs carried me all the way to the top! I couldn't believe it!? How the hell did they get up there? I chuckled as I contemplated my challenge of doing one route every day for a year – and a frog doing one route, taking the whole year to climb! Hearing this extraordinary symphony was a beautiful reminder of why earphones were not needed in nature.

The rain wasn't the only thing that cars protected me from, there was the wind too. Those eight years of cycling had prepared me for this. Last week's back-to-back windy days gave me my 71st and 72nd climb down and put me in line with the number of days in 2017 that the cableway had been closed. Reaching the

CHAPTER 14
OCTOBER - REAPING REWARDS

summit on a windy day like today was quite extraordinary. Far below, the wind danced on the ocean, often lifting it up as an adult would a child. Watching and feeling the wind simultaneously was a mesmerising experience.

As my 'mental fatigue' started redlining, Dave and Lisa stepped in to support me. It would be their 6th combo climb together, which meant they also led the pack. Lisa had 27 to her name and Dave 14. Today, we did something special though, we took time out to walk along the sky track and nestle ourselves above Platteklip with picnic goodies and laughter. We probably spent a good two hours enjoying the stillness, and clouds that flowed over Table Mountain while Devil's Peak looked like it was getting a head massage. Bliss.

A 6 am start meant that even with the pause, we were able to summit around 11 am. We ended up celebrating life's beauty together with an impromptu glass of vino. We headed to the balcony that was sheltered from the breeze and closest to Lions Head. There, Rob and Katie, a newlywed couple from the UK, took an interest in our 'pre-noon' celebrations. They soon understood why, as today's climb marked my '55th Mt Everest summit'. It was wonderful to see the love oozing out of their eyes as they shared their journey: Cape Town - Garden Route - Safari - Mauritius. And it wasn't surprising that it ended at one of the sunniest places on earth! They disappeared inside, only for Rob to re-emerge with a R200 donation - another glowing Nelson Mandela looking up at us.

The following day's climb with Heide as company was another early start and was also my 16th barefoot climb of the year. My approach now was so different compared to the beginning of the year. In the early months, I visualised 20 people climbing with me every day, but now the fewer, the better! The perks of having a stranger join alone meant I got to engage and not just guide. This was even better with conversationalists like her. Hearing about the burnout she experienced at another company reminded me how everyone was fighting some sort of battle. Heide had just started a new company which aimed to help others. She also mentored a young woman named Sipho, who was an avid hiker. Although she was originally from Pretoria inland, she was in love with Cape Town and the accessibility of the mountains.

It was a clear day, and as we neared Ubuntu Rock, she spoke about her love of mist. The sunrise had been spectacular, and we took some time to pause, where I shared the significance of the row of rocks, family rocks and pyramid. As if conjured by magic, a cloud started forming below and rose up the gorge. She got her wish! The thin veil turned into a thick dark mist and blotted out the sun. I took our group photo of the day while the mist surrounded us. Talk about instant manifestation!

Even after 284 consecutive climbs, I was still astounded by the sheer beauty of the two cliffs lining the gorge and the experiences I enjoyed between them. I wondered if anything like it existed anywhere else in the world? And did people 'complain' about how awful it was? I'd love the opportunity to host those people and challenge their distaste.

Finally, after my top photo captured a ghostly cable car emerging from the mist, she thanked me for the opportunity to be part of something special. It was a pleasure and something we both created. It was a climb that should've happened earlier in the year. I found that out after she took the time to create this special post on Facebook:

DIARY OF AN ENTHUSIAST

"The biggest treasure I knew I would find on this journey was of course Andrew. A wise & noble soul with compassion & purpose. The mindful conversations & intentional BARE FOOT steps he championed once again is an inspiration & gift that I will be forever thankful for.

Since it started in 2018, participating in 365 Ubuntu Climbs intrigued me - the need to climb with Andrew was prominent & I was determined to go up with him at least once a month. Today, for the first time, I managed to do Platteklip Gorge with him. It took me almost 10 months to create the opportunity. I've missed out

CHAPTER 14
OCTOBER - REAPING REWARDS

on so much (physically & spiritually) and have recommitted to going up once a week with him from now on. From all the walks I have done on Table Mountain, this path was a first...

With great anticipation & excitement my sunrise began with our Table Mountain Conqueror. The gorge is extraordinary, captivating, charming & majestic! Echoing bird tweets, unique vegetation & wild mist swirling around friendly dragon-like cliffs are but a fraction of the sparkle that feeds your soul. My perception of conquering one of the steepest climbs on the mountain had morphed into a fountain of appreciation - it seriously is not that hard!

May we all be inspired & focused to become conquerors, standing united as humans in love & humility. Participating in causes that carry weight, supporting those leaders who truly make a difference. Committing to opportunities as they arise. May we strive to be graceful in our passion with great examples like the Renaissance Guy."

She almost let her perceived view of Platteklip keep her away from experiencing this. Going from 'the steepest climbs on the mountain' to 'it is seriously not that hard' is because she overcame her perception and 'conquered' it in three hours. Her frame of reference is very different, and how she understands mountains and challenges in the future will change with it. I wrote conquered in quotation marks because we don't ever conquer a mountain... We simply conquer our limiting belief about climbing it in the first place.

Reading her experience reminded me how I was almost swayed out of doing this, simply because somebody else didn't understand what it meant to me and my journey. I was reminded of the gifts that awaited me when I pursued my passion and path in life.

Just as the summit was built upon the rocks further down, so were the months stacked on top of each other. They taught and guided me like some invisible teacher delivering extra lessons to ensure I passed. But what did I need to pass, what was the test? Was it just the challenge itself, or was there more?

I believe there's always more to learn than what we see on the surface. This kind of curiosity often drives me insane. This challenge and the questions that came with it were teaching me patience, and I knew the answers could only be unlocked by the key controlled by time.

October was a weird kind of month for me: the end was closer, but it felt inordinately further away than the 284 days to get here. It was like waking up after sleeping 12 hours and still feeling tired. I wondered if people's urgency to join me would increase more towards the end, or if the persistent foul weather would keep people away. Perhaps both?

Katje joined me on the next climb, she'd read an article a month prior and immediately wanted in! In her defence, her delay had been caused by waiting for others to commit to a day. In my opinion, it was better to book a day, and those that were committed would make a plan; those that weren't, would find excuses.

Again, this turned out better for me. Katje is wise and insightful. I appreciated her willingness to share her darkest stories. Because it was another blustery day, we had to climb down, and this gave us an extra two hours to chat. I was constantly astounded by the inner strength of people I had the privilege of meeting. Hearing about everyone's mountains and how they overcame them made me hopeful about humanity. Imagine if we were given the opportunity to share our pain and, in return, allowed others to share theirs. Imagine being inspired by a perfect stranger who listens without trying to fix it. It's possible: I was living that experience. Had her friends joined climb #292, I wasn't sure I would've had this opportunity for deeper conversation. How else would I have heard this insightful nugget she gave me... "We're never disappointed in others, just in the expectations we've created for them." Powerful.

After hearing all this, it felt fitting to give her the honour of selecting rock #292. My suggestion was met with deep gratitude. My climb with Katje was immediately followed by climb #293 with Heide, who lived up to her pledge and brought Sipho - the young woman she was mentoring. Sipho, in Grade 10,

CHAPTER 14
OCTOBER - REAPING REWARDS

was highly active and had little problem bounding up the mountain. Another freezing wind greeted us at the top and, crazily, 49 climbs into spring, I was still wearing ski gloves and even handed Sipho my second pair.

Being a Saturday, the mountain was alive with people pushing themselves through the pain to reach the top. Understandably, heaps of tourists who were not satisfied to come all this way and be denied the view by the wind, were crawling up. I wondered how many who asked 'how much further' had turned around to enjoy the view? At least if they were climbing down, it would force them to see how the entire path provided its own majesty.

Heide used this as an opportunity to share how the climb was a metaphor for achieving our goals. What a wonderful lesson to learn in Grade 10! I extended the same offer to Sipho that I had given Katje the previous day. Sipho equalled Katje's grateful smile with her own wide sparkly-eyed smile as she selected rock #293.

Climb #294 brought another lesson in letting go of expectations. Lisa joined and made it 28 now! She had done 'February' with me and, more importantly, had kept my spirits up during quiet periods. She also had the instinct to help on days when I was feeling rough, and the weather was beating me down.

Wessel was down from Pretoria, and joined me on my next climb. This is what he had written to me:

'I have been following your inspirational project. I am travelling to Cape Town for a meeting in Stellenbosch on 22nd October 2018 and was wondering if I could join you on a hike up the mountain on Sunday 21st of October (come sunshine or rain)?

It would feed my passion for hiking and the mountains as well as give me the opportunity to hear about your project.

I'd love to hear from you.
Wessel.'

Our correspondence made me chuckle as he asked me to please let him wear shoes! On the day of our climb, we met at the lower cable station amongst the crowds who were eager to catch the car up. We began our journey as usual by passing the family trees. He asked about the name and logo, which, funny enough, not many people asked about. After sharing how it all came about, I don't know why, but I uttered...

'I wonder if I should trademark them?'

'I'll do it for you.' he responded.

'What do you mean?' I asked.

'This is what I do – I'm a trademark lawyer and my company facilitates registering etc.' he told me.

'How much......' I asked.

He waved me off immediately and said... *'nothing, think of it as a donation.'*

What an incredible gift. And what a way to set the tone for a very memorable final climb of week 42! At every opportunity, Wessel expressed his gratitude for being part of the journey and being able to experience it all on the mountain with its greatest supporter! He thoroughly enjoyed it and selected the rock to represent climb #294, then lit up with a beaming, grateful smile. Wessel also marked off the day's climb. '0 climbs remaining' was bearing down on me with just 71 left to complete – things were getting real now!

The cold weather snap seemed to have broken, but I was about to find out how much I'd beg to have it back.

The parking lot was transforming before my eyes, and if you'd positioned the camera just right, a time-lapse video would resemble that of the tide coming in and receding. This meant the number of people at the summit was drastically increasing. Suddenly Don's scooter was my new best friend.

CHAPTER 14
OCTOBER - REAPING REWARDS

Week 43 was no joke, and did its best to try and break my spirit. With no hint of a storm passing through Cape Town, the air felt supercharged and was as far removed from winter as ever. It was as though I was transported to the desert. Being bounced between warm and bitterly cold snaps the previous months, naturally corrupted my mind to expect the pattern to continue. Monday was different. The breeze had an ominous, warm feel, the kind that demanded a sunrise climb.

Earlier sunrises meant more time in the shade. In summer, the sun rose further south, and the rim of the peak sheltered me in her protective cloak and kept me out of the sun for some time. This week, it wasn't the direct sunlight that was trying to break me - it was the heatwave. A 5:30 am scooter ride didn't even need a jacket. Parking at the lower cable station exit, with no one around, was a complete juxtaposition to the madness of the buzzing queues I'd experience later. As I walked along the road, I got that same feeling that came up whenever multiple days of storms had been forecast. This was a little bit worse. Every single day of week 43 was going to be a scorcher. I pulled out the thermometer to see what the temperature was. Six minutes after sunrise at 6:02 and it was already 27° C (80° F). I felt it, I was already sweating!

The ease of getting up at 5 am in January felt like a distant memory now as I struggled to get out of bed, even with multiple alarms being set. Late afternoon climbs were a no-go as the hot, super-charged air haunted every step up. With zero breezes to add respite, my only choice was to start early. Even at the height of summer in January, I didn't start this many consecutive climbs at 6 am.

My biggest motivator to finally fall out of bed was the thought of being in the gorge mid-morning. If I could choose one type of weather not to climb in, it would be the baking heat. I'd take cold and wet climbs any day. The problem with heat was that I couldn't dress for it, and when there was no breeze, heat exhaustion and heat stroke became dangerous possibilities. It was worse to start in cold and wet conditions, but you'd be able to enjoy it more because you could push your body's capabilities instead of fighting the energy-sapping heat.

Interestingly, heat requires your body to send more blood to the skin to help cool it off, which means there's less blood flow to the muscles.

Racing against time to beat the first bite of sun on the skin, was like being a vampire watching the deadly line of light move towards you. And the instant it touched you, it felt like someone was throwing a hot blanket over you. A 6 am start with a decent pace, meant I could get all the way up to the 'strength and power rooted in humility' rock. It's a mouthful, but possibly my favourite spot on the climb. It's the first opportunity to get close to the cliffs, or directly underneath. The ritual started on my training climbs. I began staring straight up at the cliff, admiring the flowers and bushes that had made their home inside the rock. More of nature's beautiful examples of 'no excuses.' If I were those plants, I'd probably evaluate whether I'd get enough water to grow here, how many nutrients I'd have access to, and how competitive the nearby plants would be. These plants just understood abundance and got on with it.

In January, I developed this mantra to stay grounded… *'this is a reminder of how small I am.'* It felt a bit negatively phrased, so I changed it to, *'The mountain reminds me that the same strength and power that it has, lives within all of us.'* No mountain ever brags about how big it is either, this was a reminder to maintain the strength and power that was rooted in humility. I stopped here every day and said that.

I couldn't believe that Saturday was going to be my 300th climb, it was like a mirage in the desert. I was drinking so much water on the mountain and couldn't freeze it anymore, which had been my trick to keep drinks colder for longer. I was finishing an entire bottle, and often dipped into one of the two extra bottles.

ESPN confirmed their commitment to join on the 300th climb to do a story on 365 Ubuntu Climbs which gave me a boost. It blew my mind because, in September, I'd written down that I should ask my friend who had been working for them in LA whether they'd like to join to spread the word. They beat me to it, and I was thrilled that they did. Michael was another international supporter

CHAPTER 14
OCTOBER - REAPING REWARDS

and donated some dollars to help the cause. We became friends at the age of 6, but his family emigrated in the early 90's. Thanks to Facebook, we reconnected after many years.

By Wednesday the heatwave was playing tricks with my mind! I began to contemplate whether this was worse for my body than the forced down climbs on windy days. My clothes were drenched in sweat as I arrived at the cable car. My new 'family' were always waiting with smiles and high fives and would shake their heads at my madness. Rieyaaz had been incredible. He used his influence to get more support for my cause and always scooted me to the front of the queue when he saw me.

'Why are you waiting?!' he'd ask me incredulously.

'I don't want to take advantage and just assume I can always be helped to the front,' I'd respond.

'Nonsense – You can always come to one of us in the control room and we'll make a plan for you!'

His offer was gold because the cableway experienced upwards of 15,000 visitors a day on these summer days, and an afternoon climb guaranteed a wait. With just 67 days to go – I'd need their help another 19 times. What makes this kind of generosity even more incredible, is the fact that the queues guarantee they'd have to work an extra two (maybe even three) hours making sure everyone gets down safely. The last car down is supposed to be 19:00, meaning they could very well only leave the mountain at 22:00 and then still need to get home. I sincerely hope the company appreciates their staff. The friendliness and love they've shown me have positively contributed to the Ubuntu teachings. It's not just my experience they contribute to, it's every visitor. I'll always love going home to see their beaming faces.

I became a hermit this week, and desperately hoped that no one would invite me anywhere. I used the sanctuary of my home to get extra sleep because my body was crying out like a baby for its bottle.

Lisa and Dave joined climb #299, which continued the split and made it 155 solo and 144 days joined. I can't single either of them out for this next accolade, though, so we'll just say they both became the 500th person to join. Dave couldn't make it the following day, but Lisa would be there again for another milestone, which timed her 30th climb of the year perfectly.

I can't remember where I heard this, but the theme of our chat on our way up centred around this statement: **You can't accomplish anything without the possibility of failure**. It resonated with me the instant I read it. But now that I was so far into my challenge and still 66 days away from achieving my goal, I was feeling the pressure. And even though I was doing the exact same challenge every day, the possibility of failure was always present. Just one break in this unprecedented run of successive summits was all it took. Thank you legs!

15 people joined my climb #300. This number concerned me because it meant we'd be spending more time on the mountain, in a heatwave! It wasn't just the hottest day of the whole week, it was looking to be the hottest day of the whole year. I shared this with everyone and suggested a 5:30 start. Everyone agreed, which was quite incredible for a weekend.

This is what my milestone climbs looked like in terms of participants: climb #50 – Alone, #100 – Jessie, Lisa and JP, #150 – Michelle and Nicholene, #200 – Alone, and #250 – Marzahn. This one in the heat was more than double the people of all the other five milestone climbs combined. It was a diverse group which included my cousins Louise, who was down from Durban, and Sharon (both daughters of John and Di), and her two daughters Caitlin and Courtney. Lisa was on her 30th climb, coach Karel on his 4th and was sporting his shirt with 6/365 and cap. Karel's brother, his partner Joachim, and friend Nicole also came along. Sharon's neighbour (also Sharon) joined with her twin daughters Madisson and Sienna. Dimitri from Seedspace, Donna, and finally, Shifaan from ESPN also joined.

CHAPTER 14
OCTOBER - REAPING REWARDS

Sadly, Sharon's husband Ryan couldn't join us, but created his own opportunity and organised a corporate climb on #320 later in November with Luke, Jen, Peter, Denzel, Nic, Sean, and Graeme.

Our climb was a tough one and took over 3 hours. The extra early start was an excellent move. We helped a woman along the way who had NO water. Insane! Martin and Nicole, who shared theirs, also ran out. Thankfully, the extra three bottles instead of one came in handy.

Reaching Ubuntu Rock on days like this was extra special. Four additional family stones were placed to complete three generations of stones. Only my family could top that with four generations, from my gran all the way down to my nieces; her great-grandchildren.

I wasn't sure if it was the relief of finishing the 6th consecutive climb in this heatwave, reaching climb #300, or having such tremendous support on a milestone, but this summit was extra special. It was a weird combination of exhaustion and elation all at the same time. We were at the top around 9 am, and it was still relatively quiet, so I took them to my favourite spots. The first stop was at the drop-off that allowed you to see the entire path you'd just tackled. This was followed by the spot where the monks prayed and feasted at the previous month. It was here that Karel gave me a signed copy of his new book with a personalised message in it. I'd been wondering who to choose to cross off the completed climb #300, and it felt perfect to ask him. He was very emotional while handing me the book, and expressed a deep sense of pride for what I'd accomplished since arriving dejected for our first session back in December 2017. He's a tremendous part of my story, and I'll always be indebted to him.

Everyone was buzzing with joy at the top, and nobody left early as we celebrated with some coffee. They were all keen on some pictures with me too. The cutest were the youngsters who whipped out certificates they'd made for me to sign and make official. I was hugely impressed with them, and how they made it up in this heat with their little legs. Their certificates were earned today, I hope they always look at them with fondness and a sense of accomplishment.

Climb #350 was the last milestone to complete as part of a set of seven, and it made me realise something about milestones – they were great tools to show I was on the right path, but ultimately meant nothing without the consistent actions it took to get there. Daily milestones are also powerful contributors to whittling away larger goals. This climb was another special day added to the memory bank to treasure.

65 days to go.

Today wasn't just my milestone, it was also Dexter's birthday and day two of Summer Camp - an initiative created by Harry and Dani Boden whom I'd spoken about earlier in the book. Crazy to think the climb they organised was already 244 climbs ago. They used the party as a fundraiser, too and made 400 tickets available. Climbs #299 to #301 doubled as opportunities to donate R20 in support of 365 Ubuntu Climbs. They used their existing platform and generously contributed R8,000.

I felt my act of gratitude needed to match their effort, so I decided to make the journey out to Robertson to surprise them and thank them personally. If it had been earlier in the year, I'd probably have camped for one night, but now that my legs and body were so tired, I needed all the comfortable sleep I could get! There was one problem though, taking a two-and-a-half-hour drive on a scooter was out of my comfort zone. Don came to the rescue once again and suggested we visit our friends who often spent their weekends there. The distance was close enough to spend a night and return in time for a late afternoon climb on Sunday. If I thought the hottest climb of the year was bad – we arrived in Robertson at 16:00 – and it was still 39°!

I dropped Don off and headed over to Pat Bush, a stunning venue they'd used in March 2016. Incredibly, within the first five minutes of arriving, I spotted Dani, who ran and jumped to hug me. This was her trademark greeting. Next,

CHAPTER 14
OCTOBER - REAPING REWARDS

I spotted Dexter, who was celebrating his birthday and dancing up a storm in his March 365 Ubuntu T-shirt! I was greeted by a sea of smiling faces of friends who realised I wasn't an apparition. I'd made so many wonderful friends, like Darren, Rose and DT (the one that met me at 4:30 am January 1st). It was great to be able to celebrate and show my gratitude for the support, but sad not to be able to stay and dance. I remember my legs screaming at me back in August at midnight to stop dancing. I wouldn't even have made an hour here. Harry and Dani, meanwhile, were true to their character and shook off all the praise and gratitude I shared.

'We're proud of you and happy to be able to contribute.' they said.

The time came for me to leave, so I gave them massive hugs, and slinked away like a leopard disappearing into the bush. When I got back to the house, just a 20-minute drive from the scenic mountain resort, I was greeted with an ice-cold glass of wine and the smell of a braai (our term for a barbecue). With a pool in crawling distance, I dipped my feet, and although it was nowhere near as cool as the Atlantic, it was refreshing nonetheless.

We spoke about the last time we spent a weekend together, and how much things had changed in 392 days. From eagerly waiting for three months to pass, to being 65 days away from completion - things were moving quickly!

Roux, who was also on the Safety Mountain WhatsApp group #6, saw my check-ins and check-outs every day, and, as a lover of mountains, shared his thoughts on watching my journey unfold. Perspectives from other people active on the mountains were always interesting to me because even now, at 300 climbs, I'd fall into self-doubt and wonder if what I was doing was really that much of a challenge. Then I'd see it through someone else's eyes and be reminded of how tough it was.

I was exhausted but unable to hit the hay early because I had a radio interview with Pippa Hudson on Cape Talk at 23:30. I also had a habit of passing out - just ask all the food delivery guys who were unable to get hold of me after arriving at my door. I'd hate for that to happen here! I headed to my room and decided to put my earpiece in my ear so it would ring full blast. Thankfully I did that because I started drifting off just before the call.

Who was listening to this interview so late on a Saturday evening? No idea... but being so close to the end, it was all systems go, so I needed to rustle up as much support as possible for the three charities I was working with. Anything could happen at this stage.

As the talk show host bid me farewell, the word 'bye' had barely left my mouth and I dove head first into dreamland. It was the first time all week I didn't have to be up at 4:30 or 5:00, and that was bliss. I'm sure I fell asleep smiling.

A scorching Sunday afternoon climb awaited me as we made our way back to Cape Town. I had about two hours to relax and psyche myself up for the 7th straight day of climbing in unbearable heat. I was feeling grateful that there were only 9 weeks remaining. It was mind-boggling that besides the final climb, there were just 9 Mondays, 9 Tuesdays, and 9 Wednesdays to go.

I was begging for a break from the heat, and thankfully, my calls were answered. Monday was freezing, and the wind closed the cableway, which meant I'd be climbing down for the 76th time. This was also one step closer to that 100 mark. With fewer climbs remaining, the 'what ifs' were becoming more tangible. Like a child getting closer to their birthday and speculating on what gifts they were going to get.

It was 11° at the top! Sheesh, that's a 20° change from the previous day. Driving back in Don's car, I remembered that he was moving the next day and how this would be my last time on four wheels. The cold was great if you arrived in a car, but it was highly unpleasant if you arrived on a scooter. Surely November wouldn't have too many of these?

October ended in spectacular fashion as Carl, one of my dearest friends, arrived from London with his fiancé and her family from Austria. They enjoyed

CHAPTER 14
OCTOBER - REAPING REWARDS

the beautiful Cape and found the perfect wedding venue too. It was a treat to have them in town and even more so to host them up the mountain. They'd been such tremendous hosts for my Austrian Christmas almost two years ago in 2016, now it was my turn to repay their hospitality. They were rewarded with a rare sighting of mountain Tahrs - only the 7th time I'd seen them all year. We didn't just see them, they came up close and provided Kordu and Gerhard, both avid photographers, with an endless stream of poses. Their smiles beamed gratitude and reminded me why I loved moments like these.

And then, in a moment of pure ecstasy, Carl and Maddy asked if I'd be one of the groomsmen for their wedding.

'ABSOLUTELY!' I responded. 'What an honour!'

Carl and I had struggled together. We knew what it was like to desperately wait for 'Wacky Wednesday,' - a local two-for-the-price-of-one burger special. In London he was rapidly becoming one of PepsiCo's most valued employees. How far we've come. It would be an absolute honour to be part of their beautiful wedding. A well-earned beer went down a treat at the top and, and then, we were lucky enough to witness a spectacular sunset from the cable car on the way down. I could only smile at the grace they'd been given to enjoy on this magical day.

My final climb for October was another pleasant surprise. I ran into Taahir, a man committed to providing safe trails for mountain users. He started an initiative called *Take Back Our Mountains*, which arranged hikes for groups of people from all walks of life to experience the mountain without the fear of getting mugged. A sad reality was that more hikers, climbers, trail runners, and mountain bikers were being assaulted on various trails. It's easy to sit and talk about how terrible these things are when we look at it only from our own perspective, but as I've learned, we can never understand another person's circumstances, especially when they've got a tortured mind and live in extreme conditions. That bullet hole through my pants is always a reminder of how dire people's circumstances can be and how it can push them into making bad choices. I certainly don't condone violence of any order – but I need to know all the facts before condemning people. If anything – it's our systems that are broken.

Taahir interviewed me for his page at a quiet spot we found on a path less travelled close to Waterfall Corner. A quick 5-minute walk was enough to get away from the midweek crowds, and also provided a majestic vantage point of the gorge as the final 100m vertical climb between the narrowed cliffs awaited. As a keen mountaineer and a man with a heart of gold, Taahir kept it short and punchy and posted the interview immediately to help us get more attention and, hopefully, more donations.

Once again, it was bitterly cold at the top, but it was also a photographer's dream with incredible lighting and cloud formations.

The last two days were special, and saw two amazing men tick off some climbs to count me down to #62 and #61.

My birthday month had arrived, but something about it didn't feel right.

CHAPTER 14
OCTOBER - REAPING REWARDS

OCTOBER STATS: 304 / 365

People Joined: 56 / 524

32 days 16 hours 27 minutes 07 seconds / 2,008.08km / 59,14 equivalent Everest Summits

157 solo climbs (51.6%) / 76 Up & Down (25%) TOTAL DONATIONS: R347 149.24

Jackie: 'Great sharing a bit of your journey, Andrew...thanks for always making time for a chat too!!! A pleasure meeting you, and what an inspiration you are!!! Almost there... Wishing you strength.'

Nina: 'What an inspiration you are. Wishing you all the luck in the world with the rest of your mission. Thank you immensely for your patience with me on the mountain this morning! I made it... thanks to you!'

Heide: 'Human connection, community, love - thank you.'

> *The task is not yours to finish (the job of perfecting the world), but neither are you free not to take part in it. And if not now when?* ~~
> **Jewish Rabbi Tarfon 500B.C**

CHAPTER 15

NOVEMBER – THE PERFECT STORM

My birthday month had always been a source of excitement for me, but this time it felt a little more important.

My exuberance was quickly brought down to earth as I enjoyed hosting some fresh faces. Melissa, the daughter of an ex-colleague of mine, Carey, and her boyfriend, Jandre, joined me Thursday; it was their first climb up Platteklip. Ordinarily, mountain newbies wouldn't phase me, but at this late stage of the challenge, nothing was 'ordinary.' The 11th month began with an up-and-down climb, which, at 5 hours and 1 minute, was also the 4th longest climb of the year. I didn't realise it at the time, but I'd been given a warning about what could happen if I didn't prioritise my legs.

It was also a lesson in diplomacy. While it's true I hadn't turned anyone away up until now, I needed to set boundaries and ask people to respect where I was on

CHAPTER 15
NOVEMBER - THE PERFECT STORM

the journey with my mind and body. I wanted people to consider their fitness levels and capabilities so as not to jeopardise where I was. It wasn't about the pace; it was about maintaining focus. For starters, anyone who wasn't a seasoned climber and comfortable on Table Mountain needed to join on days that the cable car was guaranteed to run. Friday's solo climb gave me time to reflect on this as I prepared for another unbelievable moment: **Huni's arrival from Iceland.**

He'd never been to South Africa, and I was excited to host and finally show him the project he'd been supporting from so far away. He's a big man – standing at six feet six inches, and it's not often I hug someone taller than me! Hard to believe we first met at a business conference a year ago. His kind and inviting face exudes peace, and he has a generous heart, demonstrated not just by his support for me – but in his dream to build a school in rural Kenya. This idea had been built on the back of trauma, a career-ending injury in professional basketball, and almost dying.

His first climb coincided with 'The 3 Peaks Challenge'. It's a gruelling test for Athletes that starts in Cape Town at Greenmarket Square. The first summit is Devil's Peak, followed by Platteklip to Maclears Beacon and finally, Lions Head. After each successful summit, climbers are required to head all the way back down into the Square, and to start from sea level. We were joined by Jana and her husband, Chris, who'd heard about me through a mutual friend.

For Huni and the athletes, the high clouds and a gentle breeze meant perfect conditions. Maclears Beacon was also part of today's climb. The last time I'd been there was 201 climbs ago for the rescue. I took them along the eastern table's front face, where the cliffs drop away from our feet, and give even the strongest stomach flutters. For the first time, I saw where the fourth fire crested and where the firemen stopped its journey. While the plentiful winter rains had brought nourishment to the scorched land and life was clawing its way back, there were still plenty of dark black patches and charred rock.

Some new friends were manning the refreshment station at Maclears Beacon. Jackie and Alex had been training for 'The Sky Run,' a race unlike any other challenge on the South African racing calendar. Participants were required to navigate and manage their gear whilst tackling the remote terrain of the Witteberg Mountain range in the Eastern Cape. The demanding race is 100 kilometres at an average elevation of between 2,200 to 2,500 metres above sea level, 4,445m of elevation gain, and a 30-hour cut-off time.

I remember our first introduction on the mountain during one of their training climbs. It was a cold and misty day, and we were all wrapped up with buffs covering our mouths and ears. They pledged to join me, and as always, I thanked them for their support and told them how excited I was for that day. Their continued encouragement on the mountain and generous donation demonstrated their commitment. It was great to see them paying it forward in other ways and helping to rehydrate the athletes. Their race was on the 17th, and I wholeheartedly agreed that they should join me once their training and race were over. I certainly couldn't keep up with them on a training 'run' up the mountain, and even if I could – it would be foolhardy.

It had been incredible seeing them train in a variety of challenging conditions, and their commitment to finishing the race within the 30-hour cut-off time was inspiring. I personally thought they were mad, but they thought that about me too (touché).

It took us two hours to complete the loop to Maclears beacon and get back to the Cable way, and as we took our time enjoying the ample light and the uniqueness of the mountaintop, I was reminded of how vast the table was. At certain points, the ocean is no longer visible, and it feels like you're on a vast grassland on the plains of Africa. I had to pinch myself to remember that there was an ocean just over the edge. The air was lightly dusted in a soft grey light and clear enough for us to see from Cape Point to Langebaan and from Camps Bay to the Heldeberg. It had been the perfect start, and Huni was over the moon.

CHAPTER 15
NOVEMBER - THE PERFECT STORM

I was excited about the new route the next day celebrating the #300 milestone the previous week. Because that climb had such a large group, and possibly the hottest day of the year, I banked my reward route up Kloof Corner and decided to use it the day before my birthday. Of course, Lisa was going to join, and after meeting Huni in LA with me, she was eager to see his friendly face again. As I'd never done this route before, I called in my trusty friends, The Mountain Slayers, to lead the day.

Alas, more unseasonably cold, wet, and misty conditions descended upon us. Part of our planned route had chains, so The Mountain Slayers and I agreed that it wasn't worth the risk, and made another plan. Instead, we went up India Venster, which made Huni happy that he got to explore a new route on his second go. He became the 4th person to do back-to-back climbs with me.

It wasn't long before the mist surrounded us, and made the idea of a view far-fetched. Up top, Huni shared what an incredible experience it had been for him. I was eternally grateful that he made the massive effort to come. The memory of our first discussion in Anaheim was still fresh in my mind. It was at this moment that we discussed the importance of making the distinction between saying you want to do something; and saying you're going to do something when attempting to reach a goal. He'd heard countless people say 'I want to' and explained that the very nature of wanting something already fulfilled the desire. You can want to achieve things, but that wouldn't make it happen. However, saying I'm going to do something was different because it created intent.

Saying 'I'm going to', entices your mind with the fulfillment of the action. It's such a simple yet profound statement. I wish I'd kept a record of all the people who 'failed' to show up and see whether they'd used 'want to' as opposed to 'going to'. In any case, that distinction was burned into my brain, and I corrected myself whenever I felt I was about to say it.

After finishing our coffees, we headed back down, and I caught up with my cousin Charles, who'd flown down from Johannesburg to join me on a climb. We were going to discuss which day would work best.

Our meeting started a series of events that would culminate in some of the greatest lessons of the year. Because he'd smoked for 25 years and avoided exercise most of his life, my mom told him flat out that he wouldn't make it. I encouraged him to use the stairmaster at the gym and always use stairs wherever he went because these actions mimicked climbing. Although he was confident he'd make it, I had my reservations. I politely expressed my new sense of self-preservation and explained that I reserved the right to tell him to turn back. He didn't enjoy that. I'll never forget the tone in my voice and the look on his face. It definitely came out harsher than intended. I knew it was going to be a long climb, and prepared for something a bit longer than my sister's climb. Nevertheless, he'd made the effort and flew down from Johannesburg, which certainly deserved an opportunity to climb. I still made sure to survey the weather apps to find the best climbing window. Monday would be my birthday, and I needed to get Huni to the airport afterward, so that day was ruled out. The weather looked a bit iffy on Tuesday, which meant a wet path and a potential downclimb, so that was also a hard no. On Wednesday, Fred, an ex-colleague, had arranged to do a team building with his brandy team, so that was also a no. Adding to this, Charles was due to fly back on Friday morning.

'I'd hate to fly all the way down here for nothing,' **he exclaimed.**

I was truly sympathetic to his situation and appreciative of his effort, but the first three days were non-negotiable, even if it resulted in a fruitless trip. We'd have to push for Thursday morning then! The south easter would pose some challenges though, and if it got strong enough, would close the cable car at 14:00. Knowing this, we'd have to start at 7 am to be safe. Eager to climb, he pleaded for me to keep an eye on Tuesday's weather for any changes. I promised I would and headed back home to join Lisa and Huni for dinner.

CHAPTER 15
NOVEMBER - THE PERFECT STORM

My 309th climb coincided with my 39th birthday and brought my total vertical kilometres of climbing up to 222 - the equivalent of 60 Mt Everests. Imagine climbing for 33 days, 3 hours, and 7 minutes to reach 55.5% of the International Space Station? With 56 climbs remaining, my mind drifted back to an earlier climb with Dani, Colleen, and Craig, where I was still fresh in the challenge and with no real clue how I was going to be tested through winter. But here I was with the belief that the hardest part of each day was getting out of bed.

Today's climb felt extra special, not because it was my birthday – but because of all the birthdays that had come before this. In 2004, when I turned 25, I watched the sunset on top of Table Mountain for the first time and sipped cocktails. It's also when I bought that fridge magnet that had the gorgeous sunset I was able to take my own picture of last month. I was struggling to find my path back then, but had the courage to pursue opportunities others advised against. If I'd never visited Cape Town back then – I'm not sure I'd be standing on top of Table Mountain now with such purpose.

All my life experiences had helped shape me, escape boredom, and led me to a path of fulfillment on Platteklip. I found the balance between empowering others, looking after myself, and enriching my life with experiences instead of 'things.'

According to Numerology, 6 is my life path number, and in keeping with that theme, on my birthday, I was blessed with 6 donations totalling R2,915.47!! It was the greatest present I could ask for.

I was smiling through the pain as I added to the 821,940 steps I had climbed so far. Lisa and Huni's energy was like nitrous. After all those years of being exhausted by self-doubt, I was being confronted with real exhaustion. I could easily have dismissed my idea as crazy and left it in my life's folder of 'what if's.' I was grateful that I was finally stepping through my own barriers.

I was constantly reminded of reasons to feel grateful. There was a mother whose child matched a new donor through DKMS Africa, a family that was given a new home by Habitat for Humanity, and under-resourced teachers who were helped by One Heart's contribution towards the education initiatives that changed children's circumstances.

The collective effort of 363 online donations, 541 fellow climbers, and countless cash donations on the mountain (now totalling R20,000!) created a profound birthday experience. This is Ubuntu. This is what it feels like. The project was nothing without these supporters, the friends who quietly reached out on some idle Tuesday, or my family, who, without saying a word, constantly shared the message and gave me the support needed to take something like this on.

Jessie had only been in my life for 13 months, but her impact on me was already immeasurable. She cheered me on, invested her time, energy, and money into this and us, all from the other side of the world. She was everything I'd been patiently searching for. There's a reason she's loved and respected by so many people - now she can add me to that list.

Up till now, only Jessie had done three climbs back-to-back. Huni was about to join her to make it two internationals - an American and an Icelander. This was proof that when something's in your backyard, it's 'always there' to postpone indefinitely. But when you've travelled from afar, you're more likely to suck the bone marrow out of the experience.

I live by that principle now. I do my best not to become complacent and embrace opportunities to do things. The truth is, the time may come when I no longer live here or may not have access to many of life's amazing experiences. It reminds me that I never watched a Premier League game while I was in London, I constantly put it off because I had 'years' ahead of me.

Huni had some Icelandic schnapps, which made for a perfect birthday toast at the summit in icy conditions. I got awesome birthday love from the staff and joked about my 'free ride' down in the cable car. It was my 232nd trip down with them, and brought my daily cost down to R2.75! It was a fantastic investment considering the cost of paying the one-way fee each day, which would have amounted to R44,080!!!!

CHAPTER 15
NOVEMBER – THE PERFECT STORM

Don's move had gone smoothly and made his first trip back 'across the border' to come enjoy lunch with us in Camps Bay. Allan joined too, making it a lovely way to round off Huni's trip. We collected his things at home for one last car ride together. I was sure the rental car we were travelling in had never had two behemoths like us in it before! Hosting Huni had been an absolute pleasure. And then just like that, he disappeared into the airport. The orphans in Kenya were the next lucky souls who would have him in their presence.

Tuesday arrived and the weather looked to be wet all day, so I informed Charles that we'd take our opportunity early Thursday. I prayed that the wind scheduled in the afternoon would stay away for as long as possible.

I wasn't alone on my Tuesday climb though. Marcus, my tattoo artist, joined me. He was an avid outdoorsman and undeterred by the wet, so we set off at 9:06. His plans to be in Johannesburg or Plettenberg Bay for his birthday fell through, so he grabbed the opportunity to climb. I've spent 11 hours with him getting two tattoos. He was the perfect person to turn my right shoulder blade into a piece of art. The tattoo was a daily reminder of my connection to something greater and an understanding of ancient wisdom. I have the face of Three Eagles, from the Nez Perce tribe, a Native American with no particular rank or prestige, whose face has seen much pain and been carved by time and deep life experiences.

Marcus is a deep thinker, a philosopher with great insights and knowledge. Today wasn't just any birthday, he'd turned 40 and chose to begin his next decade in nature. The rain didn't affect his mood – in fact, it was quite the opposite. He felt more connected, knowing the importance of rain as he embraced a new year and decade with a clean slate. A pearl he shared on the way up was that as the world below got smaller – so too did its 'problems.' Climbing Table Mountain, surrounded by grandiosity, life, and ancient rocks with knowledge none of us could fathom, has a way of reminding us of what's really important.

His intention for a meaningful climb helped him see all the faces on the rock without me pointing it out. He thought his big gulps of air and extra oxygen intake may have heightened his senses. Each step that he took had an intentional pause, not because of fatigue – but for him to reflect.

I did what few get to do with him and felt his appreciation for the experience. We went and sat at the pyramid after he placed his birthday rock next to the one I'd placed the previous day. Immediately and with intent, he scanned each stone from the past 307 climbs and pointed to a new one, describing its unique attributes. Enjoying the silence was something few could do, but we easily sat for 20 minutes, grinning like two idiots without a care in the world, just listening to the water dripping and the mountain echoes dancing through the mist.

His open mind and willingness to learn and share, allowed me to highlight all the synchronicity we'd experienced in the day. He pointed out that he placed his rock at exactly 12:12. As a numerologist, I loved numbers and we shared the exact same life path – 33/6's. I had 55 days left, and we got to the top in the 13th hour (4 for him) in 3 hours. I showed him Table Mountain's latitude, which was 33 degrees. After meditating and with the wind slamming into us, I shared that today would be my 233rd cable car ride down. Finally, we got off the cable car at 13:36! We both laughed and smiled and, without words, shared our gratitude, love, and appreciation.

Besides choosing nature as the right place to start his next chapter, he'd enjoyed the gift of all 4 elements: the mountain – earth; the rain – water; the wind – air; and the scarred path below – fire. It was a self-prescribed 'right of passage.' After our meditation, he was rewarded as the mist lifted and revealed glorious clouds with shadows across Lions Head and the Atlantic Ocean. I took note for my 40th next year.

Once again, 24 hours made all the difference. Misty, wet, and cold conditions became hot, clear skies. Lisa joined Fred's team and me as we started two hours later than planned. It was great to see the familiar faces of Sipho, Fano,

CHAPTER 15
NOVEMBER - THE PERFECT STORM

and Arthur as well as the new face of Saraah. The heat started affecting some of the team just after halfway. My eyes were met with shaking heads and cries of 'every day?' Disbelief oozed from their voices in between gasping breaths.

I missed the people from my old company and really enjoyed reminiscing with them. I heard about who else had left and how the 'restructure' had impacted those that had stayed. Needless to say, I felt that I had made the right decision.

Simply put - Fred wasn't even from my old department, and yet he'd been the only senior manager to reach out and support. And on top of that, of anyone I knew, he'd probably been through the toughest year out of all of us combined, losing his wife to cancer and with two young children in tow.

When I have groups, I encourage them to climb with intentionality:

'I don't know what challenges you're facing right now - but think of the mountain as the physical representation of that challenge. You'll see some parts are easier than others, and that perhaps just by starting, you realise it's not as bad as you thought it would be. No matter what though, it won't last forever. You WILL get to the top, and you will see the strength and power that already lives within you.'

No one's ever come back and shared whether it's helped or not. Today, though, I hope it reminds Fred that his strength, what he's endured, and how he's made it to this point is appreciated. He was the only manager supporting me, and he'd challenged the entire senior leadership team to show their support on other climbs. Out of all of them, Caroline was the only one who embraced the challenge.

I got home filled with the joys of another successful climb and the excitement of being a day closer to the end. More money was raised to empower others, and I began to embrace the idea that although this year and all its chapters were about to close, it wouldn't mean the end, I'd still be able to open a fresh new book that would contribute positively to the lives of others.

Week 45's conversations had a sense of uncertainty to them, but I remained focused on dealing with the next day.

Thursday arrived, and the afternoon weather forecast still looked bleak. Charles was happy to start at 7 am. I wish I'd captured a screenshot of the weather app showing the lovely mild green and yellow colours indicating mild breezes for early on and then the dark red ominous blocks for later in the day. It was a race against time.

I welcomed everyone to climb #312, which had an interesting start. Heide had already done 2, so she represented the 3, Carl, Maddy, and Kordu chose to join, too, which made it their second time, and Charles was on his 1st. I made a very conservative estimate with a return time of 13:00. Six hours would be the longest climb up so far. I warned Heide and Carl that it was going to be a slow one before they arrived and they still chose to come and support me.

Five minutes into the climb, and everyone else was around the corner and out of sight. We'd eventually catch up to them, but I knew my worst fears were being realised. I told Carl they had no obligation to remain with us. He considered that, and when he realised the pace would impact their lunch date with friends, he bid us farewell and pushed on. Bless Heide, she was committed to staying and helping me out. Her face spoke volumes as she sensed my unease and frustration at how things were panning out. Charles, as the editor of The Star, had published a story in the paper to help create awareness. He introduced me to Sarah, who had joined four times, donated, and wrote an article about her experiences too. He'd been full of ideas and thought I should've had a lot more support to this point. *Me too Charles. Me too.*

I was concerned about our pace though, and constantly checked Windguru. The worst-case scenario was reaching the point of no return and having to climb back down as well. Weirdly though, there wasn't a moment I felt the need to step in and command Charles down as garishly as I had on Sunday.

CHAPTER 15
NOVEMBER - THE PERFECT STORM

The heat picked up steadily, and I watched wisps of cloud pass overhead as they left the mountain, evaporating into nothing. It must have looked as though I was watching tennis. Path... Wisps of cloud... Path... Clouds. It was an intriguing battle, and I couldn't wait to see who'd win the rally! Finally, the path hit an overhead smash to win the point.

At the start of Ascension Corner, a bug flew into Charles's throat, and he let out an almighty roar followed by a wheeze. It wasn't the sound you wanted to hear from someone struggling up the mountain. He sat down on a rock, which made me think that if I had not known about the bug, I could easily have thought he was having a heart attack. Very calmly, I asked him how he was feeling and let him know that going back down was still an option. There was no point in putting his health at risk for anything. It wasn't my body, so I had to trust his honesty.

'Are we past half way?' he asked.

I was tempted to lie.

'Uh – no we're not. Forget about halfway.' I responded. *'I can tell you when we reach it, how's that?'*

'What?! You must be joking!' he exclaimed.

I wish I had been.

I think there was a bit of 'I'll show you' going on with Charles, which may have been because nobody really believed he could make the climb. His motives weren't my concern, I was more focused on ensuring he knew all the options, so he could make informed decisions. I decided not to talk about the wind factor to prevent adding to the pressure. There's a big difference between someone slacking and someone with nothing left in the tank yet giving their absolute best. I also knew that once we hit halfway, going down would be just as hard for him as finishing the climb.

I took serious heat and got some choice words from people who told me *how dangerous it would be to continue.* I disagreed. He's a grown man with a clear understanding that actions have consequences. He had all the options available at hand and, instead of asking how much longer, he kept asking about halfway. He didn't believe me that we weren't there yet, but still he kept pushing on.

Just like with Lifa, my intuition told me that things were okay. Yes, we were going slowly, but there were no alarm bells. Heide, like an absolute champ, continued to climb with us. By the time we reached halfway, we'd been on the mountain for four hours. I won't lie, at this point, I couldn't fathom going back down with him only to redo it all. At best, we could double the time, and we'd be on the mountain two hours longer than my previous longest climb. At least that previous climb had been in cooler conditions. I gingerly took out my thermometer and watched the temperature rise into the 30s.

Waves of anger and frustration swept over me. I'm sure I released an inordinate amount of both on this climb. People who climbed past, whom Charles spoke to, could sense my frustration. To his credit, though and with deep gratitude on my part – he told everybody what I was doing, which, at this point, had become quite a few people! I checked in with the tracking team on the cable car's status, and they were still open! The wind was still minimal, but midday was ringing in my ears, thanks to the noon gun. We had just two hours to get up.

Two things about this day will never make sense. Firstly, the wind forecast meant a definite shutdown of the cableway, but the wind never came. It was the first prediction of the year that was so wrong. I'd experienced the opposite plenty of times where the wind pumped after none was predicted. I was grateful that today was the first time I'd experienced it in reverse.

Then secondly, I recorded the temperature in the gorge all day, and while the thermometer reached 35°C (95°F) – it never felt that bad. I wasn't complaining at all – I was simply dumbfounded every time I measured it. I never measured it in front of him, or shared it with him. The mind is a powerful thing, and he never asked what the temperature was or complained about it, so there was no need to give him information that would just open a can of worms.

CHAPTER 15
NOVEMBER – THE PERFECT STORM

The man was pushing himself harder than he'd ever done before, and apart from pockets of pure frustration – I admired his effort. I began to wonder if I should've brought as much water as I did on climb #300, which was the hottest day of the year. Thankfully, he listened and brought extra water and juice. Still, I was getting nervous about running out before reaching the top. Heide had been incredibly patient and did her best to keep my spirits up.

'I think you're being taught the value of patience.' she said with a wry smile.

I'd been thinking about that and came to a different conclusion. Maybe if I'd been impatient throughout the year, I'd agree. This felt different. It took twice as long as any other climb up, and after having 311 climbs behind me, it was incomprehensible. I felt that the lesson was perhaps more for him than it was for me. If anything – my lesson was to broadcast the request for others to respect me and my legs as much as I had done for them all year. At least there was some shade at the end of the tunnel. At 13:29, the sun had moved enough for the cliffs to cloak us in shade.

Eventually, Heide had to call it a day, her afternoon appointments were in jeopardy, which left just Charles and I. At the halfway mark, he turned around and thanked me for not leaving him behind. I immediately picked up climb 312's stone. Until then, I hadn't been sure if he'd appreciated it, and those two simple words released some tension. I was drawing on every experience I could to stay focused on each step. It was as though all my tough days had been preparing me for this.

His dad was my grandad's brother, and one thing I enjoyed tremendously was hearing about his experiences as a child and how my grandparents helped him through some difficult times. I was already immensely proud of my grandparents, but hearing firsthand about their generosity took it up a notch.

He gave me some truly hilarious moments too.

'What's the fastest time up the mountain?' he asked.

'I think the record is something like 27 minutes,' I responded.

'I wonder what the record for the slowest time is?'

'Can we please NOT aim for that!?!?!' I begged.

Then when we were closer to the top, he gave me a zinger and he suddenly exclaimed...

'I've been divorced twice.... And this is still the hardest thing I've ever done in my life.'

Jessie went to bed as we started and woke up expecting to hear all about it. But we were still on the mountain. My concerns about water materialised at Waterfall Corner when Charles's last sip slid down his throat. I'd previously suggested pushing up to the top to get more to bring back, but he blew it off, probably worried I wouldn't come back! The location we were at would normally be 20 minutes from the top, and running dry here wouldn't stress me, especially in the shade, but it wasn't going to be 20 minutes this time, so I had no choice but to get more refreshments. I made an executive decision and decided not to ask and just told him that I was going.

Conscious of how accidents happen, I stayed focused and proceeded without letting the past six hours distract me. I'd be extremely upset with myself if I allowed it to cause a serious injury just 53 days away from the end. Everyone in my family was watching me on Endomondo now, concerned about how long it was taking, and my phone's battery life was in the single digits. While passing Ubuntu Rock, I stopped to place the day's stone and to update Safety Mountain Tracking. I preempted a future concern and explained that if my battery died, they should assume that everything was fine, and when I made it back home, then I'd check out.

By the time I reached the top, it was 14:44 and I took the opportunity to grab my photo before my phone died. As I began my descent to Charles, my eyes were blessed with an incredible sight. Seeing my shadow on the path in front of me caused me to turn around and gaze up. The sun sparkled behind the cliff and told me there was 'light at the end of the tunnel.' It gave me one of my favourite pictures of the year.

I prayed that I'd at least find Charles at Ubuntu Rock, ready to place his family stone. I filled all my bottles and took huge, grateful sips before rushing back to Platteklip. This confused everyone who'd been watching me on Endomondo and made them wonder why on earth I was going back down. As they called me to find out what was going on, my battery chose to die! Finally, I reached Charles, who was just two corners away from Ubuntu Rock. He was incredibly grateful for the water.

I'm not sure if it was stubbornness to prove others wrong or pure grit, but his perseverance and 'never give up' attitude were impressive. He finally admitted that he'd completely overestimated his abilities, which wasn't an easy thing to do. It takes character and strength to be able to admit it to others like that. His insights into what the climb was about and how it related to other areas of his life showed how much the experience meant to him. There haven't been many occasions where people have drawn deep conclusions about their experience on the mountain and related it back to their daily lives, so this made me even more proud of him.

We rounded the final corner, and only Stairway to Heaven remained. With all these emotions happening at once, I felt like I was being jumbled around in a washing machine. I experienced joy, relief, anguish, disbelief, and anger... I needed a drink! Incredibly, a woman who started maybe 30 minutes after us caught up to us. They looked at each other with a quiet desperation that said... 'I should've stayed at home.'

We finally reached the top, and then I remembered we still had to do the chains. Whatever energy he had left before that was finally extinguished. After that, there was nothing but a flat pathway. The relief was evident on his face. He made it!!

He thanked me multiple times for patiently sticking with him, he also bought me a beer as his final act of gratitude. We sat under the shade, both exhausted from the longest day of our lives. I thought about how many times I could have told him to turn around, and then he uttered these right words...

'This is the greatest accomplishment of my life.'

Ubuntu taught me another lesson – who am I to tell others what they can or can't do?

Completing Platteklip had never been an option for him before. He was never that active. He'd never climbed a mountain before. It was through 365 Ubuntu Climbs that he wrote and published an article that reached hundreds of thousands of people with the message. Unlike the majority of other journalists, he did what he'd asked others to do: **donate and climb.**

His climb was #312, and he was climber #553. No one can ever take that away from him. It made me think about how many times in the past, because of my own assumptions or selfish motives, I'd either not invited someone, or made decisions on their behalf. I would tell myself that I was either doing it for their benefit or because they wouldn't finish, but the truth is if it didn't fit my narrative, I seldom did something for others in this way.

Today wasn't about patience. Patience provided the platform for another human being to learn about themselves. I don't think I've ever been that happy to get home. I finally walked through the door at 17:44, making it just under 10 hours on the route - with an 8-hour marathon on Platteklip alone. I was exhausted and knew that I had to do it all again the next day, and another 52 climbs after that.

I finally revived my phone and let Safety Mountain Tracking know that all was 'well.' Then I told my family and Jessie that I had no energy to talk about the day, and I didn't really want to. I just wanted to be 'alone' and recharge. Everyone understood. Another day like this would break me. Finally, I waited for my Monks Chinese food order to be delivered and drank possibly the greatest glass of wine ever. I also kept shaking my head in disbelief... *'8 hours!'*

CHAPTER 15
NOVEMBER - THE PERFECT STORM

The end suddenly felt a whole lot further away.

Hearing one side of the story tells you my perspective. But I'm trying to highlight a vital lesson: barring criminal offences, there's no good or bad, it's just how we view something. Even that can change over time. What I view as a bad experience from years ago, I may look back on again and see as hugely beneficial. When I become open to learning through experiences, I don't get stuck in a negative spiral. I learn, I adapt, I grow. Climb #312 was just such an experience for me. Don't take my word for it though, here's what Charles had to say about his experience:

I heard through Andrew's mom that he was planning to hike up Table Mountain every day for an entire year.

What a crazy idea, I immediately thought. But also what incredible determination - both as a personal challenge for Andrew and as a commitment to helping several worthy causes.

I can't recall what made me decide to attempt this climb, but I gave it a shot despite being pretty unfit and in my mid-60s.

I was going to gym regularly in those pre-Covid days, and, in the days leading up to my adventure, I tried to boost my stamina by walking up several flights of stairs at nearby malls.

I flew to Cape Town from Joburg and met my burly and super-fit cousin, whom I hadn't seen in years.

A suitable day was chosen, and I was picked up from my hotel early in the morning. I brought along several litres of water.

The first part of the climb in mild weather was tough, albeit manageable. About halfway to the top Andrew suggested I could give up and walk down, but I reckoned that, having come that far and made so much effort, I should press on.

The sun was getting hotter and I was struggling to ascend the steep inclines and rugged terrain, notwithstanding all the encouragement from Andrew and some fellow climbers.

Then my water ran out, and Andrew very kindly offered to climb to the top of the mountain to get me some.

After more than eight hours I finally made it to the top. I certainly felt a great sense of achievement but I was upset that I had taken up so much of Andrew's time and inconvenienced him a great deal.

He has subsequently told me he admired my tenacity and determination not to quit.

If I'd known how tough it would be I probably wouldn't have tried. But, thanks to Andrew, I can now tell people, with considerable pride, that I climbed Table Mountain.

Charles.

"Probably wouldn't have tried." That stands out the most for me. How many experiences do we rob ourselves of because of the perception that they're 'hard'? Instead of trying to manicure life, accept that it comes with challenges. Embracing that can make all the difference in discovering what we're capable of.

Ubuntu asks us to put ourselves in someone else's shoes and see from their perspective. I'm truly grateful Charles took the time, made the effort, and spent his money to join me. Without his contribution, I'm not sure I would have learned the value of practising Ubuntu in tougher situations.

I passed out without any thought of setting an alarm, but my eyes stirred surprisingly early. It was my sister's birthday, so I called to wish her. She was already on her way to drop the girls off at school, and had me on speakerphone, so I got to chat to all of them. I told her how Charles and I took double the time it took her to get up, and they couldn't believe it. Hearing my sister's voice far

CHAPTER 15
NOVEMBER - THE PERFECT STORM

outweighed getting messages on the family chat; it was the boost I needed. It helped me verbalise my feelings about facing the mountain today.

I'd use today's and tomorrow's solo climbs to re-energize. Today, I had two choices: just get it done early or rest more to build up energy for an afternoon climb. I decided to get it over with. I felt like waiting to complete climb #313 would hamper my brain's need for rest. Years of grabbing the opportunity to go first, whether introducing myself to a large group of people or delivering prepared talks, taught me how going first or early means sitting calmly instead of worrying about when my name would be called.

The drive up seemed quicker than usual. It was another warm day, and felt hotter than yesterday, so a 7:30 start was not ideal. The device told another story - maybe it was faulty?!?! I couldn't explain it. The thermometer kept showing me numbers below yesterday's 35 and yet the heat got unbearable and made yesterday's experience so much more bizarre.

I spent 20 minutes processing everything in the stillness of the gorge, just laying in the shade next to my pyramid. I drew strength from the 308 stones (the five from this week were still on Ubuntu Rock) as the coolness of the boulder beneath me acted like an air-conditioner. I repeated my gratitude prayer, and it reminded me of what I had to focus on.

Word about my longer climb the previous day had spread throughout the team at the cableway, and Brendon was the first to ask me about it. He reiterated Charles's sentiment of what a sense of accomplishment it must've been. Charles did his own processing about the climb and sent me a beautiful message before his flight. Incredibly, his body wasn't in too much of a shock, and he didn't have much stiffness either. It was probably all the breaks that made the difference.

Now, with firsthand knowledge of what 365 Ubuntu Climbs entailed, Charles could garner more support for me through his network of journalists. These efforts would later materialise into two things I'd never dreamed of. Jonathan, a man Charles dined with the night before the climb, called me up in December.

'I've pitched the story to The Sunday Times (one of the largest publications in South Africa) and we're going to run it on the first Sunday of 2019.' Jonathan told me.

Not only did the story run, but it featured on the front page. The Sunday Times cut portions of the article out that he wasn't happy with, so he contacted me again...

'Hey Andrew, I wasn't happy with how the editor cut my article in the paper, so I've pitched the idea to Men's Health, and they love it! They want to do a four page spread. Can they send a photographer to do a climb with you in January for the March issue?' he asked.

Can they?! Are you kidding me?!?! I still had my mock 'Men's Health cover' I was given for my 21st... The one with my face on the model's body and taglines that told me how to live it up on my 21st. And let's not forget the 'Harder Abs with Andrew' as the headline article. I'd looked at it every day for 18 years, and now it was becoming a reality – but even better: I was being featured for something I was doing, not how I looked!

The two publications expanded Ubuntu's reach and raised awareness for Habitat for Humanity, DKMS Africa, and One Heart. It reached a combined total of 275,368 people. The free publicity was worth a staggering R508,814.18! If ever I needed a reminder that what we put out there comes back to us – this was it. Not just that, 275,368 new seeds had been planted.

Mistakes were still a potential threat, even after all these days on the mountain. I had some farewell drinks at Carl and Maddy, and with the wind predictions in mind, I stayed longer than usual. I started my climb at 9:40, thinking the wind would pump and I would climb down. There was no wind, though. Usually I'd be ecstatic about something like this but not today.

I felt like I was being roasted alive in the world's largest oven. The most climbing I could manage before needing water in the shade was 10 minutes. At this late

CHAPTER 15
NOVEMBER - THE PERFECT STORM

hour, there was nothing but relentless heat for at least another half an hour until I could crawl up to the section covered in shade. My cheek against the rock was bliss. 10 minutes... break... 10 minutes... break. The only comfort against the pulsating heat was the realisation that I'd get to enjoy a cable car ride down. It felt like my heart was going to explode out of my chest. Staring at the ocean, I knew there was only one thing left to do. Normally, I wouldn't swim in the arctic-like temperatures of the Atlantic, but it shimmered like an oasis in the desert and called out to me.

I scooted down to Clifton 4th Beach, and easily found some parking up front. As I hit the sand, I started undressing and just melted into the water. I may as well have dived through a portal and landed in Antarctica. Coming up for air, a loud moan escaped my lungs as I adjusted to the icy grip. My calf muscles started twitching in the water, and it felt like my body was thanking me for giving it this sweet relief. As I climbed out of the water with Table Mountain watching over me, I pondered how this was already the third longest week on the mountain, with 22 hours 28 minutes, and one more climb in hand.

Week 45 started with my birthday in gloomy conditions and finished with Lisa, Allan, Jana, Chris, Jessica, and Sacha from the UK. The combination of it being my 18th barefoot climb and four taxing days of climbing made this outing a challenging one. Jana and Chris also went barefoot after listening to me talk about it to Huni – they loved it! I had some more converts.

Sascha was doing a film shoot and had never climbed before. She was in complete awe as we steadily rose high into the sky, like Jack up the beanstalk. She soaked it all in and took time to explore the changing nuances and perspectives of the beautiful mountain. They all did a sterling job, and since it was 11/11, I planned to enjoy some bubbles and treats at the top while basking in the sunshine and toasting another testing, yet successful week.

Just 50 climbs to go now....

Climb #318 brought with it another group of three, and it was my 10th group in 14 days for November. After meeting Rod and Rina, I realised this wasn't the 'usual' group. They heard me on the radio back in June and donated immediately. Their message read:

'Respect for your hikes and the causes you are supporting Andrew, we salute you.'

They got my contact details in an automated thank you email and expressed their desire to join. I couldn't help but overflow with gratitude and give them my best bear hug. On Saturday, they were going on a three-week trip to Vietnam to visit their daughter, so rather than delaying the climb even more, they decided today was the day.

Massimo made it a trio of participants. I'd met him through his generosity with DKMS Africa. In 2013 I was the Western Cape's highest fundraiser for the Cape Town Cycle race, and Massimo donated a 'dinner for two' at his restaurant in Hout Bay as a prize. I was privileged to receive that for two years running. I met him briefly at the second dinner with my friend Dave, but this was our first real opportunity to chat properly. He's a leukaemia survivor and has supported DKMS Africa for years, it's how he heard about my challenge.

He climbed, donated, and clearly went away deep in thought. Barely a day later. He contacted me with a proposal. He wanted to push himself to climb for a week and use his restaurant as a vehicle to advertise and encourage patrons to sponsor. His restaurant was already a shining example of how businesses could use their existing networks to uplift the communities they served. Many of the proceeds of the meals purchased at his restaurant went to animal shelters, DKMS Africa, pizzas to local organisations like Amoyo, or feeding firefighters who were battling regular mountain blazes in the area. The menu also detailed exactly who your meal purchase would benefit. And, of course, he was donating a portion of his profits too! This is a man who is truly living his second life to the fullest and with purpose.

CHAPTER 15
NOVEMBER - THE PERFECT STORM

He was due to climb with me on Tuesday, the 4th of December, but he felt sick, and with the rain forecast, we agreed it was best to delay it by a week and start on the 11th, which would be my 20th barefoot climb. This meant he'd finish on climb #350! It created another exciting future prospect to look forward to, and it was just three weeks away.

November overtook February and May with the longest unbroken run of cable car rides back down – 12 had been moved up to 16 now. It was as if nature was giving my legs a pardon for time served, and it didn't go unnoticed.

My 78th climb back down was far better than expected! In fact, it was the second fastest time for the year. I really loved the down climbs, and because of my training, I came into the year with zero apprehensions. The beauty of late afternoon climbs, besides 80% of them being in the shade, was that Table Mountain's shadow was cast over Devil's Peak in front of you. The outline of the cable station on the shadow was clear, and thanks to Platteklip, the flat top was broken by the gap.

What was more surprising than such a long unbroken run in November, was the fact that my 36th wet climb took place in week 47?! I honestly thought the last time I'd put the cover over my bag and wear my jacket would be in October. Stupidly, because of YR and believing it to be infallible, I left my pants at home. They got the morning rain spot on, but the afternoon was dead wrong. It caught me, and a host of tourists completely off guard too. Thankfully it wasn't the same freezing air we experienced up until September, but seeing them drenched in shorts and t-shirts made me more grateful to have had my K-way jacket to keep me dry.

Now, on a completely unrelated note, I have to share this... Once on my own, on a warmer day, I took a breather in the shade of a small cave. If anything it was just a mildly concave wall offering protection. While sipping water in the humid conditions, I heard a snake hiss. I moved faster than Usain Bolt out the blocks and launched out of the cave like a long jumper. I SHAT myself and scanned the shadows expecting to see a tongue flickering at me, but I saw nothing. Whew...I stood rooted to the spot even though I didn't hear that sound again. I grabbed my bag which was still 'inside' on a ledge and dashed back out.

Is there such a thing as too much time in nature? Maybe it was just the sun and the heat messing with my mind.

DT laughed at my self-assessment and replied flatly... *'What makes you think it was really there to begin with?'*

Fair point DT!

We've enjoyed some great catch-ups throughout the year, usually over our shared love of curated burgers. Tonight though, I was cooking for him. The memory of him sending me off on Day 1 as fresh as if it happened that morning. Our catch-up was also an opportunity to hear how his back was doing. It had acted up throughout the year and punctuated just how fortunate I was to have a healthy body.

It was another timely reminder to stay focused as the end of the year loomed like final exams. I must admit, I felt like I'd already written them.

November was packed with birthdays. In three days, I'd have Dave's on the 21st, Aunty San's on the 22nd, and Lisa on the 23rd – all three great cheerleaders and supporters. I also got a present on Sans' birthday. Rondebosch Boys' Annual Grade 9 'rite of passage' send-off had some unforeseen circumstances, the speaker due to address them cancelled at the last minute, which left Rondebosch without a speaker.

I met Tracy, the organiser, on Platteklip. The purpose of the talk was to help these youngsters get the most out of their 10 days in nature while away from their moms and beds. Having been at an all-boy school myself, I felt honoured and saw it as an opportunity to plant some more seeds.

CHAPTER 15
NOVEMBER – THE PERFECT STORM

Unfortunately, I learned more about what I did wrong in this talk than anything else. Walking away, I felt like I'd done a terrible job. I realised this when some of the parents came and asked me questions I should have answered already... Like WHY I was climbing every day?!?! I know I had less than 12 hours to prepare but it was no excuse. It was a painful but valuable lesson in being prepared.

I was asked back in January 2019, so I had a chance to redeem myself. I'd be addressing the seniors as they started their final year of school – inviting them to collectively choose what they'd like their legacy to be and to become intentional about making it a reality.

There was another 'flop' on Lisa's birthday. Dani and Lisa are dear friends and go way back. Lisa introduced Dani to Harry (Dani and Harry are now married). Since Lisa's birthday fell on a Friday, Dani wanted to join and had invited 150 of her students from SAE - a creative institute offering bachelor degrees across audio, animation, and film. Dani ended up being called into a 9:30 budget meeting, so she couldn't make the birthday climb. She was gutted to miss it but proclaimed that some of her students were still keen. Only one turned up!

Back on the mountain, and it was another scorcher. Christian, the one student to arrive, was starting to take serious strain. Partly because he was carrying the dead weight of his media gear, which was useless because he'd forgotten his memory card in the morning rush. The perspiration was dripping from his forehead, and when we got to Ascension Corner, he let out a huge sigh.

'I'm not going to make it. I think I need to turn around.' he said.

He shrugged off my invitation to head back down with him, and left me alone to catch up with Lisa and Allan. It was a gorgeous day, so we took some time to enjoy summit #327, which was Lisa's 36th and Allan's 8th. Next, we headed down to Camps Bay for lunch and an ocean view. I loved the scooter and the ease with which I found parking.

Oddly, I was about to experience my first fully solo weekend since September 22nd, already 63 climbs ago. Made more surprising after the manic start to November where I only had four days alone out of 17. The drastic return of winter weather evened the month out a bit. Even as I celebrated the end of week 47, it felt like the calm before the storm.

Over the weekend I had a wobble and began to question whether I'd complete the challenge. It could've been the fatigue playing tricks with my mind or the unresolved feelings of inadequacy; either way, it wasn't fun. It was going to take everything to prevent my old mindset from derailing me. The little hiccup created a moment of clarity and put some things into perspective. Originally, my plan was to finish the challenge with a solo climb, just as I had my 1st and the halfway climbs. This was of course until David, who had joined on climb #233, proposed another idea....

'I think you should let the people that have supported you, join your final climb, and then you do your final solo climb on January 1st 2019.'

He was right, it did seem a bit crazy to punish people like Jessie and Lisa who'd championed the cause, and then deny them the opportunity to participate.

That night, Astrid invited me back to the Women's Property Network with the hopes of getting some more donations, so why wouldn't I return the favour? Not that I needed any more convincing, but this definitely sold it to me.

'As you close the chapter on a remarkable year, it will give you an opportunity to reflect on what you've achieved and carry that energy into the new year. What's one extra climb anyway?'

David was right. The more I thought about it the more I loved it. That would make it 366 climbs and would cover a leap year. I decided that even if the cable car was working, I'd start week 48 with a down climb. My gut told me that I needed the extra time to centre myself. Then I saw Achmat on his way down Ascension Corner, what a treat bumping into him! Incredibly, he was

CHAPTER 15
NOVEMBER - THE PERFECT STORM

on climb #117 for the year! It was a quiet climb which I loved. And for the first time I chose a rock from Stairway to Heaven. It blew my mind that I could still find new places! While walking along the front face of the mountain to get my top photo, a mongoose scurried across me. I'd never seen one at the top, only down on the road! This reminded me of what the mongoose represented, and what it meant to my journey.

'The mongoose is a sign of courage. It's a reminder that we should pursue our goals and passions.'

His presence brought my focus to how far I'd come since first seeing him, and made me reflect on the past 330 climbs as well as their purpose. He reminded me why the next 35 days were as important as those that led up to this point.

My intuition must've been in top form because the cable car had closed! The universe must have known I needed the extra time on the mountain. Just before I reached the junction at the top, the cloud that had enveloped me disappeared, and I was greeted by the most exquisite clear blue sky. But behind me, was a tidal wave of clouds, and the further away I walked, the more dramatic it became. It seemed to flow down into Platteklip and disappear below the summit. A gigantic flowing tidal wave of clouds hurtled down the Twelve Apostles towards Camps Bay. I felt a different kind of bliss. It was exquisite. I felt like bursting into tears. It was as if my eyes had never seen something so beautiful. It left me feeling satisfied, content, and happy as I descended back to earth.

The following day was a complete contrast. I arrived at a feisty mountain shrouded in dark clouds. I parked under the tree next to the reservoir at the start of Platteklip and it started drizzling. This left me no choice but to cover my bag and put my rain jacket on. It wouldn't stop! It was the 27th of November and just three days away from December, and I was being rained on again?? I passed about eight unprepared climbers, who must have had a change of heart or come to their senses, because I didn't see them again, on top, or on my way down.

Seriously though, it was one of the coldest and wettest days combined, which eclipsed the climb Ally had organised back on the 27th of September. Realising the synchronicity of these two days, I went back to check all the others - the 27th hadn't been a kind date to me!

The 27th of January was the second windiest day of the year.

On the 27th of July the cable car was shut down.

The 27th of August and April were wet.

The 27th of October was the hottest day of the year.

The 27th of November and September were cold and wet.

Maybe December would give me something else to add to the list? Mmmm we'll see.

There was zero visibility, and I was alone at the top. The freezing air, a moist phone screen, and ice-cold fingers made it almost impossible to take my picture, but finally, I managed to swipe the camera on.

I was 330 days in with 80 "down climbs" under my belt, and my legs screamed in displeasure. I hadn't felt like this after 16 consecutive days of shutdown-induced "down climbs" in July. The fatigue caused me to slip quite a few times but, thankfully, caused nothing more than heart flutters. I was reminded how quickly it could happen and became eternally grateful that I'd remained injury-free. The incessant rain had also drenched my shoes to such a degree that I was sloshing in my socks. That second pair would come in handy.

Urgh, I really needed to be more mindful... It was my 5th trio of downclimbs for the year. November joined September, August, July, and January with its challenges all occurring around the 27th...(except for July) that pesky date! I had to laugh, I'd been completely out of sync with the cable car and could have avoided this if I'd chosen to do a combination of morning, afternoon, and morning climbs instead. I guess you win some, you lose some.

CHAPTER 15
NOVEMBER - THE PERFECT STORM

Although dry, it was a bitterly cold afternoon and caused my eyes to tear. I couldn't help but marvel at nature. The winds had been exactly the same over the past two days but produced completely different experiences. It was a lesson to acknowledge your own experience and not take someone else's as gospel.

Learn to ask better questions, Andrew.

I was the last person climbing down and enjoyed the dry rocks. I did, however, fall over.... at the EXACT SAME place I did the previous Sunday???!! Just three minutes away from reaching the road, I began to think about how sore my feet were.

I got soaked the previous day and it dramatically softened my skin. I left my wet shoes and socks on long after I finished, and it didn't do me any favours either. When I got back down the scooter had been blown over and the side mirror had broken off... eish...

It was great leaving after 17:00 and still having 10 minutes to spare to enjoy the sunset. With my eyes still watering, I reflected on my chat with Achmat at the start. The scale at which three consecutive climbs back down had impacted me compared to 16 consecutive days in July show how a lack of rest can catch up to us. It's crazy to think that was already 115 days ago.

My ankle was okay, tender and tight yes, but not immobile. I tested it by walking up my eight flights of stairs at home.

Just 33 more climbs Andrew.

Avril wanted to join me on climb #222, but had been away on a spectacular trip to Egypt and Jerusalem. The number 222 has a special meaning for her, so after missing it, she asked me to remind her when climb 333 was near. Fittingly, our birthdays were just four days apart.

She had arrived, ready for her climb. Besides her massive smile, she was holding a R333 donation neatly broken up into 3 groups of R111. I loved the intentionality.

What a magical start! I'd been unable to travel all year, but my gift was being able to listen to people like her share their stories. What a trip she had too! 111 kept popping up which was why she was drawn to join climb #222 while she was overseas. Now she had made it to climb #333.

Along the way, I got to see Don with his pooch and two other friends – they were some of my favourite locals. After asking how I was doing, they reckoned I didn't look like I was taking strain. I also met Susanne, who curiously asked more about what I was doing and then echoed Don's sentiments. I'm glad my outsides weren't reflecting my insides – otherwise I'd probably have looked like Gollum!

Avril had been on a year of spiritual growth and her insights were beautiful to listen to. She helped distract me from what I was going through. She was patient with me as I took more breaks and slowed the pace. She had the honour of choosing the day's stone and asked to place it with its brothers and sisters, while also taking a moment of silence.

It was a magnificent cloudless day with showers of sunshine beaming down on us. We had some time to spare after our climb and enjoyed a coffee as I delighted her with some interesting numbers. Not only was this climb #333, I told her, but the date, the 29th of November 2018, had three 11s in it. It was also her third climb with me.

Most people were just starting to catch the cable cars up, while we enjoyed a quiet ride down with Abdulladein. He was all smiles and made me laugh by calling me 'Mr Andrew.' All the staff were more excited about the final climb than I was! The conversation was impossible to avoid, especially as the numbers around my neck kept getting ticked off.

'I'm putting in a request to work on the 31st! I have to be here for the end.' said Abdulladein.

I shook my head. Usually on New Year's Eve, people wanted nothing to do with work. This was quite a different year, though, and by being there, he would

CHAPTER 15
NOVEMBER – THE PERFECT STORM

become part of history and could participate in the celebrations. Then again, Mother Nature would determine this, and we'd only know on the day, but I was hoping for clear weather so everyone could join and I'd have my perfect bookend sunset celebration at the top.

The last day of November. One more month (and one day!) till completion.

Virginia, in Florida, was one of the most vociferous long distance supporters I had. She introduced me to her friend Betsy who was in town for a few days. Today was the only day she could make it, but had sadly injured her ankle and was now on the fence. I knew I'd explained what the climb entailed and strongly advised her not to do something that would only make it worse. She was still interested in meeting though, perhaps before the climb.

In the end, we didn't connect which was a pity. The hour delay also added some extra heat to the climb. Honestly, I was battling to keep up with mother nature's crazy and extreme temperature fluctuations, which were so rapid they happened over days – not weeks. I knew being on the mountain every day heightened my awareness – but I still didn't recall the last four months of the year getting so crazy, so quickly!

I regularly saw Kathy guiding people up the mountain. Today was her second time. Her first was climb #167, and today was climb #334 – they were exactly 167 days apart! Talk about consistency. I wish I had known it at the time so I could have told her! Anyway, Kathy, when you read this I hope it puts a massive smile on your face.

Kathy has an adorable and energetic pooch called Pondo who enjoyed the Fynbos and made light work of the mountain. I'm pretty sure he could have pulled me up like a reindeer if I had joined us with a rope??! Today, though, even he seemed to struggle with the heat and sought shade as much as we did. The conditions inspired us to get to the summit as soon as possible. Today marked the end of 11 months.

It would be one hell of a finish, and there was a month jam-packed with exciting events ahead. It was finally time to start preparing for the day when I'd be able to get the luxury of some rest.

NOVEMBER STATS: 334 / 365

People Joined: 56 / 580

36 days 00 hours 28 minutes 34 seconds / 2 198,86km / 64,98 Everest summits / 171 solo climbs (51.6%) / 82 Up & Down (24.6%) TOTAL DONATIONS: R372 068.44

Connors: 'Can't think of a better way to help this great cause than by donating on this amazing individual's birthday! Hope, trust and know you are going to have an epic one my friend!!'

Nynke & Sander: 'Without probably knowing it, we climbed up the mountain with you and heard about your amazing challenge! All the best for the last climbs to come!'

Helenski: 'I'm in awe of the physical demands you have placed on yourself to raise the funds needed for such amazing recipients. Keep strong. Keep climbing. :-)'

Clouds come floating into my life, no longer to carry rain or usher storms, but to add colour to my sunset sky.
~~ Rabindranath Tagore

CHAPTER 16

DECEMBER - 31 DAYS TO EMBED THE LESSONS

My last climb on the 1st day of the month started off perfectly. The UTCT (Ultra Trail Cape Town) race was in progress, with four routes to choose from: 21km, 35km, 65km, and the insane one... the 100km! The three longest races all included Platteklip in their gruelling route.

I now understood why all the markers were placed on Thursday. There was a constant stream of people because each race started at a different time. This was to prevent a bottleneck up the narrow path. The entire section was made visible by a line of bright coloured shirts snaking all the way up.

My experience of UTCT was far different from last year. I had just come back from the States, and I was battling to sleep. Wide awake at 03:00, I made my way to the lounge to watch a movie. At around 04:30, I started seeing a crazy number of lights dotting the Lions Head slopes. It was the 100km athletes already 6km into their race, all dashing to beat the 17-hour cut-off time. That was during my final month of my training. I'd completed two climbs back-to-back up Table Mountain and planned on resting for the weekend.

This time, I was surrounded by athletes as I kicked off climb #335. Lisa, Heide and her friend Raymond had also joined. We were all surprised when the sound of bagpipes echoed through the gorge. At first it didn't seem possible but the cheers and energy flowing down with the hauntingly beautiful music provided a dramatic soundtrack to the grey overcast conditions and inspired all the weary legs to push ahead. The previous day had been a scorcher so the athletes must have loved the cooler conditions.

Bagpipes are not exactly the world's most beloved instrument, so the man playing them certainly came with some bravery. But, to his credit, his audience was charmed by the tunes and high-fived him every time he took a breather, or to sip some water. He was stationed at Rockfall Corner, perfectly nestled in the cliffs which created a powerful ambiance and stirred the quarter Scottish blood that ran through my veins.

His effort to climb up the mountain with bagpipes before the first athletes passed him was rewarded as the crowds shared their appreciation. As soon as he stopped, the gorge erupted with cheers, hollers, and grateful rounds of applause. There was a total field size of 1,750 athletes across the four routes, so I'd say at least 1,000 of us were inspired. What a way to kickstart the final month!

Stefan and Ally added to the celebratory start of the month with a housewarming party in Noordhoek. I knew I'd need a late afternoon climb after the party. For Sunday lunch Richard, Conrad, and I made a phenomenal choice and got a roast from the Vredehoek Spar. I felt the urge to stay as they settled into a chilled afternoon with flowing vino, it was incredibly hard to leave them. But Sarah, Warren, and Marie-Lou were joining my climb, and obviously, I couldn't miss a day.

CHAPTER 16
DECEMBER - 31 DAYS TO EMBED THE LESSONS

Even though the cable car's siren went off as we started up Platteklip, it ended up being a phenomenal climb. They all had an option to not climb if they wanted, but all of them chose to stick with it. Sarah was in South Africa on business from the US, and it was great to be able to thank her in person for the epic hand-crafted goodie bag that she and her husband put together for me. Matt was horrified when, in South Africa, he heard I'd never tasted maple syrup before. He declared he'd send a care package to rectify that "problem," which would also include some creative artwork of me climbing the mountain. It's crazy to think it was delayed at customs because of the honey and not the maple syrup, but I'd already waited 39 years. What's another few weeks? I eventually got to have my first maple syrup experience–and I loved it!

I'd last seen Warren in June when he invited me back to update his network on my progress. They both shared their insights on watching my journey unfold. Marie-Lou, an English expat, is connected to me via Donna, who was part of climb #300. It was great seeing new networks of friends develop. I was fascinated by the stories Marie-Lou told as she shared her adventures of becoming a mountain guide in Brazil.

We saw Tahrs at the bottom, which was a well-deserved reward for not bailing on the climb. It was just the eighth time this year, and reminded me I'd last seen them 33 days ago, high up on the path around Rockfall Corner. Watching them skillfully navigate the cliffs was a treat.

While collecting more trash at Waterfall Corner, we came across a woman who was resting. She asked if I always picked up trash and how often I climbed. One of the benefits of doing this all year was how easily I could share the 365 Ubuntu Climb's story. She donated R100 on the spot and her friend grabbed the online payment details. And this was all from seeing me pick up trash.

Sarah gave me some great feedback on how I present and talk about the project... She said the message had become more refined and eloquently expressed compared to the beginning of the year. I appreciated her observation.

It was a 4-hour climb so we descended in the fading light and finally walked back to our cars and scooter in the dark. This group has definitely been one of my favourites. Sarah and I headed to Beluga, where she spoiled me with a delicious sushi dinner.

She and Matt introduced me to Jeremey Jensen, the creator of 'The Adventurepreneur Podcast' based in the States. We'd conducted an interview back in March, and they'd been pushing him to find out what the next step was because he'd delayed the upload of the interview but it worked out for the best. I felt it was the best interview of the year. I was grateful to Sarah, and glad that I was able to thank her in person for setting me up to be interviewed on an international podcast that's hosted legends like Alex Honnold.

I was down to just four weeks.

It was wonderful getting Jeremy's feedback about the project and my progress. He's a fantastic interviewer and asked some deep questions about Apartheid and how it shaped me. His podcast is available on iTunes and on his website. His theme is all about sharing the stories of unconventional problem solvers, change makers, and entrepreneurs. It really digs into building businesses, projects, lifestyles, and adventure-centric brands outside.

He breaks it down like this...

'Adventurepreneurs are thrill seekers, explorers, fun hogs, thought leaders, influencers, and lifestyle designers. They are the people brave enough to rise above the traditional definitions of success. They are often misfits and risk takers, living life on their own terms.

The show was created for the adventure community and those looking to live a fulfilling adventure lifestyle. Whether you want to learn the tricks of the trade, be inspired, have a good laugh, be more productive, or start living the life you've always wanted, The Adventurepreneur Playbook can and will help you kick ass along the way.'

CHAPTER 16
DECEMBER – 31 DAYS TO EMBED THE LESSONS

What a privilege to be his 21st guest and complete the first podcast with two different perspectives on the same challenge. The 13th of March and climb #72 felt so far away, having just completed December 2nd and climb #336.

My biggest laugh of the year, though, happened after dinner with Sarah and when a literal sign showed the universe's sense of humour. 'Out of Order' in front of the lift.

'Really? You decide to do this in December?' I said out loud as though someone had just hung the sign to mess with me.

All I could do was laugh. At least it only took 1 minute and 36 seconds to get up. Although now it would probably take me twice as long. I felt like I was transported back a year to where I was climbing the stairs and 'pretending' like it was climb #336. Mercifully, it only took a couple of days to repair.

I'd already visualised the tears and emotions I'd experience when conquering my final summit. I imagined walking along the top towards the cable station one last time as an exquisite sunset dressed the sky. My family, Jessie, and friends were all around me. Visualising it with such intensity inspired two important things: it motivated me to stay healthy and uninjured for the next 29 climbs, and I immersed myself in that emotion on each remaining climb. There was no way I'd let a single minute go to waste on the mountain. I used every moment to embrace what had become my spiritual home and expand my gratitude.

On Wednesday Fred joined me again. It was crazy to think that his last climb was already four weeks ago! It was a subtle reminder of how quickly things were moving toward the end – whether I wanted it to or not. Starting week 49 was a scary prospect, not because of what was left – but because of what had already been done. Massimo was due to join for his week-long challenge, but with two days of rain forecast and him already feeling under the weather, he decided to postpone it until the 11th of December. His decision gave me two days to create my 172nd and 173rd solo climbs, and unbeknownst to me, my fourth and third last climbs alone.

There were two days of rain that drenched me on the scooter even before I made it to the mountain. Sarah decided to join me one last time before heading back to the USA, and I got to reward her with a trip to Silverstream, which produced a thunderous roar through the mist from all the rain that had fallen. I never thought I'd see it like that again. Not in summer! I picked climb #341's rock from the stream realising I'd missed all previous opportunities to do so. It was a fitting way to help me 'complete the set.'

It's amazing how doing things you really don't feel like doing often brings the greatest experiences. The truth is, that morning, I woke up to a cancellation and hoped Sarah would too, so I could roll over and go back to sleep and do an afternoon climb. Seeing Silverstream in full flow one last time made it all the more worthwhile.

My uncle Mark from Durban is a pilot for SAA and came down for the 7s rugby tournament and also got the opportunity to climb. Miraculously he picked the one dry day that was sandwiched in between two rainy days. Nobody else joined us so we had some quality time to catch up. It reminded me of the chats we had when his international flights brought him to London while I was living there. He became my "mule," bringing me things like South African sweets I missed from back home, doing the exchange as we enjoyed curry and pints. Besides my grandparents' rocks which were going to be placed on their birthdays later in the month, Mark was the final family member to physically add his stone to the pile.

I wasn't sure what was going on with my brain but I'd left the keys in the ignition of the scooter three times the past week. The first time, I felt my empty pocket and ran back in a panic, the second time, I was incredibly lucky because someone handed the keys to security, and the third time, I was fortunate they were still there when I returned! There was a feeling of panic and terror at the top of the mountain when I reached into my bag to grab the keys and they weren't there. It's the kind of self-inflicted torture I can do without. I think the mental toll was playing its part, I had to become even more vigilant on the mountain to avoid injury.

CHAPTER 16
DECEMBER - 31 DAYS TO EMBED THE LESSONS

At least my key episode gave Lisa and Karel a laugh during our Sunday climb. The wind was pumping and forced Adele to pull out before one step was taken. The windy conditions, a bad knee, and a downclimb were a recipe for a disaster. She'd flown down from Johannesburg especially for this climb, so I made an exception and opened up Monday's solo slot for her to enjoy the experience and claim her number. It was the least I could do for all her support, which included printing the pictures for the Kingsmead Fundraiser, buying a shirt, and donating multiple times. Her contribution was immense.

Along the way, we came across a group of extremely nervous climbers making their way back down. They hadn't prepared for the cable car to close, but Karel was an absolute champ and helped them down safely. It was about a third of the way down when I made the decision to eject myself from the situation. Not only did I have plans to celebrate Stan and Tamzyn's wedding, but the pace was dangerously slow, especially for a descent. Karel waved us off and said he'd happily stick with the lady.

Lisa and I continued. It was my 84th trip down, and I was feeling it. Meeting Lisa in 2010 had been a revelation, not just because of the lengths she'd gone to in supporting me, but of how she stepped out of her comfort zone and pursued growth. It had been a privilege to watch her push herself and explore her capabilities so intensely. Just one year into her money coaching, I was blown away by her ability to hold space for others in a way that inspired them to step up and succeed.

It taught me to help people recognise their overwhelming fears. It also empowered me to support and help them navigate this complex journey while feeling understood, accepted, and without judgement. It was a lesson in attunement.

It was the perfect mindset to enter the wedding with. Steef picked me up, and together we headed to a magnificent setting out in the farmlands north of the city. The location provided one of the most iconic views in the world. Table Mountain, Devil's Peak, and Lions Head rise above the brown dusty land and act as a conduit to the African sky. It was the perfect way to celebrate the end of weeks ending 'forty-something' and enter the '50s. There certainly wasn't much dancing from my side, but it was a great evening that gave both Kathy and me an opportunity to meet in something other than our mountain gear.

Massimo's Week

Things always work out for the best. Because of yesterday's wind, Adele and I would be climbing alone today. She'd experienced some tough months, and being alone on a mountain had a cathartic, cleansing effect that allowed her to release some pent-up emotion. She had been staying with family, and they all caught the cable car up with her husband Clive. He had a difficult year and spent a week in the ICU. It was a massive scare for them that I could never comprehend.

At the summit, everyone was rewarded with a majestic sunset, capped off with a thin sliver of the waxing moon, which hung like a balloon in the sky. Adele earned her beer and became the 604th climber on my 344th consecutive day. It was another memorable start to the week. It certainly set the tone for what was to come.

Massimo's week was a mixture of early and late starts, hot climbs, and wintery weather. We kicked it off with my 20th barefoot climb and Kathy's first after she finally broke through the preconceptions she'd held about not being able to complete the route barefoot. Massimo brought 'Socks,' his energetic sheepdog. It highlighted a thought at the beginning of the year: *If I had a dog, would they have been able to join me every day?*

Milli, a lovely woman from New York, joined me while her husband waited patiently back at the hotel. It was such a shame that he suffered from vertigo, a family trait that seemed to be getting worse with age. Meeting Milli was another great introduction, thanks to Richard. Besides the great company, I was left with more smiling Mandela's at the end of the climb. Massimo was ecstatic to have had the first one of the week under his belt. It was exciting to

CHAPTER 16
DECEMBER – 31 DAYS TO EMBED THE LESSONS

hear how he'd placed table talkers on each table to invite his restaurant patrons to contribute in some way. If all went well, Massimo's week of participation would culminate on climb #350. I decided to host a dinner at his restaurant as a token of my appreciation.

My favourite moment with him was on Wednesday when we started late in the afternoon to give my friend Rose an opportunity to join us after work. The cableway closed at 20:30, so a 17:30 start was more than enough time for all of us. Sue, one of the Heritage Day participants, joined us again and brought her son Matthew for a wonderful, cool climb. Matthew, who was still in school, was already a talented photographer and filmmaker. Now that he was on holiday, he could focus on his passion. He asked for permission to film the route and interview me at the end. He then created a wonderful promo video as part of his donation to the project. It was inspiring to see someone exude so much passion at a young age and create videos of such high quality. His journey will definitely be one to follow.

This, however, was not why it was my most memorable day with Massimo and Rose. Table Mountain was showing off tonight, and the five floodlights that illuminate the city's protector were on. It's an awe-inspiring sight, which I hope everyone gets to see sometime. I appreciated the thought that the city council put into the impact that the lights had on the natural rhythms of the plants and animals in the area, which is why they put them on sparingly. I waited for 346 climbs to see this splendour from up close, and that made it so much more special.

With just 19 climbs left, these things were a wonderful distraction, but the major question on everyone's mind was still... 'What next??' I was certainly getting close enough to think about it and doing everything I could to keep myself grounded in the present moment. I was just as focused on the 12th of December as I was on the 1st of January. Falling short wouldn't be wasted at all, but the job wasn't done until the final steps were taken at the top on December 31st. 970,900 steps would be climbed to get there.

I'd been engrossed in a book called *Destiny versus Free Will*. It shares how gratitude builds both the immune system and the nervous system. It was my first year of intentionally practising gratitude, and I directed it toward my body's amazing handling of such an extreme challenge. It proved to me how powerful the practice really is. It's a fact I've learned through experience.

The lesson was reinforced beautifully when Lisa brought Nershen along with Massimo and me for Thursday's climb #347. He'd studied what I'd just learned and gave me a deeper explanation about it. The synchronicity was incredible. I no longer questioned these events, I simply thanked the universe for bringing these experiences in such perfect order and embedded them in my psyche. Happily, I had no appointments after this climb, and while Massimo was headed back down to the restaurant, the three of us sat up top, discussing life and gratitude in more detail. Our continued discussion gave him the idea to host a workshop where all proceeds from ticket sales at R365 a piece would go to 365 Ubuntu Climbs.

The workshop would be about creating a balanced mindset to support wealth creation – something 99.9% of us want! He was inspired by what I'd been doing and created his own act of service. Thanks to Astrid, we secured a venue free of charge for December 29th, which would help us raise a further R6,000!! Not only that but the participants would be educated on dealing with trauma and would get an opportunity to invest in our country's future.

Friday's climb brought with it one of the friendliest smiles I'd seen all year. Lindisa worked in the café at the top of the mountain and always checked in on my progress and how I was feeling. One day, she casually said that she'd never climbed the mountain, so naturally I invited her to join. As per usual, all I could do was extend the invitation and it was up to the individual to make their own decision. Lindisa was one of the few who kept her word and showed up. She shared a great insight at the top and said that without us pushing her, she would've stopped more often and climbed far slower. Massimo brought both his dogs while Kathy had Pondo again. I was starting to look at the pets as my reindeer, and dreamed of attaching leads to my waist for them to pull me up the mountain!

We celebrated up top and Lindisa became the fourth successful staff member to join. It was only fitting that she crossed off a climb to reveal only 17 climbs remained. Lindisa's beaming smile while crossing the climb off just perfected the top photo. Looking at it, I'm flooded with gratitude, ecstasy, love, pride.

Massimo is a fascinating man. An Italian who lived the corporate life in London and also met his wife there. He'd since built a life of memories in three countries. They first tried their hand in the hospitality industry in France, but after a holiday to Cape Town, felt inspired to make it home. I always loved hearing stories of foreigners moving to South Africa, especially when they showed a greater appreciation for what we have than most locals. Still today, you wouldn't be able to pay Massimo to leave Cape Town.

Massimo started a restaurant in Hout Bay, and 10 years later, it's still thriving. In a city where restaurants open and close faster than the weather changes, it's a remarkable feat, made even more so that it's not even in the busiest part of the city. They're a benchmark of what's possible when a business owner embraces purpose, quality service, and employee care above the bottom line. He's created a family environment in his restaurant where staff often sing and smiles greet you in every corner. The food? Man, my mouth is watering as I type this... It's exceptional! I believe they're a living example of the concept, 'The more you give, the more you get.'

While other restaurants try gimmicky promotions that offer Instagram 'influencers' free meals, he creates local polls that highlight the positive contributors in the community and gets people to vote on which of them should eat for free.

Having him join for six days straight gave me a bit of anxiety, but luckily, Socks and Lola's energy rubbed off on me. Massimo's a truly inspirational man, and his contribution to the world is immense, that's why it blows my mind he was able to find the time to participate and help us raise even more money.

Massimo's 5th climb was an important one. Thanks to DKMS Africa, I'd been introduced to The Western Cape Transplant Society. It worked out perfectly that their climb tied into Massimo's week. They brought 10 people along, some with kidney transplants while others were Leukaemia survivors. Virginia, an employee at DKMS Africa, brought her son and his friend. Lisa, Nicole from Climb #300, and Craig (the birthday party donation champ) all joined, too. It was a day brimming with inspiring stories of cheating death. Purpose and intent guided us up for the 349th time.

It all started at the bottom after the society grabbed a picture of the four athletes and I. Massimo shared this powerful insight.... 'How many people do you see? I count 9 – Andrew, 4 transplantees, plus 4 donors. Without them, we wouldn't be here.' Climbing with the people we aimed to empower was important for creating the impetus to push through the gruelling two weeks ahead. Pain is temporary, empowering another life is generational.

Craig shared how my year of climbing had inspired him to live with more gratitude, mindfulness, and humility. It was his final opportunity to climb before heading to Dubai for a well-deserved vacation with his family. It wasn't just about the money raised and the beneficiaries, it was also about the interactions, the lessons we were all learning, and how they were being incorporated into their daily lives. This year has been a phenomenal gift with powerful experiences of giving and receiving. Craigs donations, checking up on the tougher days, and participation, had been an amazing pillar of support.

We took quite a long time to get to the top and enjoyed a celebratory drink together. Lisa and Nicole drove me to the airport for the special arrival of Jessie. It was incredible to think there'd be no more climbs without her. She was here! What a first New Year to spend together! I was so excited for her to meet Caroline, her family, and spend more time with the parents.

CHAPTER 16
DECEMBER - 31 DAYS TO EMBED THE LESSONS

Sunday's climb up Ledges with the Mountain Slayers was a tough one. Massimo politely declined, so we were unable to celebrate his successful week. We did, however still have climb #350's dinner celebrations at his restaurant, and with Jessie here, it was the perfect opportunity for two amazing souls to meet.

Climb #350 was the final milestone on an unexplored route called Ledges. It was my last chance to enjoy a different perspective of the mountain during my challenge. The route had the potential to stoke Jessie's mild fear of heights, so it meant that just like back in July, she'd get her first Sunday 'off.' She'd never done the route and chose to stay home. It was a justified call.

My brain was beginning to lose it a bit, though, not only had I left the scooter keys in the ignition three times, but I also hadn't processed Miriam's breakdown of the climb via text message. It was as if my eyes had blacked out the parts where she detailed the length of the climb. I wasn't sure how I even accepted her message:

'Ledges on its own, isn't much of a hike so we're first going to do Knife's Edge up Devil's Peak.'

Yup. Devils Peak is the other 1,000m high Peak that flanks Table Mountain, so I was expecting a 5-6 hour climb on Devils Peak, Ledges, Maclears Beacon, and then a walk across the top to the upper cable station? I clearly wasn't thinking very well... I wasn't even close!

It turned into a mammoth 13km route and an almost ten-hour day in searing 34-degree heat with little to no wind. My sense of humour failed as the climb kept going and going, and by the time we made it to Devil's Peak, I realised I'd created the longest possible route up Table Mountain. Maybe back in April, this would've been okay.

Knife's Edge is a beautiful experience, and it's been on my 'to do list' for ages, but my timing was horrendous. My first mistake was listening to 'Ledges is not enough of a hike' from someone nowhere near as bushed as I was. I should've asked more questions to save myself an agonising day. My second mistake was that it was Jessie's first day in the city. That coupled with an idealistic view of how long I thought the climb would take, and you've got Jessie alone in Cape Town all day. I had no idea when we'd be finished either because I'd never done the route. To top it off, my battery died midway through the afternoon. She was understandably not amused by this. In hindsight, I should've just said I'd be gone all day. This wasn't exactly the great start I was hoping for to express my gratitude for flying out for the third time in a year.

The climb was brutal. We hacked through overgrown sections and steep climbs along the spine of Devil's Peak and still had to climb down to the Saddle and then up a tricky section on Table Mountain's east cliffs above Newlands. It took every ounce of my remaining leg strength to climb two mountains in the blazing heat.

We'd already been on the mountain for five hours and not even half way up Table Mountain when I had another brain meltdown like I did on climb #312. This was worse though, because it was self-inflicted. The route was tricky, with many steep cliffs dropping away below us. The views were exquisite and one of the only rays of light helping me through. Most of the climbing and scrambling was manageable until we made it to the reason it's called 'Ledges.'

Everyone removed their backpacks while one person climbed up the 30-foot face of exposed rock with a rope. One by one, we attached our bags so he could haul them up the cliff face. Because I'd never done the climb, my hand kept reaching out, looking for holds, I may as well have been in the dark. My other three limbs clutched tiny ridges on the rock face. I imagine rock climbers who'd scale it with ease, laughing uncontrollably at the descriptions I'm using. That feeling of falling, though... my stomach seemed to squeeze the life out of the surrounding organs.

I was hot, tired, and my mind kept asking, 'how much longer?' All I could think about was Jessie being alone. Then I got myself into one of those tricky positions where I felt like I wasn't secure enough to let go with one hand to reach higher. It was a small moment of panic where I felt like I'd been hanging forever. I'd watched almost everyone else successfully navigate the section, but now my face was up against the wall and unable to see the holds I'd been suggesting from below. My hands are sweating just thinking about it again. I didn't have any other option, not this late in the afternoon. I had to retreat to find a more secure route for my attack. Just the smallest route change made all the difference, and I finally pulled myself up to the next ledge. My heart was racing as I swung my backpack on my shoulders.

It was the last nerve-wracking section to climb. Tiny gullies filled with water and what felt like the grass plains of the Okavango delta awaited us. It took us 4 hours and 45 minutes to get to the saddle between Table Mountain and Devil's Peak, and then 8 hours and 1 minute to reach Maclears Beacon.

Those three hours scratched my legs, cooked me alive, filled my stomach with butterflies, and made me chastise myself for leaving Jessie alone. And there was still another hour of walking left where I'd be able to contemplate it all. While putting one foot in front of the other, I tried to draw some positives from the situation. My time at Zebula helped me prepare mentally for this challenge, but this hike today... It was just as important and would help me close the year off with the right perspective. Now my mind and my body were both ready. Any concern I may have had about how I'd feel at the end had been nuked. I was finally ready for the year to be over.

Massimo completed his last climb alone with the dogs, barefoot, and managed a 1 hour and 5 minute summit! I'm so proud of him and grateful for his contribution. He's been a tremendous companion and injection of energy. I'm honoured to have him as part of the story. His fundraising efforts at the restaurant and the contributions of his patrons added another R7,200 to the mix!

This is what he shared:

Early in 2018 I read something in social media about this man who was going to climb our mountain every single day for a whole year. I didn't really think much of it, apart from looking at Platteklip Gorge and thinking that it was too hard. The cable car has always been my method of reaching the top.

Later in September I had just celebrated the 5th anniversary of my bone marrow transplant (by running for as long as I could on a treadmill in my restaurant, raising funds for DKMS Africa!) when I read about Andrew again, who was now on the 9th month of daily climbs. I noticed one of the 3 charities he was raising funds for was DKMS Africa. I contacted him on FB and decided to join him for one day.

What an experience it was. We met at 6.30 by the lower cable station along with 3 or 4 other 'strangers' who had also heard about Ubuntu 365. After a couple of km on the flat road we started the climb. Luna, my border collie was with us. Andrew was the perfect guide, and stopped for a chat every few minutes, or to tell us anecdotes from his last 10 months, and how on certain days he also had to hike back down because of the bad weather. But Andrew was also interested in each of our personal stories, and curious as to why we followed him.

Step by step the summit got closer, and the moment you reach the top you forget all the pain and just enjoy the view. You take in the feeling of having walked all the way up and soon start crossing paths with the 'normal' tourists who took the cable way up. Soon you can't help but feel just a bit cooler than them.

When I went home that night I started thinking about how I could use my connection to DKMS Africa to help Andrew, both financially and by spreading the word about his epic year, so I suggested that I join him for a whole week.

We planned it for the beginning of December but then I got a bad chest infection and had to move it to just before Christmas. The most amazing day was when 3 other 'transplantees' joined us (2 bone marrow and one kidney). It ended up being one of the best weeks of the year. Every day different people joined us, and Luna and Socks, my border collies came along too.

By then I fully understood why Andrew was doing it, and as crazy as it may seem to some, I can see how the commitment to do things like these can be used to

CHAPTER 16
DECEMBER - 31 DAYS TO EMBED THE LESSONS

inspire others. I am glad Andrew's work didn't finish after 365 climbs, this is just the beginning of what he can and will do.

I am very proud of my week of climbing and can only imagine how Andrew feels about his whole year.'

Dinner ended up with just Lisa, Jessie, and I as the others faded after an epic day on the mountain. I was grateful to Massimo and congratulated him on his fantastic achievement over the week. I also introduced him to Jessie. His food is always fantastic, but that night, it was extra delicious.

December felt like the equivalent of two months in one. It was as though I was adding a 13th month to match the number of full moons in the year. It was the only month that I surpassed the 90-hour mark, missing 100 by just 25 minutes.

After 12 consecutive days with people joining, I completed my second last solo climb and was grateful again for the sanctity of Platteklip. I was exhausted. The 350th climb drained the physical reserves. More people had joined in this month than the previous three combined, so my brain was just as knackered.

Jessie's arrival was perfectly timed again. My sister and her family arrived a week later, and my parents the following week. Their collective presence energised me enough to complete another day.

Jessie and Roy from Business Matters joined me on the last rainy day of the year and got to experience the mountain in a new way. Tourist season was in full swing and Jessie and I were using a rented car. This reminded me of how glorious Don's scooter had been the past few months.

With my 350th climb completed, I was mentally on the final stretch but still maintained my strategy of sucking the bone marrow out of each and every one of the remaining climbs. I'd always known the year would end at some point and had always been preparing by enjoying every day for what it had to offer. My gratitude had been steadfast, my legs unwavering, and my focus razor-sharp. The final countdown with just 12 days had begun...

Climb 353 – Wednesday, December 19th

We started at sunrise with Toren, Carmen, Roland and Jessie making up group 179. Toren's a deeply insightful man who I met through Summer Camp. Carmen was proudly sporting her Ubuntu shirt, and together we celebrated hitting R400k in donations!!! I loved how people had come out and pushed the limits of their own physical capabilities and collaborated with strangers to empower others. I'm so grateful for the support. I remember how I felt in January, I was apprehensive and uncertain as to whether this idea would gather support. I had high hopes of raising millions of Rands, but just as December had accumulated 10x the money invested compared to January, this year would be a first in a lifelong commitment to supporting these organisations.

Climb 354 – Thursday, December 20th

Our sunset climb brought me one of the greatest compliments all year. I was climbing with Nicole's new friend Natasha, when she paused on the last corner before Halfway Rock and said...

'You remind me of Nelson Mandela – not just in height (he was 1,85m), but because you also lead from behind.'

It was the greatest honour to have my name associated with Mandela in that way. I was doing what I'd done all year, and not that I ever needed justification to do it, but these conversations were always memorable and insightful. For example, I told her the story of my sore throat and she responded by expressing how important it was to hear as a reminder in her own life, as she reflected on how her own sore throats were linked to a lack of confidence in being vocal.

Our conversation reminded me of a lesson in diplomacy I encountered in February, and it highlighted the important relationship between teamwork and Ubuntu. Her words also tell us how vital it is to share our lessons with the world.

CHAPTER 16
DECEMBER - 31 DAYS TO EMBED THE LESSONS

Climb 355 – Friday, December 21st

The summer solstice arrived and brought the 13th full moon of the year along with it. I really wanted to give Jessie the experience of watching it rise, and with both evenings of the weekend busy, tonight was going to be the night.

Jessie, Lisa, and Nicole made the trek up with me. I also got to test my second 'Plattekliphenge' theory which believed the sun set between the cliffs. To find out, we did something I'd never done before and continued to the higher point directly behind the gorge exit. It was the perfect spot with 360 views of the gorge. A drone would've captured a stunning photo of the sunset with the cliffs on either side, just as I'd done for the shot in the middle of Winter.

On our way up, we passed a woman wearing a Habitat shirt from the States. This reminded me of how important it was to find my inner voice. This would empower me to help the thousands of people the project was aimed at, and would plant the seeds in new hearts for future daily acts of Ubuntu.

Climb 356 – Saturday, December 22nd

On my 21st barefoot climb, I finally met Jack, the man who introduced me to barefoot climbing. He was always in the zone, zooming up and down with classical, rock, or other music to motivate him. It was a treat to finally speak to him. I must've seen him at least 50 times throughout the year in his red shorts and with earphones in. He's such a champ and shared how he'd broken toes chasing guys up and down the mountain to keep up.

I'd decided to do the last climb of the year barefoot, too, bringing it to a total of 22 climbs without shoes.

Gerhard, a friend from high school, finally managed to join after fretting all year over whether his knee would cope. Chantelle also joined again. She contracted mumps after joining me 217 climbs ago! I managed to convince her to climb barefoot which provided the impetus for Tammy and Max to join. Eventually,

Jessie joined the party at Waterfall Corner and took her shoes off too. Lisa, as always, did it from the start.

Jack and I spoke about climbing barefoot, reminding me of lesson four – putting things into form with application and patience. The daily practice provided me with countless opportunities to learn and helped me move closer to mastery, which is, after all, why we continue to practise something even once we know it intimately.

Climb 357 – Sunday, December 23rd

It was great finally having Harry join. I was grateful that I spoke at the 8 o'clock club in October and met him there. The turnout was tremendously low (just ten people), but it was the first time every person in the audience asked me a question. Climbing with me definitely gave him a true sense of what I was doing and would help him when analysing the data. He's a fitness expert and was surprised that a guy my size could manage so well and complete this challenge injury-free.

Our pace was slower than expected, so Lisa's friend, Lizelle, left us behind to ensure she made her lunch appointment. Before she dashed off, she pulled me aside to tell me about her sister, who had committed suicide exactly two years prior. She was dedicating her climb to her. Unbelievably, this happened at Josh's Rock. You never know how your actions may impact someone else, but by acting with love, kindness, and compassion, you're sure to touch somebody going through a difficult time positively.

According to the data, climbing has positively impacted my health. It's the fittest I've ever been, with a resting heart rate as low as 40 beats per minute but averaging 46 in December. It reminded me of the importance of sticking to a plan, the simplicity of creating a vision, and how much 'easier' things become when we have a road map to follow. I also heard a magic quote from Marie Forleo that summed up my understanding. It read, *'To be responsible, keep your promises to others. To be successful, keep your promises to yourself.'*

Climb 358 – Monday, December 24th – Christmas Eve

Caroline was so upset that she couldn't climb again. Seeing someone who wanted to do something mentally but physically couldn't was hard for me. She was still eager to be part of it one more time, so we came up with a solution: She could catch the cable car up and walk down with Jessie, Krissy, and I. Terence and Katie climbed up with us and took the car down. I managed to get her straight to the front instead of waiting two hours in the queue.

Allan and Lisa joined again and in searing heat until halfway. Katie and Krissy gained a different experience now that they weren't waiting for Mom anymore. I was happy to climb down again for the 85th so they could see what it entailed. Incredibly, it would be the last up-and-down climb for the year! December may have had crazy weather, but the wind had stayed away and gave my legs an early Christmas present. I'm grateful that I spent my final descent with Jessie, Sis, and Krissy. Caroline did amazingly well but started shutting down again from the contour path. Her legs felt like jelly, but luckily, we made it back down just before dark.

We also gathered an unexpected bonus of collecting another person for the group at Waterfall Corner. JD was the first person I'd met from Alabama, and was working at the US embassy in Chad. He shared how expensive Chad is, explaining how the government officials send their kids to school in Europe while everyone else struggles back at home. It breaks my heart to keep hearing stories of governments keeping their own people in poverty.

JD was a great conversationalist. He listened intently and shared his thoughts about people from Alabama who never left their state. We gave him a lift back into town in the Brown's car, newly dubbed 'the party bus.' He was appreciative and happy, considering it was his first day in Cape Town, but also completely in awe of the mountain and the Ubuntu experience.

That evening, we enjoyed the most spectacular sunset. I'd completed 51 weeks; now, there was just one more to go.

Climb 359 – Tuesday, December 25th – Christmas

Eight of us arrived for a chilly 6 am start. Being in the festive spirit, Jessie and I wore Santa hats and brought Lindt balls to hand out to the staff. They showed their appreciation with the warmest smiles. After handing them out at the top, we arrived at the bottom with an entire unopened box and just knew that Christopher should be the one to enjoy it. As a security guard, he often works 12-hour shifts and always with a beaming smile.

It was unbelievable how the weather felt more like the coolness of August than the start of summer. We had a fabulous lunch planned out in Noordhoek with Donald and his sister.

Kathy, Toren, Blake, Roland, Carmen, Lisa, Jessie, and I enjoyed our climb and took some time to relax on top of the mountain and enjoy some Christmas treats. I'd gained some wisdom over the year by trusting my intuition and not trying to control milestones or landmark occasions. I allowed things to unfold naturally and in their own way, and that way I had the perfect collection of people with me to celebrate the Christmas Climb.

Blake was supposed to join the previous week but woke up with a back spasm. He apologised for ditching me last minute, but all it did was serve as another reminder of how even the fittest of us are susceptible to injury. It made me even more appreciative of my smooth run of injury-free days. It's also a grim reminder of what can still go wrong six summits before the end. Now, it felt like my gratitude ritual carried the power of each day completed with it.

It was one of the most unique Christmas experiences of my life, and wonderful to see how I could build an 'Ubuntu family' outside of the one I was born into.

Climb 360 – Wednesday, December 26th

We stayed in Noordhoek, which meant no alarm and more time with Don before returning to Cape Town. It was just perfect waking up to the soft sound of the rain which flirted all day. Jessie felt really nauseous, so we left around 13:00 to book into an Airbnb flat in Kloof Street. It was the first time I'd been alone since Monday the 17th. I was excited for what I knew would be my last solo climb before the end. It also ended Jessie's eight consecutive days of climbing and Lisa's six.

Lisa had planned to join today, but since Jessie and others pulled out, I asked her to let me make it a solo climb for a mental break. I'd been looking to immerse myself in silence a little more. I loved having others join and adding to the excitement of getting to the end, but today's quiet solo climb was exactly what I needed.

It was oddly warm but with some mist just past the halfway point. Thankfully, there was no rain. I shared another video on how grateful I was to be born in Africa and how it helped me understand and feel Ubuntu. The challenge I'd taken on had been a lot about feeling. Feeling the mountain... Feeling people's struggle... Feeling connected... Feeling grateful.

I saw Bulelani for the first time in ages. He'd been sick, and once again, he shared my message. A cute little Indian boy came up to me and asked some questions. He also got a picture with me in the cable car.

I timed my climb perfectly today and arrived home around 17:30. It was pouring rain on the mountain, and there was a greyness I'd become accustomed to. As I type this, I can actually feel being back in it: the patter on my rain jacket; the water dripping on the rocks around me; the cold air on my cheeks. Three hundred and sixty felt like I'd come full circle, yet I still had five more climbs.

Today's solo climb gave me the freedom to take it all in. I felt like the same person and yet wholly transformed. Like all the butterflies I saw on the mountain, I truly understood what it meant to 'cocoon' myself for a year. I took everything that I was, melted it down into a goop, and worked tirelessly each day to transform that goop into what would become a butterfly. I pushed to become a more enlightened individual with greater compassion, a desire to learn, and imbued with the spirit of Ubuntu. It's as though the caterpillar always knows how to fly, but has to choose to transform to fulfil that desire, knowing it will bring beauty to the world with its transformation. I, too, felt like I had all this knowledge before I started – but by taking this year to push the limits and test my beliefs, I'd built myself a platform to soar from and a place to return to when my wings got tired.

These thoughts reminded me of the lessons I'd learned about constructive power and its use in August. My perceived strengths over others were just an opportunity to ground myself in Ubuntu and do my best to give my brothers and sisters a helping hand.

Climb 361 – Thursday, December 27th

Ally was really being screwed, first by her clients in September and then by her health. She was still dealing with the after-effects of the flu and could not join me on a climb again. Darren and Rose came along, which was great. I was pleased to see that Darren's injury had healed. As a fellow sportsman, I know what it's like when injuries force you to remain indoors to heal - especially when it's as serious and requires months of rest.

Tamzin brought some of her Joburg friends. Jodene, who was one of them, was another great conversationalist. Tamzin suggested that once I finished my gratitude ritual, everyone should get to say what they're grateful for.

Today's climb took my mind back to September, a month teaching me about unconditional love, and reminded me that we must show unconditional love to others and ourselves. It was interesting watching the quality of my answers evolve. I learned to surrender and let go more freely. I know that to keep that momentum going, I'll need to work on my journey of life every day.

Climb 362 – Friday, December 28th

I had the most wonderful climb with Sharni, Lisa, Terence, Krissy, and Warren. Jessie didn't come because there was a chance we'd have to climb back down, and she wanted to keep her legs for Monday. Her legs still felt the eight consecutive days on the mountain and Monday's climb down. She couldn't fathom how I managed 16 days in a row.

Ironically, the wind wasn't too bad, and we caught the cable car, but my gut taught me that being safe rather than sorry is always best. Sharni was bedridden five months prior, but we still managed to climb up in under two hours. It was beautiful, and our group photo had us looking straight into the sun, making everyone laugh and squint. It still came out perfectly! I was happy to start a bit earlier in the afternoon so that most of the second half of the climb would be in the shade. I was feeling more and more blessed as the journey continued.

Today, Lisa's 50th climb reminded me of the incredible support I've received throughout the year. She's been one of the standout pillars of strength through wind, rain, heat, early starts, and massages. She definitely puts the 'U' in Ubuntu.

Climb 363 – Saturday, December 29th

Louise brought a large crew, including her bestie Sarah, whom Jessie called 'sandwiches' after hearing about her love of food. It was an impressive turnout, considering they were all British, on holiday, and had to start at 6 am. It was also my late gran's birthday, which meant placing the final family stone. It was hard to believe it was a year ago that I left Johannesburg and landed back in Cape Town, excited to finish my final preparations. Now, I was relieved to be finishing.

Sarah had never been up to the top, even after the three attempts when her boyfriend led her. She'd been apprehensive but determined to smash it this time around, and she did! I was also delighted to see Ally's smile. After all the support, encouragement, and missing an opportunity for a birthday climb - she finally made it! It was a satisfying feeling when people like her got their climb number. I also felt honoured to enjoy the experience with them. One of the more interesting aspects of this challenge was hearing all the different perspectives on the same thing.

Nershen's workshop was as amazing as I'd imagined it would be. My biggest breakthrough was learning that even the most heinous things have a positive side and that my mind finds positive things in negativity far easier than it does finding negativity in positive experiences.

Today had highlighted a massive shift for me - my focus had moved from a positive mindset - to a balanced mindset.

Climb 364 - Sunday, December 30th

The penultimate climb brought out an all-star cast. Massimo, Terence, Krissy, Jessie, Lisa, Dave, and seven other friends made it the second time a group of 13 had done the climb. My legs were like lead, and I was really struggling. I was right at the back and found it interesting how few people checked in to see how I was doing. I think people just assumed that I was physically crushing it when, truthfully, I was so ready for it to end. That morning, when I woke up, all I wanted to do was turn over and go back to sleep. I had to recall the memory of a year earlier when I felt the same way to do Devil's Peak in the wind and ended up having the best climb. It was the last Sunday. It signalled an end to week 52. The project I cared so deeply about and felt immensely proud of - was coming to an end. Having the end so close may be why my body was feeling so exhausted.

Ben brought his Canadian mates, Yule and Attanas, along. Attanas, a budding videographer, asked if it was okay to document the climb and interview me at the top. Yule asked some great questions while he filmed it. Later on, when I got the six-minute video, I was blown away by it! What an amazing gift.

CHAPTER 16
DECEMBER - 31 DAYS TO EMBED THE LESSONS

The interview sparked some questions of my own, which I'd like to pose to you, the reader:

Have you felt overwhelmed by the problems of the world?
Have you felt overwhelmed by your own life?
Have you felt disconnected?
We have a common hardship if you answered yes to any of these questions.

I felt overwhelmed until the universe gave me a gift and retrenched me. It also gave me an idea that would instil the feeling of 'Ubuntu' in me for life. And you can feel it, too.

To add to Ben's amazing gift, while I sat drinking a mochaccino, a raven perched right above me, and spoke to me while opening its wing. There was a powerful message in that for me.

Transformation. Perspective. Ubuntu. Love. Support. Community.

Having Jackie and Alex join helped drive that message home. We'd passed each other on the mountain so many times and ultimately developed a friendship. Our bond grew stronger when they completed their sky run before the 30-hour cut-off and tackled the beast that is Platteklip soon after.

Massimo whipped his shoes off again to experience the magic of a barefoot climb. Lulu and Socks were with him and provided a wonderful addition to the group. Dave was disappointed that he couldn't make the final climb. As one of the major supporters, it was a real shame. But he was with us today, giving us a chance to chat about all the different experiences we'd had along the way. It was like watching someone flip through a book's pages.

Having such an important group together pushed me closer to the realisation that I only had one climb left. I thought I had experienced everything. I was wrong.

In one of the most unexpected experiences I've had on the mountain, I met a woman, Louise, who'd dined with an acquaintance the previous night and spoke about climbing Table Mountain. She recognised me when I passed her on the mountain around halfway because she'd followed me closely. It was a seemingly innocuous interaction, it felt like many of the other interactions I'd had encouraging people to push on and reach the top.

At the top, I randomly walked past her and congratulated her on a fantastic achievement. The unexpected part of the experience came when she shared her hijack horror that almost took her life a few months earlier. Her eyes pooled up as she spoke about the difficulties she'd experienced in battling to find a way back to the light. She suddenly shared what she'd learned from me, and cried tears of gratitude. I had no idea how to respond, but something made me reach out and hold her. I imagined connecting our hearts and sharing the day's achievement, with the hope it would inspire her to get through her experience and choose light instead of darkness.

It was a tear-jerking moment. We never know what our actions can do for others and how it might give them the courage they need to push through their mountain. The world can feel like a dark and lonely place – all we can try to do is shine the spotlight on the beauty around and inside each other. Here is Louise's experience in her own words:

> My 60th birthday was on the 2nd of October of that year. It had been three months since the incident, and I was already walking in Newlands forest. I remember praising myself, thinking, "I'm such a superstar!"
>
> That day, I made myself a promise that I would climb Table Mountain by the end of the year. Before I knew it, it was the 30th of December 2018, and my emotions were all over the place. Although I was filled with excitement and nerves, doubt was my greatest fear.
>
> Early on the morning of December the 30th, I awoke, thinking, "What am I doing? Will I be able to do it?" I was filled with questions and hesitation.

CHAPTER 16
DECEMBER - 31 DAYS TO EMBED THE LESSONS

My son and daughter-in-law fetched me before sunrise that morning. We double-checked our supplies and water and headed off for Table Mountain. The drive felt like it took forever. My heart was pounding, and I was nervous, but excited.

When we arrived, I gazed up at the mountain. It was enormous!

By sunrise, we started climbing. My heart was thumping, and I felt the fear starting again. I thought, "Breathe! One step at a time" and that's what I focused on. When we were halfway up the mountain, Andrew Patterson came walking past us! I have admired, followed and supported Andrew ever since he started his journey to raise funds for UBUNTU! He was and still is, a huge inspiration to me.

Before I knew it, we were on top of the mountain. We rejoiced and enjoyed the most magnificent, picture-perfect day, atop this most amazing mountain, with our beautiful coastline below. I thought, "Wow! I did it! What a blessing." Suddenly, I felt Andrew's massive hand on my arm. My heart skipped a beat at the surprise of his recognising and speaking to me. I don't recall the exact words we exchanged, but I remember him saying that what I had achieved that day was equivalent to what he had done the whole year! The rest is a blur. All I remember is sobbing in Andrew's arms, until my son, Neal, came to the rescue. Neal and I then went for a stroll around the mountain and found a spot for breathing and reflection before we all headed down the mountain by cable car.

You never know what someone else is going through. When I encouraged her at the halfway point, I had no idea what stresses she had to overcome just to attempt to climb. Seeing people's achievements through their lens has become one of my greatest lessons to learn.

I was exhausted, but excited for our family dinner at Massimos later that night. I was thrilled that the others who hadn't climbed and already met him would get to meet the special man. It was the first time I had Jessie and the entire family together with me. It was the perfect time to express my gratitude to everyone for helping me get to this point. Their contributions and commitments had been the best Christmas, and birthday presents rolled into one.

These humans had supported a crazy idea that had the power to bring people together through effort and not just a hashtag. They'd all been my teacher in one way or another, and had been herculean in their long-distance efforts to get others involved and supporting me. My gratitude left them in tears of joy.

I might not say 'I love you' every day. I might not be the best at communicating my feelings, but I make sure to let people know how impactful they've been in my life. We never know when our last chance is to let them know what they've done for us.

Climb 365 – Monday, December 31st

The final day had arrived. The weather gods were smiling down on us, so it looked like I'd get my perfect bookend to the year with a sunset at the top.

Jessie's friend arrived from London in the morning and then headed off to get some party goodies for the night's celebrations. I had an interview with Sarah-Jayne King on Cape Talk at 13:30 and got a chance to talk about my journey. This would be our fourth chat and to her credit, she stuck to her word and set it up before I'd completed the challenge. Initially, I hesitated because I thought my final day would be too chaotic, but I'm glad I agreed.

As I sat in the studio with her beaming at me, live on air, she said… 'You did it!' I was taken aback and struggled to find the words to respond. I'd never had a more significant New Year's. It was the beginning of a life of service. That stood out as my passion and purpose to follow. The focus was not that the year was coming to an end – it was a year filled with lessons that would support me on a new journey of purpose.

CHAPTER 16
DECEMBER - 31 DAYS TO EMBED THE LESSONS

Jessie spoiled us by booking different Airbnb's for the duration of her stay. Initially, I was peeved to be moving around and checking in all the time until I remembered how shocking the December traffic in Sea Point was. I saw it again as I headed home to collect my '1/365 1st January 2018' Ubuntu Shirt to wear. I also spent some time alone in my flat, sitting down on the floor in a heap. Thoughts of all the energy, pain, elation, gratitude, love, people, strangers, weather, lessons, beauty, storms, wind, laughs, tears, money raised, and people empowered washed over me. I could feel what it would feel like to say, 'I climbed Table Mountain every day for a year,' and was looking forward to using that to inspire others.

The weather was extremely generous, so I could push the last climb out to 17:00. Even with a three-hour climb, we'd still get to the top before the sunset. It was another roasting hot day, and the sun beat down on us while we were still on the road to Platteklip. Mom, Dad, Caroline, and Abby caught the cable car up and took all the champagne and snacks for the celebrations with them. The staff were impeccable as they scooted them up to the front so they wouldn't get caught in the queue.

I'd originally wanted to do this solo, but I was glad David came up with this brilliant alternative. My aim was to avoid the limelight seekers. I'd received messages like 'Okay Andrew I'm finally ready to climb with you' from someone I'd met in June. I kindly declined and let them know the previous day was the last day he could join.

The final day was perfectly scripted... 12 people joined us from the start while Achmat waited for us on the mountain. Jessie, Lisa, Terence, Krissy, Katie, Allan, Sage, Oyke, Simon, Warren and my family all linked arms and joined me as I shared the opening gratitude speech. Steve and Roxanna, two special guests from the UK also joined us.

Everything was coming together to make this one of the most inspiring climbs of my life. It was also my 22nd barefoot climb and I loved that Krissy went barefoot from the start too. Her and Katie climbed behind me and asked lots of questions. I responded and asked what they'd learned most from their first climb.

Krissy felt it was important to take her time and not rush the journey. Katie said that as a runner, it was far different to anything she'd done but really enjoyed it and didn't find it too difficult.

The shade provided us with some much needed relief from the heat of the contour path. From there I looked back to the safety of the road that had always been the starting point - this was the 365th time I looked back. I wasn't searching for its security, I was looking for a marker of how far I'd travelled. The road held a special significance so I looked back at it a final time before turning my gaze up to the view of the path which wound its way between the cliffs. The rocks beneath my feet were still warm from the day's sunshine, encouraging my legs to keep going.

Every turn, every waterfall, and every tree lined the path as if it were the end of a marathon with crowds stacked each side cheering and whooping with delight. I extended both my hands and high-fived my daily cheerleaders, who were there for me no matter the weather. Ascension Corner whispered its congratulations through the leaves. I kept moving, step by step, to another tough moment where I placed my hand on Josh's rock. I'd now lived 205 days without his heartfelt messages of support and encouragement.

I passed the fragment from the rockfall that I always showed people, and waved goodbye to the trees it decimated. We finally reached halfway, and then the 'Strength & Power' corner, where I craned my neck one last time in admiration. I closed my eyes and held a thought for a moment... *'The same strength and power that resides in you, is in all of us - keep it rooted with the same humility.'*

I still hadn't found the right rock to represent climb #365. It needed to be a triangular rock that would act as a capping stone to the pyramid. Finally, near Guardian Rock Corner, I came across the perfect rock! My eyes must have sparkled at the sight of it.

CHAPTER 16
DECEMBER – 31 DAYS TO EMBED THE LESSONS

Our late start had left us alone between the cliffs, and just the echoes of our voices danced around and mesmerised my ear. Hail Corner, Heart Trio Corner, and Waterfall Corner beautifully welcomed my feet. The rocks were already cooling down and acted like air-conditioners, while my lungs and legs burned for the final time. No matter how many times I'd climbed here, it was a tough workout to reach the top.

Achmat finally reached us, he was doing his second summit for the day and wanted to support me and be part of the experience. He got to us just as we reached Ubuntu Rock. He had already done 137 summits for the year and would be part of our celebrations.

Reaching Ubuntu Rock for the last time was an incredible feeling. It was Monday, so I took week 52's rocks across with eight final rocks to form an almost perfect pyramid. I sat on my haunches with my bare feet on the cool rock and stared out into the splendour that is the Cape. I couldn't stop smiling. My heart couldn't either. I closed my eyes and felt the mountain living and breathing around me. I could almost hear it cheering me on for the final six switchbacks. Almost everyone had gone ahead and left me to my own devices. Little did I know of the magic that lay ahead.

As I climbed the last few corners, an eerie silence enveloped me. We'd taken just over 2 hours and 30 minutes to get to this point. Heaving and puffing, I made the final corner and was greeted by one of the most magical sights I'd ever seen... my family and friends beaming and cheering me on.

Katie had made me a banner to walk under and everyone was at the end cheering me on. It was even better than I'd imagined at the start of the month. In my vision, I'd been overwhelmed with gratitude and crying tears of joy, but now all I had was pure delight, relief, elation, bliss, inner peace, and gratitude. My parents were in tears. I'll never forget what it felt like to hug them, knowing it was finally over, and never forget their words of pride that filled my ear. Being able to hug and share it with everyone made it the perfect ending. It felt a bit like a movie, like I was outside my own body watching it all unfold.

We found my cousin and his girlfriend at the top. We missed them climbing up, but I'm grateful they were part of the celebrations on the balcony. They must've driven right past us to the start and kept one step ahead of us.

The top was quite extraordinary. Only the tip of Constantiaberg Mountain was visible. The air was warm, it was just right. Clouds flowed over the twelve apostles, but there was hardly any wind. Honestly? I couldn't have pre-ordered more perfect weather if I'd tried.

The staff allowed us to take over the balcony and pack 24 people into where the previous day's interview took place! To add to my delight, Dex and Lou caught the cable car up and joined in the celebrations. They congratulated me and then headed off to their New Year's party in Hout Bay. Just epic. EPIC!! It was another perfect bookend, just like when DT came to wish me well on the very first climb.

Roxana had found me online in October and asked to join a climb in December. There was a very important purpose behind her request. She'd lost her 12-year-old son 12 years earlier through a hit and run. Her life had been tumultuous, to say the least. At 6, he'd told her that she should become a teacher. She'd since become one and graduated the same time he would have. At 12, her daughter told her, *'Mom you're not living your purpose and you're using me as an excuse to live.'* Purpose was something Roxana had never considered. Then she heard my story through Lianne and Clare, who'd joined climb #78. And here she was, all the way from Chiswick, England.

Our timing had been off over the weekend, and we also missed each other the previous day. I could've enforced my rule, but her story wasn't that of someone who was looking for the limelight. Quite the contrary. Both she and Steve oozed warmth and authenticity. They were genuinely grateful for being included in the final climb. That was evident in every step they took and how they engaged with everyone.

CHAPTER 16
DECEMBER - 31 DAYS TO EMBED THE LESSONS

I couldn't begin to imagine the heartache they'd experienced in their lifetime. Meeting them was another incredible experience that showed me the kind of strength people possessed and how they could turn adversity into something meaningful. We're not condemned to walk in pain, but rather to use it to fuel parts of us we never knew existed.

I took my final step and my last photo of my bare right foot to close the chapter. It was very different compared to the dark first step I'd taken on January the 1st when I was full of purpose and drive. Here I am in the light, surrounded by loved ones and even more excited. The contrast was incredible:

From the dark, to the light.
From being alone, to being surrounded by my greatest supporters.
From climbing in shoes, to being barefoot on the rugged surface of the mountain.
From understanding the journey at the bottom, to celebrating it at the top.
From pre-sunrise, to sunset.
From the beginning, to the end.

I had two perfect book ends to my story.

I'm profoundly grateful to have learnt what living in gratitude means and how it creates a beautiful life.

As the champagne bottles popped, the sun dipped further down, and all those that joined me on the day, got to experience the gift of watching a sunset from the top.

My final photo at the top was perfect, and captured the cable car reflecting the last rays of the sun against the backdrop of a perfectly clear sky. The sea was the calmest I'd ever seen. The final climb with group 195, took 2 hours and 52 minutes. The challenge covered a distance of 2,429 km, which is about 85% of South Africa's coastline. It's also the vertical equivalent of 71 Mt Everests, and connected 744 people to make a difference in thousands of lives. Stories were shared, experiences were learned, hardships were endured, beauty was felt, and abundant love was transmitted.

At the end of the challenge, the donations reached R535,639.15. We added 60 new donors to the DKMS Africa registry, built a new home, renovated the Habitat for Humanity orphanage that helped abandoned children in Khayelitsha, and delivered books to four primary schools.

It was impossible to feel happier.

Jessie rented a large place on Airbnb, so the whole family could braai, congregate, relax, and enjoy a celebratory cake from Charly's bakery on the 1st of January. The Airbnb house was perfect. It had a pool, braai area, and a spare room for mom and dad to relax in. Jessie's thoughtfulness and attention to detail was incredible, and I loved being on the receiving end of it. She was already adding tremendous value, and the family was happy to have her become the final piece of our family puzzle.

It was fitting that my final climb was on my grandparents' wedding anniversary. It would've been their 70th.

I finally got to bed around 1 am, but I wasn't done just yet.

CHAPTER 17
SAYING GOODBYE TO AN OLD FRIEND AND MENTOR

Our celebrations eventually ended around 1 am, and my alarm buzzed at 6 am. Everyone thought I was crazy to go back and climb Table Mountain again.

'You're done Andrew! You did it!'

I certainly had. This just felt right. I started the challenge with a solo climb up and down, and did the same with the halfway mark climb, so it felt fitting to end on the same note. It wasn't like one extra day would make it crazy, so I may as well go and do it again. I was living the, "What is the one degree more you can do?" It would be a time to absorb what I'd achieved in 2018.

It was a clear, hot morning, so I headed off in the quiet of the storm with all the party animals finally sleeping from the night before. I was travelling from Newlands, and decided to park at Deer Park to take a new route up and down and break up last year's route. It was also only 132m above sea level and added nicely to my last climb's elevation gain. Why do things the easy way, right??

It was the first time in a year that I wasn't taking a photo of the mountain with the cable station in the background. The decision to take this route almost killed my shins on the way back down and gave me a dose of mini shin splints for a couple of days afterwards, but unlike last year – my legs were about to get something they hadn't experienced since December 2017: rest.

The climb started on the tarmac before reaching the pump station on Camissa River. I arrived at the beautiful twisting gravel roads used by mountain bikers to crunch their way up to Tafelberg Road, where the tour buses turn around. It was far different from last year's weather, this time, it was much warmer, with hardly any breeze to speak of. I wondered if I'd want to stop at certain rocks to ponder the varied experiences of the year?

Our braai was only starting at 13:00, so I had more than enough time to make it up and down and drive back before lunch. 20 minutes later, I reached the same road I'd walked for a year, and was hypnotised by the beauty and scale of the mountain in front of me. My gratitude prayer had an extra element today…

'I'm grateful for the opportunity of my lifetime.'

I kept waiting for floods of tears with emotion to come. I reached the waterfall and dad's rock, where I smiled, but nothing. I made it up to the shade of the trees, thought about my meltdown, and smiled again. I reached the contour path, and finally looked down further than the road, searching through the trees to spot the houses near where I parked. I was definitely feeling the extra 200m climb in my legs… but still no sadness. I passed each of the 38 corners one by one, and said hello to the family stones.

I'd just completed 365 days of gratitude and searched for the uniqueness in each moment. I'd taken every step as if it were my first, and lived the year on purpose. I'd seen what I needed to see. Felt what I needed to feel. Been open to a new experience every day instead of viewing it as a chore. That's why there was no anguish. No goodbye tears. No feelings that I'd be 'missing out'. I had 365 experiences at each point, instead of taking one day to try and cram

CHAPTER 17
SAYING GOODBYE TO AN OLD FRIEND AND MENTOR

everything into what was less than 1% of a year. It was like trying to read the last page of a book instead of savouring every page.

I was happy to climb at my own pace. December was a busy month – 27 days with 163 people, and only four days alone was mentally exhausting. To put that in perspective, that was three more people than November, October, and September combined.

There were not many people on the mountain today. Most would have opted for a lay-in after a late night. It felt good to have made it even though I only had five hours of sleep. I was climbing in the heat because of my extra snooze and the later start. I'm also sure that I missed Achmat. I saw him right at the top, waiting for someone else. It was bittersweet knowing I wouldn't be seeing him and his spirit that much anymore. But as with everything, there are seasons, and the next one has arrived.

I didn't need to get my picture up at the top, but all year, I'd been admiring a rocky outcrop just below the cliffs. It's visible from the place where I sat with the monks 93 days ago. One of the rocks juts out, so I decided to try and get to it. I clambered down and tried to figure out a route. It was a perfect day, and the view delighted my eyes whenever my head popped up. Alas, I couldn't find a safe route down, so I settled for a slightly sheltered spot to sit and admire Cape Town one last time on this challenge.

There was silence. I had nothing but my thoughts, admiration for the views, gratitude for being able to do this challenge, and excitement for all that still lay ahead. Two crows glided effortlessly on the breeze above me without moving their wings. Just their tail rudders moved them from side to side. They seemed to be checking in on me every now and then.

My aim was to grab the opportunity of a lifetime during the lifetime of the opportunity. I'd done exactly that. It was over, and my legs were the happiest part of my body. I could hear them waiting for the final descent. I wonder how many chances I'd squandered because of fear and lack of belief? Perhaps I squandered a chance to learn something, grow, or become part of something far bigger than myself? Maybe this year had squeezed all those missed opportunities into one.

It had been a humbling experience to watch people participate. All 744 climbers. Every cash donation. Every online commitment. All the companies supporting the initiative to make a difference. All from one thought.

It had been a blessing to hear other people's experiences and what the journey meant to them - that was something I couldn't buy. Never again would I underestimate the power of my words and their potential to lift someone's spirits and fuel their weary 'legs' as they climbed their own personal mountain.

Challenges will always exist. My biggest mountain of all, was still self-doubt, and would surely be a daily climb for a long time to come. Completing this hasn't eradicated it, but given me a view of what I can achieve when I finally overcome it. Just like Table Mountain will always remain, so too will self-doubt, but I now have the belief and the tools to summit it every day, no matter what other ideas I have in the future.

Thinking and actions are the only two things we have direct control over.

I'd like to leave you with this message from the video I made yesterday:

'It's hard to put into a few words what this year meant to me, only to realise it's actually already in the name that I used for the challenge: Ubuntu.

That's what this was all about. Community. We're either finding ways to improve it and build it up for everyone – or we're destroying it.

Ubuntu was at the heart of this challenge and all of you who supported me with your donations have created a community based on love and empowerment. We've chosen to do something about the problems instead of moaning about them. The climbers, the supporters, the donors, the sponsors, the interviewers, the sharers – you've all helped one man spread a message of hope, that's inspired action, and encouraged people to make magic together.

CHAPTER 17
SAYING GOODBYE TO AN OLD FRIEND AND MENTOR

I cannot thank you enough. I am eternally grateful. Thank you.

This is not the final chapter of this book, it's the first chapter of a new one. It's the start of another journey, and a life of service.'

As I sat staring out over the city for the last time during my challenge, a simple thought entered my mind.

I am enough.

Remember back in June when I met Charlotte and mentioned that the discussion we had about depression would lead to my greatest lesson of the challenge? Well... here it is 204 days later.

I was all smiles as I walked back down, each painful jolt on my joints and legs reminded me that I needed to appreciate what I'd accomplished. 'I am enough' permeated through my mind as I sat with the Ubuntu Pyramid, which was safely tucked away in the shadows of the East Cliff. Every stone represented a climb, and told a story. It was a beautiful piece in my 3D puzzle of purpose and discovery. Having the belief that I am enough is the most powerful tool I have to fight depression.

365 Ubuntu Climbs doesn't define me – it's an expression of who I am, and what I'm capable of. It's such a simple distinction that's had a profound impact on me mentally, and led to the question that would push me even further in life:

What am I made of?

I reached the final steps of the path at 10:30 am. It was a place where I'd said 366 gratitude prayers. David was right to encourage me to do my final solo climb today, and finish with a down climb where I'd have the opportunity to sit and absorb it all.

I asked a couple from New York about to start their climb to take a photo of me. They snapped one which was far better than the selfies I was trying to attempt. I didn't envy them one bit as the sun began to intensify. Thankfully, they had plenty of water and looked fit, so I bid them farewell.

The steep decline on the Jeep track started to create painful shin splints. I wondered if my body was reminding me of the contract we had! Finally, I reached the bottom and gazed back up at the mountain one last time. As I was about to switch off my tracker, I saw that it was on 10,53 km, 03 hours, 23 minutes, and 46 seconds.

The best part of getting back down? I'd be joining Jessie and my entire family for a relaxing day of braaing by the pool. Donald and his sister Heather were on their way too. Jessie's forward thinking and booking the perfect Airbnb for the family was genius.

In closing...

I know things aren't easy for anyone, but at some point, I had to decide to stop running away from challenges and start facing them head-on. I now realise I don't have to do this alone. I hope this book has provided you with some insights into what can be achieved when you take on a new perspective and show compassion. Most importantly, I hope you understand how the world can become a better place by simply practising the principles of Ubuntu.

We can't always help everyone, so it's important to focus our efforts on providing solutions that give a hand up – instead of a handout. I have no doubt that you've got some ideas stewing inside you, perhaps you've been putting them off. My idea was 37 years in the making, and came to life when I began to confront the world outside of my comfort zone. It had been a tremendous journey, and I'd slowly come around to the fact that the journey was where all the magic happened.

Your journey won't be easy, but it will be fulfilling. No amount of money in the world can buy that.

I hope one day to read about how you took your first step.

FINAL THOUGHTS

I have no idea where this journey will take me, but isn't that what makes life so incredible? How boring would it be if we knew what would happen and exactly when?!

18 months prior to my challenge, I'd left corporate life with an idea and a plan to add value and make a difference in South Africa. We reached people across the land, the continent, and the oceans. People's hearts opened and touched the lives of those who had been caught up in vicious cycles of poverty. We let them know they hadn't been ignored, and we extended our hands to them.

One day, you and I will have an opportunity to sit next to each other, and I know I'll see the same sparkle in your eye that exists in mine. Your strength and power may not be geared toward climbing a mountain every day, but perhaps you'll express your compassion in other ways. Maybe you'll teach and expand young minds to believe in themselves, become leaders, and spread the principles of Ubuntu even further.

You may be about to become a parent. This could be the perfect journey for you to share your wisdom, nurture happiness and health, and create an environment for your children to thrive and become great one day.

Or you might have been sitting on an idea for years that you know deep down is something this world desperately needs – but like me and the adult elephant tied to a chair, you may be letting the childhood memories or debilitating beliefs hold you back instead of taking that first step.

One step. That's all it takes to create momentum.

There's no magic word or spell I can give you to suddenly transform your life. I do hope though, that through the examples given over the course of this book, you can see how life works for us. I believe seeds are buried deep within you, and once you start watering them, life becomes exponentially better.

Bad and good are sides to the same coin, and in order to grow sometimes, we have to experience the pain of being in a dark room in search of the light switch. We're going to stumble, and all of us do. I'm still stumbling.

Nelson Mandela said... *'After climbing a great hill, one only finds that there are many more hills to climb.'*

Now... I get it.

People say I've conquered Table Mountain, but I think that's inaccurate. The only thing I've conquered is my belief in what I thought was possible. There's a perfect prayer for this from Chief Dan George (born Geswanouth Slahoot):

Oh Great Spirit whose voice I hear in the winds, I come to you as one of your many children. I need your strength and your wisdom. Make me strong not to be superior to my brother, but to be able to fight my greatest enemy, Myself.

The mountain was there long before me, and it will be there millennia after my bones have turned to sand. But that's the thing, our mountains will always be there. We always experience strife, difficulties, and challenges beyond our comprehension. That goes for social challenges too. We can all take a moment to stop, think, feel, and breathe.

Challenge your mindset on what you think is possible in society. Perhaps you heard about this story and didn't believe I'd do it, or you wanted to participate but didn't. I'd like you to create your own 365 Ubuntu Climbs for South Africa, and simply swap the country's name to wherever you are if you're outside of South Africa.

Here's the thing, I completed all the climbs... that part isn't dependent on the support of others, but the overall success and the social impact depend on people's involvement. Every little bit counts. It's not about how much someone contributes... It's simply about getting involved. That's what makes us human beings.

Our potential is limited only by our minds. I hope you find the spark that sets your soul on fire and unleashes your potential with a thunderous roar across our spectacular planet.

And if you feel doubtful about taking that step, remember this...

I pursued something that initially had little support, because I believed in what it could do for others. I also knew I would come out the other side a profoundly changed man.

As I finish this book, I'm in Oregon to visit Gram, one of Jessie's friends' grandmothers. I mentioned that today's youth felt more disconnected because of technology, and she corrected me with a beautiful explanation...

'They don't feel more disconnected, they just have more access to the problems of the world.'

That's why we feel so overwhelmed, we're connected to problems on the other side of the world. I hope this understanding helps you shift the focus away from the problems, to what you can do.

I used to say how embarrassed I'd be if I raised more money off the mountain than on it. That almost happened after I received an email from Cornelia in June. I appeared in the March issue of Mens Health Magazine, and afterward received even more support from a company called *Beautiful News SA*. They set up an interview, and posted my images in Uber cars, on electronic billboards at petrol stations, with SAA on their inboard flights and at Airports. I'm not sure which of these is responsible for what followed, but honestly, at first, I thought it was a scam.

It turns out, Cornelia had shared my story with the creator of the meditation practice she follows. Commonly referred to as Suma or Supreme Master Ching Hai, she's a Vietnamese spiritual leader of the Guanyin Famen (Chinese) or Quan Yin Method transnational cybersect based out of Taiwan. She founded the

Loving Hut vegan restaurant chain and vegan Celestial Shop fashion company under the Supreme Master Ching Hai International Association.

The reason I thought it was a scam? When she heard about what I'd done, she pledged to donate $27,000!! It wasn't a random amount, as Jessie had pointed out, she was doubling the amount raised through Backabuddy! This meant that together with the direct donations to each charity, and the cash we'd collectively raised, we came in at just under R1 million.

The cash injection added 60 new donors to DKMS Africa, enabled One Heart to Deliver literacy aids to 12 of the poorest primary schools, and helped Habitat for Humanity build a new home for Baphumelele Children's Home, which is a place of safety for orphaned and vulnerable children from the Cape Flats.

And to think, this almost didn't happen. I almost listened to someone with zero understanding of who I am and what my purpose is. This is what I'm most proud of.

How is THAT for a bit of Ubuntu Magic!

ACKNOWLEDGEMENTS

Writing this book has been an incredible journey, and I owe its existence to some remarkable individuals. First and foremost, my deepest gratitude goes to my wife, Jessie, whose unwavering support and belief in me serve as my guiding light. Her profound encouragement provided the cocoon which helped me delve into the intricacies of crafting this memoir. Jessie not only offered me the time to explore the depths of my storytelling, but also her belief in me has been a constant source of inspiration, making this journey richer and more meaningful.

I'd like to acknowledge the countless publishers and literary agents who ghosted me with rejections and pushed me to reconnect with the core of my writing — inspiring others facing their own mountains to climb. You allowed me to find, in my opinion, the best people to publish my book.

Scribe Media helped me create the core essence of my book. Their free workshops during lockdown and writing guide helped me recognize that it wasn't just another self-help endeavour but a living testament to the boundless potential unlocked by following one's heart.

Special thanks to Lisa Thompson-Smeddle, founder of One Heart for Kids, for her incredible work in tackling illiteracy. She introduced me to Zainab Karriem, MD of Imprint Publishing, whose generosity and belief in my story resulted in the sponsorship of publishing my book.

To Zainab's editor, Matthew Hodges, whose intimate knowledge and fellow love of Platteklip Gorge (not something many people share with me) brought a unique dimension to the editing process — thank you.

I extend my appreciation to my family, especially Mom, Dad, and Aunty San, whose encouragement began in my early twenties while reading my London updates via email. Your words planted the seed for my professional writing journey, which ultimately led to the creation of this book.

Lastly, to every reader who holds this book, my gratitude is boundless. Just like the people who climbed and donated during my challenge — you are actively participating in the creation of a community centred around the power of collective action. A significant portion of the profits from this book will go towards teaching kids to read in South Africa, embodying the true spirit of Ubuntu. The goal of this book is to support communities and help you on your own personal journey. May its words kindle a flame, inspiring the pursuit of your ideas that ultimately reveal the extraordinary potential that resides within you. Take action — because you are undeniably worth it.

ABOUT IMPRINT PUBLISHING

It was Lisa Thompson-Smeddle from One Heart for Kids and her incredible work in rural areas eradicating illiteracy that got noticed by the Department of Basic Education (DBE) and then asked to work on an audacious project to revolutionise South Africa's education system. When South Africa eradicates its corrupt officials it will actually happen - but this project introduced me to Zainab Karriem, MD of Imprint Publishing. In one of our meetings while back in South Africa 2022, I had resigned myself to the fact that no publisher was going to pick my book up and I'd have to self-publish. Hearing Zainab talk about printing, I wondered if she knew a decent printer to get quotes for my book.

Zainab told me about the perfect printer that actually uses its profits to support an orphanage! I was overjoyed, and in my enthusiasm, she asked if she could read my book. I thought nothing of it and emailed it through. Five days later on the 27 March 2022, Zainab messaged me on the Sunday morning telling me she'd just finished it. What followed was her desire to sponsor the publishing costs — everything up until printing — because she loved it so much and wanted to support me in getting my story out. All those ghosted emails. All the rejections. All the time wondering if it would ever happen. All vaporised in an instant that overwhelmed me with joy and gratitude. Overcome with tears I couldn't even tell Jessie, I had to hand over the phone for her to read the message.

Even in my most perfect scenario of what I could've wanted in a publisher — I would have come short. Our values perfectly align and I'm truly grateful to have a publishing partner with such heart.